ATLAS OF Heart Failure

Cardiac Function and Dysfunction

SECOND EDITION

ATLAS OF
Heart Failure

Cardiac Function and Dysfunction

SECOND EDITION

Editor

WILSON S. COLUCCI, MD

Professor of Medicine and Physiology
Boston University School of Medicine;
Chief
Cardiovascular Medicine
Boston University Medical Center
Boston, Massachusetts

Series Editor

EUGENE BRAUNWALD, MD, MD (HON), ScD (HON)

Distinguished Hersey Professor of Medicine
Faculty Dean for Academic Programs at
   Brigham and Women's Hospital and Massachusetts General Hospital
Harvard Medical School;
Vice President for Academic Programs
Partners HealthCare System
Boston, Massachusetts

b

**Blackwell
Science**

Developed by Current Medicine, Inc., Philadelphia

CURRENT MEDICINE, INC. ─

400 MARKET STREET, SUITE 700 • PHILADELPHIA, PA 19106

Developmental Editor .... *Danielle Shaw*

Director of Product Development .... *Lori J. Bainbridge*

Editorial Assistant .... *Lisa Janda*

Art Director .... *Paul Fennessy*

Designers .... *Christopher Allan and Christine Keller-Quirk*

Illustration Director .... *Ann Saydlowski*

Illustrators .... *Paul Schiffmacher, Lisa Weischedel and Debra Wertz*

Production Manager .... *Lori Holland*

Production Assistant .... *Amy Watts*

Indexing .... *Larry Meyer*

Library of Congress Cataloguing-in-Publication Data
Atlas of heart failure : cardiac function and dysfunction / Wilson S. Colucci, editor.
   Eugene Braunwald, series editor.–2nd ed.
              p. cm.
       Includes bibliographical references and index.
       ISBN 0-632-04381-4
       1. Heart failure. 2. Heart failure–Atlases.
       [DNLM: 1. Heart Failure, Congestive atlases. 2. Heart–physiology
atlases. 3. Heart–physiopathology atlases. 1999 C-421]
RC682.A818 1999
[RC685.C53]
616.1′2–dc21
[616.1′29]
DNLM/DLC
for Library of Congress   99-26627
                                                              CIP

   ISBN 0-632-04381-4

Although every effort has been made to ensure that drug doses and other information are presented
accurately in this publication, the ultimate responsibility rests with the prescribing physician. Neither
the publishers nor the authors can be held responsible for errors or for any consequences arising from
the use of information contained herein. Products mentioned in this publication should be used in
accordance with the prescribing information prepared by the manufacturers. No claims or endorse-
ments are made for any drug or compound at present under clinical investigation.

Printed in the United States by Quebecor

10   9   8   7   6   5   4   3   2

CONTRIBUTORS

AINAT BENIAMINOVITZ, MD
Assistant of Clinical Medicine
Department of Medicine
College of Physicians and Surgeons
  of Columbia University;
Division of Circulatory Physiology
Columbia-Presbyterian Medical Center
New York, New York

ROBERT J. CODY, MD
Professor of Internal Medicine
Associate Chief
Division of Cardiology;
Director
Heart Failure and Transplant
  Management Center
University of Michigan Health System
Ann Arbor, Michigan

JAY N. COHN, MD
Professor of Medicine
Cardiovascular Division
University of Minnesota Medical School
Minneapolis, Minnesota

WILSON S. COLUCCI, MD
Professor of Medicine and Physiology
Boston University School of Medicine;
Chief
Cardiovascular Medicine
Boston University Medical Center
Boston, Massachusetts

MARK A. CREAGER, MD
Associate Professor of Medicine
Harvard Medical School;
Medical Director
Vascular Center
Cardiovascular Division
Brigham and Women's Hospital
Boston, Massachusetts

JORGE A. CUSCO, MD
Department of Internal Medicine
Orlando Medical Center
Orlando, Florida

MICHAEL M. GIVERTZ, MD
Assistant Professor of Medicine
Boston University School of Medicine;
Clinical Director
Cardiomyopathy Program
Boston University Medical Center
Boston, Massachusetts

JOSHUA M. HARE, MD
Assistant Professor
Johns Hopkins University
  School of Medicine;
Department of Medicine
Cardiology Division
Johns Hopkins Hospital
Baltimore, Maryland

ARNOLD M. KATZ, MD
DMed (Hon)
Professor of Medicine
University of Connecticut
  School of Medicine
University of Connecticut
  Health Center
Farmington, Connecticut

CARL V. LEIER, MD
Overstreet Professor of Medicine
  and Pharmacology;
Director
Division of Cardiology
The Ohio State University College
  of Medicine
Columbus, Ohio

CONTRIBUTORS

DONNA MANCINI, MD
Associate Professor
Department of Medicine
College of Physicians and Surgeons of
  Columbia University;
Columbia-Presbyterian Hospital
New York, New York

MICHAEL O. OSAYAMEN, MD,
  PHARM D
Resident
Department of Internal Medicine
University of Minnesota Medical School
Minneapolis, Minnesota

MARC A. PFEFFER, MD, PHD
Professor of Medicine
Harvard Medical School;
Physician
Cardiovascular Division
Brigham and Women's Hospital
Boston, Massachusetts

THOMAS S. RECTOR, PHD
Senior Research Associate
Cardiovascular Division
University of Minnesota Medical
  School
Minneapolis, Minnesota

DOUGLAS B. SAWYER, MD, PHD
Assistant Professor
Department of Medicine
Boston University School of Medicine;
Physician
Boston University Medical Center
Boston, Massachusetts

MARK R. STARLING, MD
Professor of Medicine
University of Michigan Medical School;
Chief
Cardiology Section
Veterans Affairs Medical Center
Ann Arbor, Michigan

JAMES B. YOUNG, MD
Head
Section of Heart Failure and Cardiac
  Transplant Medicine;
Medical Director
Kaufman Center for Heart Failure
Cleveland Clinic Foundation
Cleveland, Ohio

PREFACE

Heart failure is a common clinical syndrome that has enormous impact on the prognosis and lifestyle of patients. In the United States, more than 4 million people have heart failure and more than 400,000 new cases are diagnosed each year. This diagnosis is associated with a 5-year mortality rate of approximately 50%, and the morbidity of the syndrome has a major effect on the quality of life and productivity of afflicted patients.

In recent years, impressive strides have been made toward understanding the pathophysiology of heart failure at all levels, from molecular changes to the integrated circulatory system. It is now apparent that many forms of *primary* cardiomyopathy, such as hypertrophic cardiomyopathy and some forms of dilated cardiomyopathy, are genetic in origin, and rapid progress is being made in identifying specific molecular defects that cause a variety of inherited heart muscle diseases.

Likewise, it is now clear that profound *secondary* changes occur in previously normal myocardium in response to abnormal mechanical stresses and neurohumoral stimuli that result from common cardiovascular conditions such as myocardial infarction, valvular heart disease, and systemic hypertension. Collectively referred to as "remodeling," these secondary changes in myocytes, fibroblasts, and other constituents of the myocardium result in myocyte hypertrophy and apoptosis, interstitial fibrosis, chamber enlargement, and abnormalities of systolic and diastolic pump function. These structural and functional changes determine the timing and extent of the myocardial dysfunction and thereby play a central role in defining the time course and severity of the clinical syndrome.

Advances in understanding the pathophysiology of heart failure have been paralleled by an impressive expansion in modalities available for treatment. Only a few years ago, a monograph dealing with this syndrome would have focused on therapies directed at the short-term improvement of hemodynamic function. Although short-term hemodynamic stabilization continues to be an important goal of the in-hospital management of patients with heart failure, it is increasingly apparent that hemodynamic improvement is only one aspect of successful long-term therapy.

There is now evidence that therapy of heart failure with at least two types of neurohormonal antagonists, converting enzyme inhibitors and β-adrenergic blockers, improves clinical status and reduces mortality. Furthermore, it appears that the early treatment of patients with left ventricular dysfunction can slow or prevent the progression of disease and the development of heart failure. Several new factors, including inflammatory cytokines, endothelin, and oxidative stress, have been identified that have the potential to mediate the development of myocardial failure and have led to promising new therapeutic approaches.

This volume is divided into three sections that address normal cardiac function, mechanisms of dysfunction in heart failure, and therapeutic approaches to managing the syndrome. The first section provides a state-of-the-art review of the mechanisms that regulate myocardial function, beginning with molecular and cellular events in the cardiomyocyte and progressing to the level of tissue/organ mechanics and systemic circulatory regulation. In the second section, pathophysiology is presented in four chapters that address the etiology of the syndrome, the molecular and cellular basis of myocardial failure, myocardial remodeling, and the critical roles of the circulatory system and neurohumoral mechanisms in the pathophysiology of heart failure. The third section is devoted to the clinical management of patients with heart failure; six chapters discuss the clinical assessment of the patient suspected of having heart failure, clinical indicators of prognosis, management of the hospitalized patient, conventional therapy for the ambulatory patient, new pharmacologic approaches, and cardiac transplantation.

As understanding of heart failure advances, new approaches to the prevention and treatment of the syndrome will emerge. Conversely, it is likely that lessons learned from prevention and treatment trials will continue to foster insight into the mechanisms that determine this syndrome. The complexity of this intersection of basic and clinical information presents a challenge to both the clinician and the investigator but ultimately promises that additional exciting progress will occur in both arenas. We believe that this volume of the *Atlas of Heart Diseases* will serve clinicians, investigators, and teachers who are interested in heart failure by synthesizing and presenting information that is relevant to all.

Wilson S. Colucci, MD

CONTENTS

CHAPTER 5

CARDIAC REMODELING AND ITS PREVENTION

Marc A. Pfeffer

CHAPTER 6

NEUROHUMORAL, RENAL, AND VASCULAR ADJUSTMENTS IN HEART FAILURE

Jorge A. Cusco and Mark A. Creager

SECTION III: MANAGEMENT OF HEART FAILURE

CHAPTER 7

ASSESSMENT OF HEART FAILURE

James B. Young

CHAPTER 8

PROGNOSIS, USE OF PROGNOSTIC VARIABLES, AND ASSESSMENT OF THERAPEUTIC RESPONSES

Michael O. Osayamen, Thomas S. Rector, and Jay N. Cohn

Physiology

MOLECULAR AND CELLULAR BASIS OF CONTRACTION

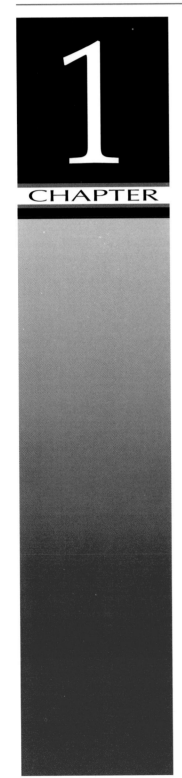

1

CHAPTER

Arnold M. Katz

The ability of the heart to meet the changing demands of the circulation involves three fundamentally different mechanisms [1]. The work of the heart can be regulated by changes in its ability to empty and fill (organ physiology), to utilize chemical energy for the performance of mechanical and osmotic work (cell biochemistry), and to replace its constituent parts (gene expression). Each of these control mechanisms operates over a different time course.

As an organ, the heart adjusts to changing preload (venous return) and afterload (arterial impedance) by length-dependent mechanisms: the Frank-Starling relationship, or Starling's Law of the Heart [2]. These physiologic mechanisms, which allow increased preload or afterload to augment the heart's ability to eject blood, provide beat-to-beat adjustments that enable the heart to meet short-term changes in hemodynamics and to equalize the outputs of the two ventricles.

The second mechanism relies on biochemical changes to modify the ability of individual cardiac myocytes to contract and to relax, and thus to alter the heart's ability to empty (inotropy) and fill (lusitropy). Most of these cellular mechanisms, which enable the heart to meet such sustained hemodynamic demands as those caused by exercise and emotion, influence the interactions between the cardiac contractile proteins by modifying the many membrane ion pumps, ion channels, and ion exchangers that regulate the inotropic and lusitropic properties of the heart [2]. The calcium fluxes involved in excitation-contraction coupling and relaxation, in turn, are influenced by a variety of signaling cascades. These cascades are initiated by the arrival of an extracellular signal, usually a chemical transmitter or hormone, at the cell surface, and generate a diverse group of intracellular messengers that modify cardiac function.

The third and most complex of the mechanisms by which the heart adjusts to the changing demands of the circulation involves growth abnormalities that modify gene expression in the cardiac cells. The resulting molecular changes provide long-lasting adjustments in response to such stimuli as endocrinopathies (*eg*, altered thyroid function), aging, and chronic hemodynamic overload. Although an understanding of this third mechanism is still in its infancy, rich and subtle molecular changes caused by growth abnormalities in the diseased heart are likely to play an important role in such common clinical conditions as heart failure [3].

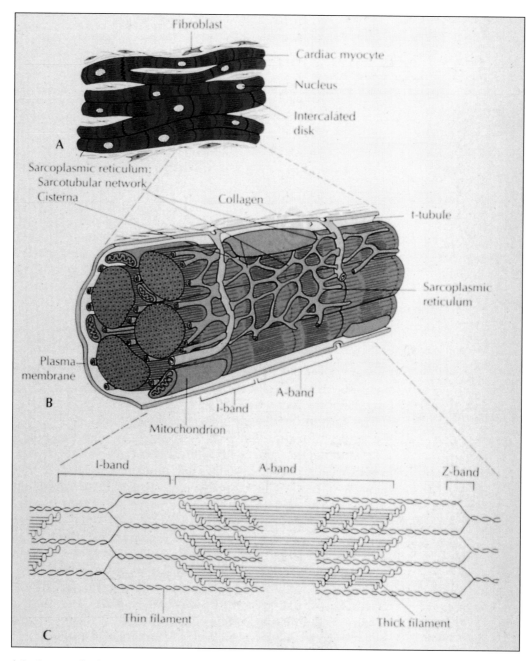

FIGURE 1-1. Structure of the heart. The heart is composed of both myocytes and nonmyoctes. **A,** Nonmyocytes include connective tissue cells (mainly fibroblasts), vascular smooth muscle cells, and endothelial cells. Whereas large cardiac myocytes make up most of the heart's mass, the majority of the cells of the heart (approximately 70%) are smaller nonmyocytes. The large, branched cardiac myocytes, which are enmeshed in a collagen network, are separated longitudinally by intercalated discs, which represent specialized cell-cell junctions. The intercalated discs provide strong mechanical connections between adjacent cells and contain gap junctions that provide low-resistance pathways for electrical conduction.

B, Cardiac myocytes that are specialized for contraction contain myofilaments whose organization in a regular array of thick and thin filaments gives rise to the characteristic striated appearance. Also prominent within these cells are two membrane structures: energy-producing mitochondria and the sarcoplasmic reticulum, which regulates cytosolic Ca^{2+} concentration. The latter is an intracellular membrane system that contains the calcium channels that initiate systole by delivering activator calcium to the myofilaments, and calcium pumps that, by removing calcium from the cytosol, dissociate this activator cation from its binding sites on the thin filament.

Myofilaments contain about 70% of the protein of the cardiac myocytes, and most of the membrane surface is found in the mitochondria. Other important membranes include the plasma membrane, which is continuous with the transverse tubular membranes (t-tubules) that extend toward the center of the cell and carry depolarizing currents into the myocardial cell.

C, Each sarcomere, which is delimited by two Z-bands, contains one A-band and two half I-bands. The A-bands are made up of thick, myosin-containing filaments into which thin filaments interdigitate from the adjacent two half I-bands. The latter are made up of actin and the regulatory proteins, tropomyosin and the troponin complex. Bisecting each Z-band is a lattice of axial and cross-connecting filaments that includes the overlapping ends of thin filaments from adjacent sarcomeres. (Part B *adapted from* Katz [4]; with permission.)

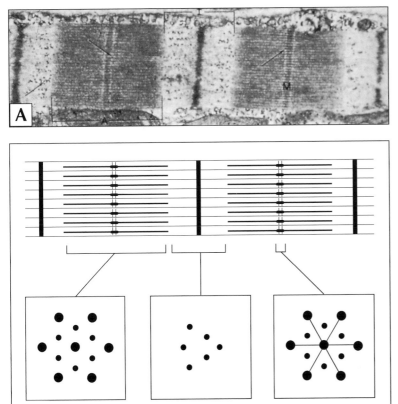

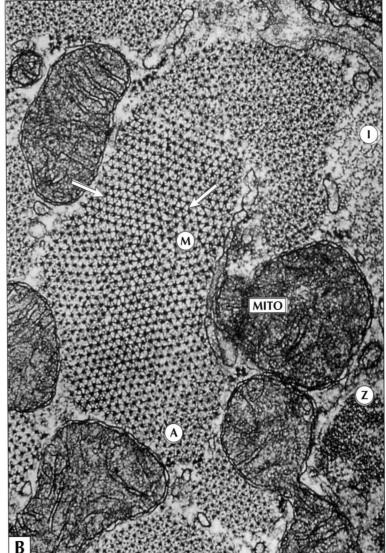

FIGURE 1-2. Sarcomere structure. **A,** A longitudinal section of two sarcomeres of cat atrial myocardium shows the characteristic cross-striations created by the regular array of myofilaments. The A-band (A) is made up of closely packed, myosin-containing thick filaments. In the center of the A-band is the M-band (M), an electron-dense region that contains thin radial filaments running transversely to the long axis of the sarcomere. The I-bands (I), which are made up of the thin actin-containing filaments, are bisected by the Z-bands. Glycogen granules are present in the cytoplasm and between myofilaments (*arrows*), and mitochondria are seen below. Cross-sections of the myofilament at different levels of one of the sarcomeres show relationships between the thick and thin filaments. The A-band is a hexagonal array of thick filaments containing thin filaments that lie at the trigonal points of the array. Thin filaments in the I-band, where thick filaments are absent, are less ordered. Thin radial filaments connect adjacent thick filaments within the M-band at the center of the A-band. **B,** A transverse section through a cat right ventricular papillary muscle shows myofilaments cut at the level of the M-band, A-band, and I-band. *Arrows* point to the radial filaments between the thick filaments in the center of the M-band. Several energy-producing mitochondria (MITO) are also seen. The Z-band (Z) at *lower right* appears as a dense network. (*Adapted from* McNutt and Fawcett [5]; with permission.)

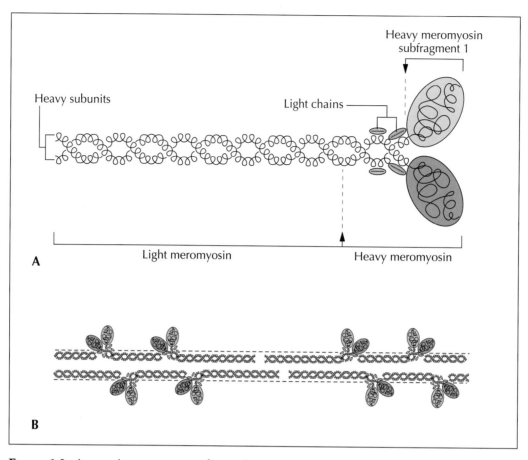

FIGURE 1-3. A myosin monomer and myosin aggregates. **A,** Each elongated myosin molecule consists of two heavy chains and two pairs of light chains. The "tail" of the molecule (*left*) is a coiled coil in which α-helical regions of the two myosin heavy chains are wound around each other. Each of the paired "heads" of the molecule (*right*) includes the globular region of one myosin heavy chain along with two myosin light chains. The latter, which are members of the same family of calcium-binding proteins that includes troponin C (*see* Fig. 1-4), play an as yet incompletely understood role in regulating contraction. Whereas enzymatic cleavage at the point indicated by the *lower arrow* yields heavy and light meromyosins, enzymatic cleavage of heavy meromyosin at the point indicated by the *upper arrow* yields the heavy meromyosin subfragment 1. Both the actin-binding and adenosine triphosphatase sites of myosin are within the myosin head, which corresponds to the cross-bridge that projects from the thick filament.

  B, The thick filament is an aggregate of individual myosin molecules. The "backbone" (*dashed lines*) is made up of the tails of the individual myosin molecules; the cross-bridges correspond to the myosin "heads," which have opposite polarities in the two halves of the thick filament (*right* and *left*). The bare area in the center of the thick filament is devoid of cross-bridges because of the "tail-to-tail" organization of myosin molecules. (*Adapted from* Katz [2]; with permission.)

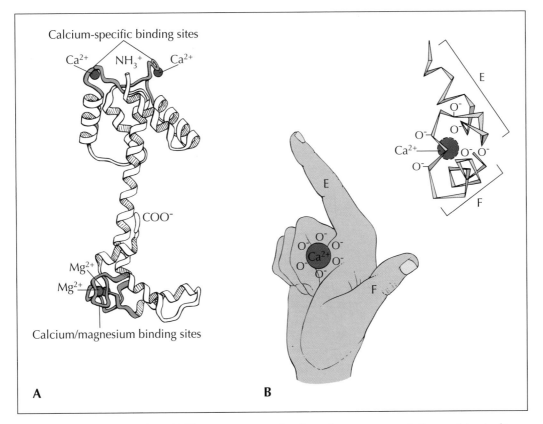

FIGURE 1-4. Troponin C. **A,** Ribbon representation based on x-ray crystallographic studies at 2.8-Å resolution shows the dumbbell-shaped molecule that contains four calcium-binding sites. The upper helical portions contain two calcium-specific binding sites, and the lower part of the molecule contains two nonspecific calcium/magnesium-binding sites. The latter probably have no role in excitation-contraction coupling, because the concentration of cytosolic Mg^{2+} is so much higher than that of Ca^{2+} that these sites remain occupied by Mg^{2+} during physiologic changes in cytosolic Ca^{2+} concentration. In skeletal troponin C, both calcium-specific sites bind calcium ions to initiate contraction. In cardiac troponin C, one of these sites has lost the ability to bind calcium, so that binding of only one calcium ion is required to initiate contraction.

B, Each calcium-binding site contains two α-helical regions (E and F) that are separated by a nonhelical loop. This structure, which localizes six oxygen atoms (O^-) so that they tightly coordinate a calcium ion (Ca^{2+}), resembles a right hand and so is sometimes called an "E-F hand." (Part A *adapted from* Herzberg and James [6]; part B *adapted from* Katz [2]; with permission.)

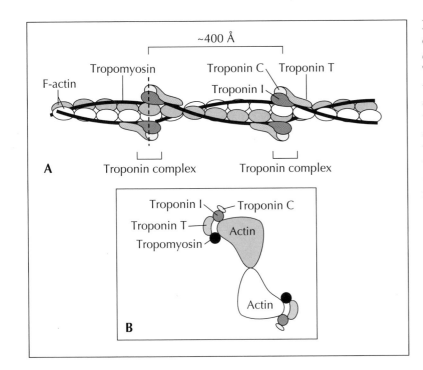

FIGURE 1-5. Structure of the thin filament. **A,** The "backbone" of the thin filament, seen in a longitudinal view, is F-actin which contains two strands of actin monomers (*light grey and white*). Troponin complexes, each made up of one molecule each of troponin C, troponin I, and troponin T, are distributed at approximately 400-Å intervals along the thin filament. Elongated tropomyosin molecules (*solid*) lie in the grooves between the two actin strands. **B,** A cross-section of the thin filament at the level where the troponin complexes are located shows probable relationships between actin, tropomyosin, and the three components of the troponin complex. The strength of the bond linking troponin I and actin varies, depending on whether Ca^{2+} is bound to troponin C. (*Adapted from* Katz [2]; with permission.)

CONTRACTION AND RELAXATION

CONTRACTILE PROTEIN INTERACTIONS

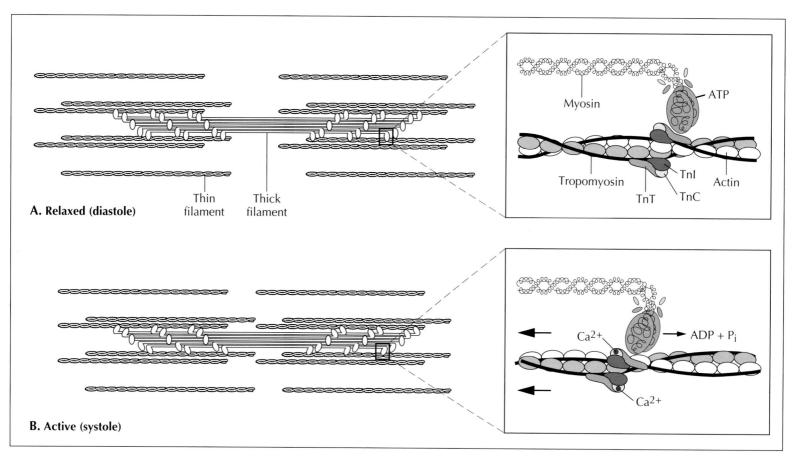

FIGURE 1-6. Cardiac contraction is brought about by interactions between actin in the thin filament and myosin cross-bridges that project from the thick filament. **A,** In relaxed muscle, where troponin C (TnC) is not bound to calcium, the "relaxed" conformation of the troponin complexes and tropomyosin prevents actin in the thin filament from interacting with the myosin cross-bridges. As a result, actin is unable to convert the chemical energy of the adenosine triphosphate (ATP) bound to the myosin cross-bridges into mechanical work.

B, In active muscle, Ca^{2+} bound to TnC has shifted the troponin complexes and tropomyosin to an "active" conformation that enables actin to interact with the myosin cross-bridges. Release of chemical energy when actin stimulates hydrolysis of myosin-bound ATP enables the cross-bridges to "row" the thin filaments toward the center of the sarcomere. TnI—troponin I; TnT—troponin T.

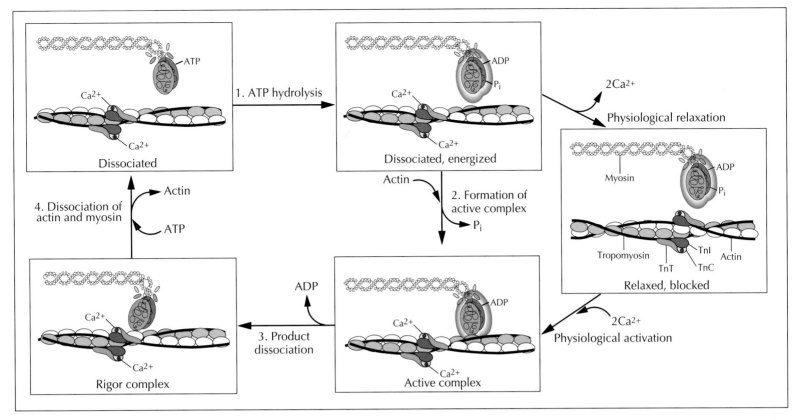

FIGURE 1-7. Reaction mechanisms of actomyosin adenosine triphosphatase (ATPase). The four steps to the *left* show the reaction in active muscle, where Ca $^{2+}$ is bound to troponin C (TnC) and the regulatory proteins do not interfere with the interactions between actin and myosin responsible for the contractile process. Beginning at the *upper left*, adenosine triphosphate (ATP) bound to myosin dissociates the thick and thin filaments. **Step 1,** Hydrolysis of this bound ATP by the ATPase site on the myosin head transfers the chemical energy of the nucleotide to myosin, which energizes the cross-bridges (*upper right*). **Step 2,** Actin interacts with the energized myosin cross-bridges to form an active complex (*lower right*) in which the energy derived from ATP is retained in the actin-bound cross-bridge, whose orientation has not yet shifted. **Step 3,** Dissociation of adenosine diphosphate (ADP) from the cross-bridge leads to the formation of the rigor complex, which causes the muscle to contract by allowing the chemical energy derived from ATP

hydrolysis to perform mechanical work (the "rowing" motion of the cross-bridge). **Step 4,** The thick and thin filaments are again dissociated when a new molecule of ATP binds to the rigor complex. This cycle of activity continues as long as Ca $^{2+}$ remains bound to the regulatory proteins and actin is free to interact with the myosin cross-bridges. **Physiological relaxation** (diagram at the *right*) occurs when Ca $^{2+}$ becomes dissociated from TnC and the positions of tropomyosin and the troponin complex on the thin filament shift so as to prevent active sites on actin from interacting with myosin cross-bridges. Even though the latter are still energized, they are unable to interact with actin so that the muscle remains in a relaxed state. **Physiological activation** (diagram at the *right*) occurs when Ca $^{2+}$ binding to TnC causes allosteric effects that rearrange the proteins of the thin filament to expose active sties on actin. This allows actin to form the active complex with myosin.

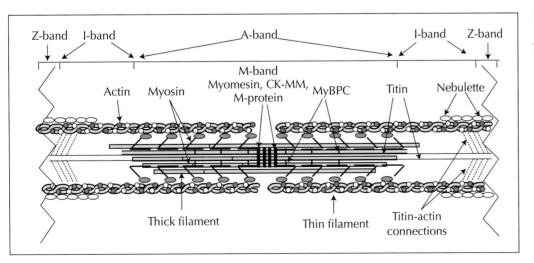

FIGURE 1-8. The thick and thin filaments of the sarcomeres in the heart are supported by a cytoskeletal lattice [7,8] that includes the giant protein titin, which extends from the Z-band into the thick filament. Titin is connected to myosin near the center of the thick filament by myosin-binding protein C (MyBPC) and near the Z-band to the thin filaments by titin-actin connections. Several proteins that make up the M-bands at the center of the thick filament include myomesin, M protein, and the MM isoform of creatine phosphokinase (CK-MM). Nebulette, a protein related to nebulin in skeletal muscle, connects the ends of the thin filaments to the Z-band [9].

EXCITATION-CONTRACTION COUPLING

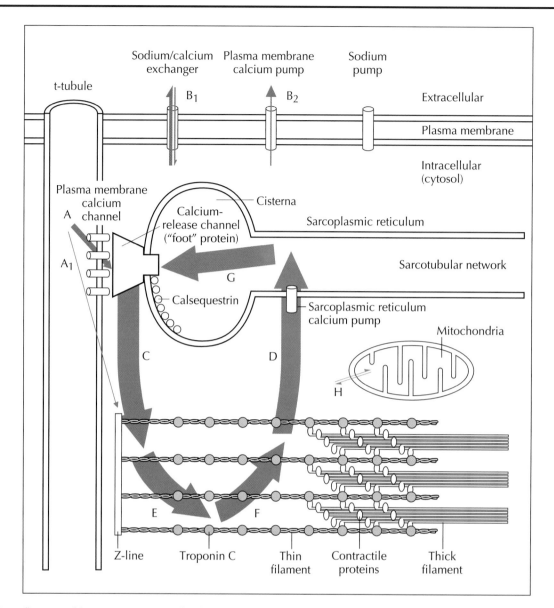

FIGURE 1-9. The calcium fluxes and key structures involved in cardiac excitation-contraction coupling. The directions of the *arrows* indicate the "energetics" of the calcium fluxes: a *downward arrow* describes a passive, downhill calcium flux, and an *upward arrow* represents active, energy-dependent calcium transport. The thickness of each arrow indicates the magnitude of the calcium flux. Two calcium cycles regulate excitation-contraction coupling and relaxation. The larger calcium cycle is entirely intracellular and involves calcium fluxes into and out of the sarcoplasmic reticulum, and calcium binding to and calcium release from troponin C. The smaller "extracellular" calcium cycle occurs when this cation moves into and out of the cell, and involves calcium fluxes between the cytosol and extracellular fluid across the plasma membrane. In the extracellular calcium cycle, excitation-contraction coupling is initiated when an action potential opens plasma membrane calcium channels to allow passive entry of calcium into the cell from the extracellular fluid (*arrow A*). Much of this calcium binds to intracellular calcium release channels, where it triggers calcium release from the sarcoplasmic reticulum. In the adult mammalian heart, only a small portion of the calcium that enters the cell directly activates the contractile proteins (*arrow A_1*).

The extracellular cycle is completed when calcium is actively transported back out to the extracellular fluid by way of two plasma membrane fluxes mediated by the sodium-calcium exchanger (*arrow B_1*) and the plasma membrane calcium pump (*arrow B_2*). In the fetal heart, where the sarcoplasmic reticulum is less well developed, the extracellular calcium cycle plays a more important direct role in excitation-contraction coupling.

In the intracellular calcium cycle, the sarcoplasmic reticulum membrane regulates two calcium fluxes within the cell. Passive calcium release through channels in the cisternae (*arrow C*) initiates contraction (*see* Fig. 1-6), and active calcium uptake by the calcium pump of the sarcotubular network (*arrow D*) relaxes the heart. Diffusion of calcium within the sarcoplasmic reticulum (*arrow G*) returns this activator cation to the cisternae, where it is stored in a complex with calsequestrin and other calcium-binding proteins.

Movements of calcium into and out of mitochondria (*arrow H*) represent yet another intracellular calcium cycle, but in the normal heart these fluxes are slow and are of little functional importance. Under conditions of calcium overload, as occurs in the ischemic heart, calcium uptake by the mitochondria can help buffer the cytosolic Ca^{2+} concentration.

Calcium released from the sarcoplasmic reticulum initiates systole when it binds to troponin C (*arrow E*). Lowering of cytosolic Ca^{2+} by the sarcoplasmic reticulum calcium pump, by causing this ion to dissociate from troponin (arrow F), relaxes the heart. The ratio E:F, which is the Ca^{2+} affinity of the calcium-specific binding site on cardiac troponin C (*see* Fig. 1-4), is lowered when troponin I is phosphorylated by cAMP-dependent protein kinases, and is increased by α-adrenergic agonists, thereby potentiating or attenuating relaxation, respectively. (*Adapted from* Katz [2]; with permission.)

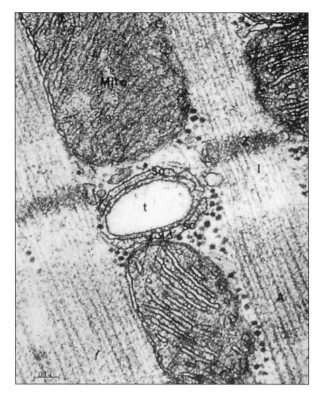

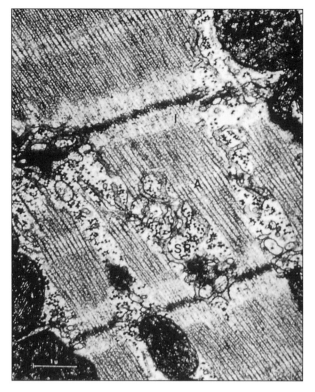

FIGURE 1-10. Cross-section of the triad in rat ventricular muscle. The large central structure is a cross-section of the transverse (t) tubular system, which is surrounded by two cisternae (sc), each of which partially envelops the t-tubule. The cisternal membrane does not contact the t-tubule; instead, excitation-contraction coupling depends on electron-dense "foot" proteins that lie between these two membranes (*arrows*). A—A-band; I—I-band; Mito—mitochondria; Z—Z-line. Scale bar = 0.1 μm. (*Courtesy of* Judy Upshaw-Earley and Ernest Page, Chicago, IL, and *adapted from* Katz [2]; with permission.)

FIGURE 1-11. The sarcotubular network (SR) of rat ventricular muscle in a "grazing" section over the sarcomeres. The dark granules near this structure are glycogen. The faint linear structure composed of two parallel lines, crossing the SR (*lower right*), probably represents a microtubule. A—A-band; Mito—mitochondria; I—I-band; Z—Z-line. Scale bar = 0.1 μm. (*Courtesy of* Judy Upshaw-Earley and Ernest Page, Chicago, IL, and *adapted from* Katz [2]; with permission.)

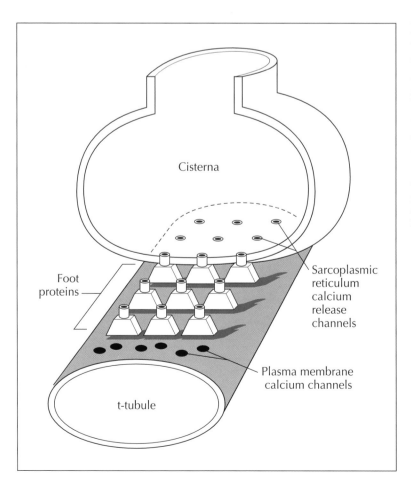

FIGURE 1-12. Schematic diagram of a triad (*see* Fig. 1-10) showing the foot proteins, which are now recognized to be intracellular calcium release channels that control the flux of activator calcium from the cisternae to the cytosol [10]. These sarcoplasmic reticulum calcium release channels (also called *ryanodine receptors* because they bind tightly to this plant alkaloid) are opened during the plateau of the cardiac action potential when a small amount of calcium enters the cytosol (*see* Fig. 1-9) from the t-tubule through the plasma membrane calcium channels (also called *dihydropyridine receptors* because they bind with high affinity to this class of calcium channel blockers) [11]. There are approximately twice as many sarcoplasmic reticulum calcium release channels as plasma membrane calcium channels [2]. (*Adapted from* Katz [2]; with permission.)

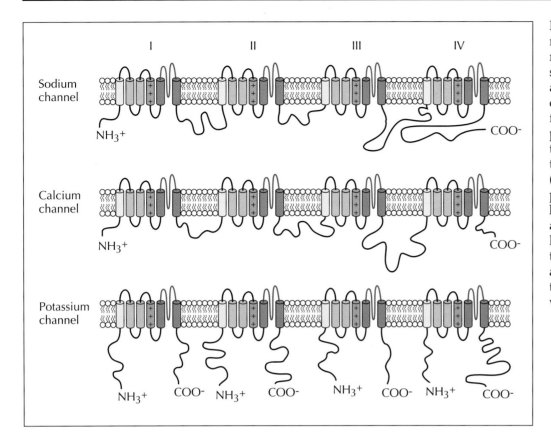

FIGURE 1-13. Molecular structures of the major subunits of voltage-gated plasma membrane ion channels. The large (α) subunits of sodium and calcium channels and the smaller subunits of potassium channels are members of an extended family of plasma membrane ion channel proteins. In sodium and calcium channels, these subunits are covalently linked tetramers made up of four domains (numbered I to IV). Although most potassium channels also contain four homologous domains, unlike the sodium and calcium channels these are not covalently linked. Not shown in this figure are the β-, γ-, and δ-subunits, which are associated with and regulate many of these channels. (*Adapted from* Katz [2]; with permission.)

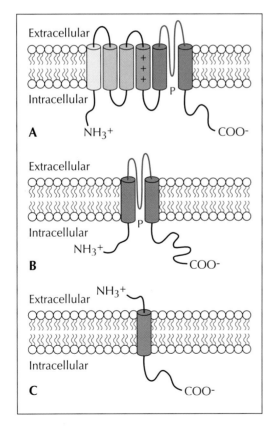

FIGURE 1-14. Potassium channels are more diverse than either sodium or calcium channels, and include three distinct structures [12]. **A,** The "Shaker" class of potassium channels, which includes the outwardly rectifying channels that repolarize the mammalian heart, is made up of four domains like that shown in Fig. 1-13. The presence of several members of the class, whose domains differ in their amino acid structure, probably allows various patterns of mixing and matching to provide a diverse group of channel structures. **B,** Inward rectifying potassium channels, which generate currents that contribute to the plateau of the cardiac action potential, are much smaller and contain only two membrane-spanning α-helical domains. However, these smaller channels are related to the Shaker class of channels in that their structures are analogous to the S_5 and S_6 transmembrane segments and the intervening peptide chain that make up the pore region of the larger ion channel. **C,** A third class of very small potassium channels, called *minK* (minimal K), includes only a single membrane-spanning domain. The role of these channels in the heart is not yet clear; they probably serve to regulate the larger channels depicted in *A* and *B*. (*Adapted from* Lester and Dascal [13]; with permission.)

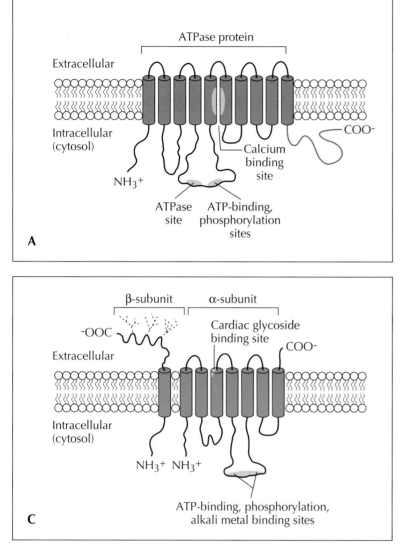

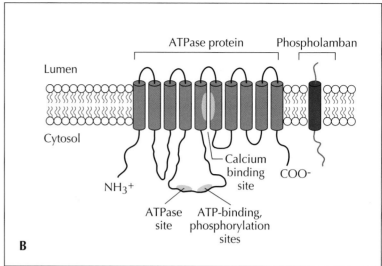

FIGURE 1-15. Cation pump adenosine triphosphatases (ATPases). Like many other structures in the heart, the cation pumps (called *P-type ion pumps*) are members of an extended family of related proteins. The calcium pump ATPases in both the plasma membrane (**A**) and the sarcoplasmic reticulum (**B**) consist of a single peptide

chain believed to contain 10 membrane-spanning α-helices (shown as cylinders). The ATP-binding and phosphorylation sites are at the cytosolic side of the membrane, whereas calcium gains access to a high-affinity cation-binding site that is probably within the bilayer and includes several membrane-spanning α-helices.

Portions of the C-terminal region of the peptide chain of both calcium pumps play important regulatory roles. In the plasma membrane calcium pump, this regulatory segment is a part of the peptide chain of the ATPase protein, whereas in the sarcoplasmic reticulum calcium pump an analogous peptide chain has become a separate regulator protein called *phospholamban*. Functional calcium pumps are dimers of the structures shown in this figure, whereas phospholamban forms a pentamer. The sodium pump (**C**), also called the *Na,K-ATPase* because it is activated when both of these alkali metal ions are present together, contains two subunits. The larger α-subunit, which is a P-type ion pump related to the calcium pump ATPases, contains ATP-binding and phosphorylation sites on the cytosolic surface. Sodium gains access to its binding site on the cytosolic side of the pump from which it is transported out of the cell, and potassium that is transported into the cell binds to the extracellular surface of the pump, near the cardiac glycoside-binding site. The role of the β-subunit is not well understood.

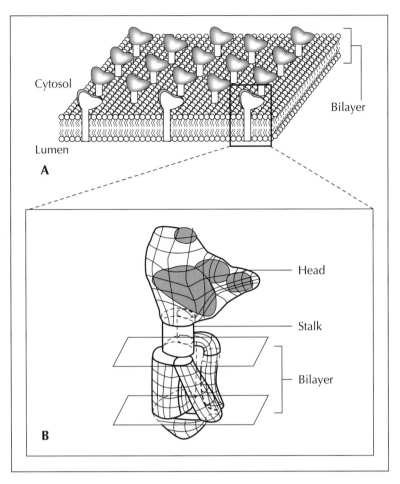

A

B

Head

Stalk

Bilayer

Cytosol

Lumen

Bilayer

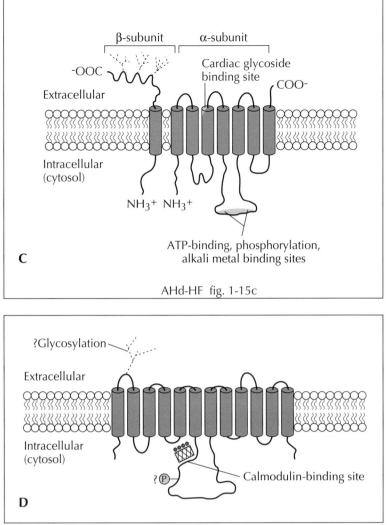

C

β-subunit   α-subunit

-OOC

Cardiac glycoside
binding site

COO-

Extracellular

Intracellular
(cytosol)

NH_3^+ NH_3^+

ATP-binding, phosphorylation,
alkali metal binding sites

AHd-HF fig. 1-15c

D

?Glycosylation

Extracellular

Intracellular
(cytosol)

? (P)

Calmodulin-binding site

FIGURE 1-16. Orientation of the calcium pump in the sarcoplasmic reticulum. **A,** The sarcotubular network contains a densely packed array of calcium pump ATPase molecules. (Note that the orientation of the pump is reversed from that in Fig. 1-15*B*.) **B,** Each subunit of the calcium pump ATPase resembles a bird whose "head," which projects into the cytosolic space, contains both the ATP-binding and phosphorylation sites. **C,** Each subunit of the calcium pump ATPase is a large peptide that includes 10 α-helical transmembrane segments (cylinders labeled M1 to M10) and five α-helices that make up the stalk (cylinders labeled S_1 to S_5). The large cytoplasmic loop between S_4 and S_5 contains the ATP-binding and phosphorylation sites. The calcium-binding site lies within the membrane bilayer and appears to include the M4, M5, M6, and M8 membrane-spanning α-helices [14]. **D,** Structure of the sodium-calcium exchanger showing 12 α-helical transmembrane segments (represented as cylinders), a possible glycosylation site on the extracellular surface, and phosphorylation (P) and calmodulin-binding sites within the cytosol [15]. (Part A *adapted from* Katz [2]; part B *adapted from* Toyoshima and coworkers [16]; with permission.)

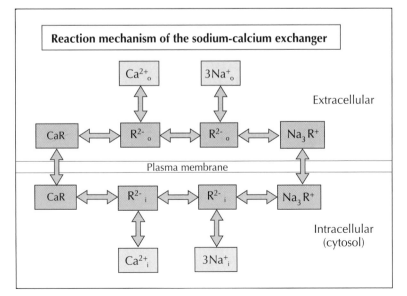

Reaction mechanism of the sodium-calcium exchanger

Ca^{2+}_o $3Na^+_o$

Extracellular

CaR R^{2-}_o R^{2-}_o Na_3R^+

Plasma membrane

CaR R^{2-}_i R^{2-}_i Na_3R^+

Intracellular
(cytosol)

Ca^{2+}_i $3Na^+_i$

FIGURE 1-17. Reaction mechanism of the sodium-calcium exchanger. The exchanger, labeled *R* and assigned two negative charges, can move either three sodium ions or one calcium ion in either direction across the plasma membrane in exchange for either three sodium ions or one calcium ion that cross the membrane in the opposite direction. Because a net movement of positive charge accompanies the flux of sodium, the sodium-calcium exchanger generates a small membrane current and so is electrogenic. The rates of sodium and calcium transported by the exchanger in either direction across the plasma membrane depend on the relative concentrations of these ions on either side of the membrane and on transmembrane potential. The positive inotropic effect of the cardiac glycosides, which directly inhibit the sodium pump, is mediated by the sodium-calcium exchanger. Because digitalis increases Na^+_i, the exchanger will carry more sodium and therefore less calcium out of the cytosol. By increasing cellular stores of calcium, this effect allows the cardiac glycosides to augment myocardial contractility.

DUAL ROLE OF ATP IN MYOCARDIAL FUNCTION

SUBSTRATE EFFECTS (ATP<1 μM)

Actomyosin ATPase (contractile proteins)
Ion pumps (sodium and calcium pumps)

ALLOSTERIC (REGULATORY) EFFECTS (ATP 0.1 TO >1 mM)

"Plasticize" actomyosin
Accelerate ion pumps (sodium and calcium pumps)
Accelerate ion exchanger (sodium/calcium exchange)
Accelerate ion fluxes
  Plasma membrane sodium and calcium channels
  Sarcoplasmic reticulum calcium release channels
Inhibit ATP regeneration
  Glycolysis
  Glycogenolysis
  Oxidative phosphorylation

FIGURE 1-18. Dual role of adenosine triphosphate (ATP) in myocardial function. ATP has two fundamentally different effects on myocardial function [17]. *Substrate* effects are seen at very low ATP concentrations, below 1 μM, which saturate the substrate-binding sites that provide energy for ion pumps and the contractile proteins. These substrate effects require that ATP be hydrolyzed to release its chemical energy. ATP at much higher concentrations exerts quite different *allosteric* effects, which do not require that ATP be hydrolyzed and therefore can be mimicked by nonhydrolyzable ATP analogs. The allosteric effects seen at normal cytosolic ATP concentrations, which are in the millimolar range, generally stimulate ion pumps, ion exchangers, and ion channels; therefore, ATP can be regarded as a "lubricant" that increases both active and passive ion fluxes. Attenuation of these allosteric effects inhibits the calcium fluxes involved in both excitation and relaxation (*see* Fig. 1-9), and thereby reduces contractility and slows relaxation in the energy-starved heart. Because ATP binding to myosin cross-bridges also dissociates actin and myosin (*see* Fig. 1-7), a fall in ATP concentration directly inhibits relaxation of the contractile proteins. Other allosteric effects seen at normal cellular levels of ATP slow energy production by inhibiting glycolysis, glycogenolysis, and oxidative phosphorylation. Attenuation of these inhibitory effects enables a decreased cellular ATP concentration to promote ATP regeneration in the energy-starved heart. ATPase—adenosine triphosphatase.

CELLULAR REGULATION

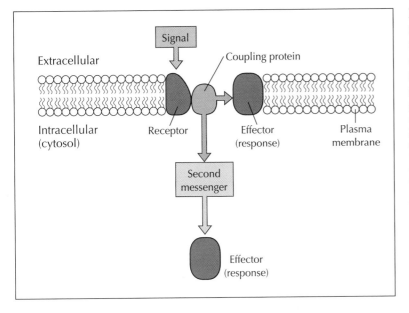

FIGURE 1-19. Most signals that impinge on the heart modify function by initiating complex multistep responses. For example, the signal generated by the arrival of a neurotransmitter at the extracellular side of the plasma membrane is commonly "recognized" when the transmitter molecule (ligand) binds with high affinity to a specific receptor. In most cases, the response to the signal requires that the ligand-bound receptor activate a coupling protein, which is a member of an extended family of GTP-binding proteins. By interacting *directly* with an effector molecule, *indirectly* by initiating the production of a second messenger, or both, the activated coupling proteins then evoke a response. Specificity in the responses to the many signals that influence cardiac function reflects the high affinity of the ligand for a specific receptor, the ability of a given ligand-receptor complex to activate a specific coupling protein, and the affinity of the activated coupling protein for specific effector systems in the cell.

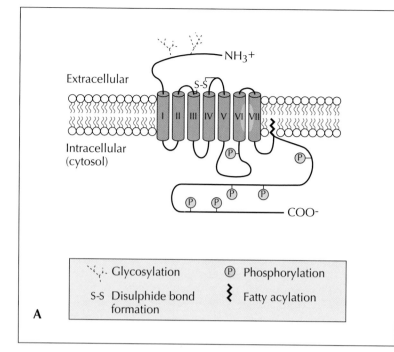

A

Glycosylation
Phosphorylation
S-S Disulphide bond formation
Fatty acylation

B. DIVERSITY OF THE KNOWN LIGANDS FOR CLONED G-PROTEIN–COUPLED RECEPTORS

Biogenic amines	Epinephrine Norepinephrine Dopamine Acetylcholine	Histamine 5-Hydroxytryptamine Adenosine
Tachykinins	Substance P Substance K Neuromedin K	
Glycoprotein hormones	Thyrotropin Follicle-stimulating hormone Lutropin/choriogonadotropin	
Polypeptide hormones **Brain/gut peptide hormones**	Parathyroid hormone Angiotensin Arginine-vasopressin Vasoactive intestinal polypeptide	Bombesin/gastrin-releasing hormone Thyrotropin-releasing hormone
Arachidonic acid derivatives	Thromboxane A_2	
Sensory stimuli	Light (ie, retinal) Odorants	
Miscellaneous	Thrombin Endothelins Platelet-activating factor N-formyl peptide	Mating factors (yeast) cAMP (Dictyostelium) Cannabinoids C_{5A}

FIGURE 1-20. The seven transmembrane domain receptors. **A,** Like many other proteins in the heart, these receptors are members of an extended family of membrane proteins that share a number of structural features. These include the seven α-helical transmembrane segments (represented as cylinders), a large N-terminal extracellular loop containing glycosylation sites, a fatty acylation site within the bilayer, and a C-terminal intracellular loop containing phosphorylation sites. The most highly conserved peptide sequences are in the transmembrane segments, whereas diversity is greatest in the hydrophilic connecting loops. **B,** Several of the ligands that bind to these G-protein–coupled receptors are listed. (*Adapted from* Lefkowitz [18]; with permission.)

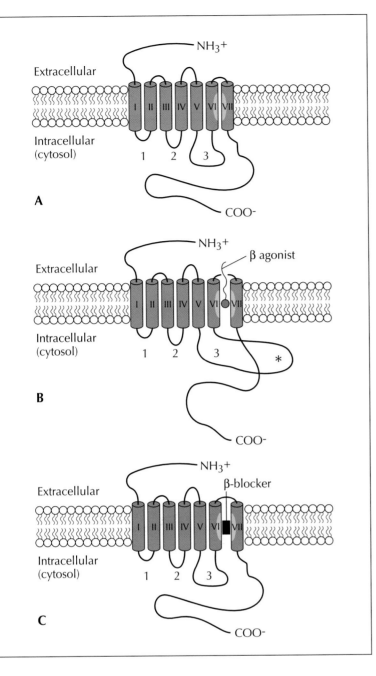

FIGURE 1-21. A, β-Agonists and β-blockers bind competitively to β-adrenergic receptors in the plasma membrane. The receptors are members of the family shown in Fig. 1-20 and contain seven membrane-spanning α-helices (cylinders labeled *I* to *VII*), three intracellular loops (labeled *1* to *3*), a large cytosolic C-terminal peptide chain, and an extracellular N-terminal region.

B, Binding of the β-agonist to the receptor site, which probably includes several of the membrane-spanning domains within the bilayer, activates the receptor. Activation, depicted as a conformational change in the large intracellular cytoplasmic loop labeled *3* (*asterisk*), increases the affinity of the receptor for binding to a coupling G-protein.

C, Binding of a β-blocker to the receptor site competitively inhibits agonist binding to this site. However, unlike the agonists, β-blockers are unable to activate the β-receptor and so block the response by preventing the receptor from stimulating the G-protein [2]. (*Adapted from* Katz [2]; with permission.)

COUPLING PROTEINS

SOME MEMBERS OF THE FAMILY OF GTP-BINDING PROTEINS

G_α PROTEIN	EFFECTOR	RECEPTORS	ADP-RIBOSYLATION BY
G_s	Adenylyl cyclase (+); K^+, Ca^{2+} channels (+)	β-Adrenergic	CT
G_i	Adenylyl cyclase (-); phospholipase C (+)	mChR; α_2-adrenergic	PT
G_o	Neuronal Ca^{2+} channel, others	mChR; α_2-adrenergic	PT
G_k (G_{i3})	Atrial K^+ channel (+)	mChR	PT
G_q	Phospholipase C (+); phospholipase A_2 (+)	mChR; α_1-adrenergic	Neither

FIGURE 1-22. The G_α-proteins are members of an extended family of coupling proteins. Different members of this family in cardiovascular tissue are ADP-ribosylated by different bacterial toxins. Whereas some of the G_α-proteins, *eg*, the stimulatory G_s that mediates adrenergic stimulation, are ribosylated by cholera toxin (CT), the inhibitory G_i that mediates parasympathetic effects is ribosylated by pertussis toxin (PT). Thus, whereas CT generally modifies activator responses, the PT modifies inhibitory responses. GTP—guanosine triphosphate; mChR—muscarinic cholinergic receptor; - —inhibits; + —stimulates. (*Adapted from* Fleming and coworkers [19].)

DIRECT AND INDIRECT ACTIVATION

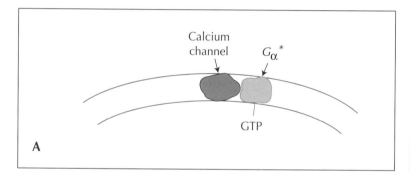

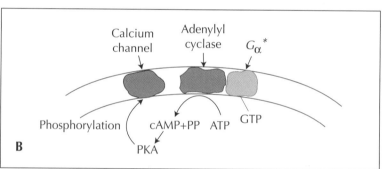

FIGURE 1-23. Direct and indirect activation. Two very different mechanisms, direct and indirect, allow the activated G_α*-GTP complex to mediate the response to β-adrenergic agonists. **A,** In direct regulation, activated G_α*-GTP binds to the effector, here shown as a plasma membrane calcium channel, to modify cell function. **B,** In the indirect mechanism, activated G_α*-GTP binds to and modifies an enzyme, such as adenylyl cyclase, which catalyzes the formation of a second messenger such as cyclic adenosine monophosphate (cAMP). In the latter mechanism, it is the second messenger that interacts with the effector to modify cell function (*see* Fig. 1-19). ATP—adenosine triphosphate; GTP—guanosine triphosphate; PKA— cAMP-dependent protein kinase; PP—pyrophosphate.

RECEPTOR DESENSITIZATION AND RESENSITIZATION

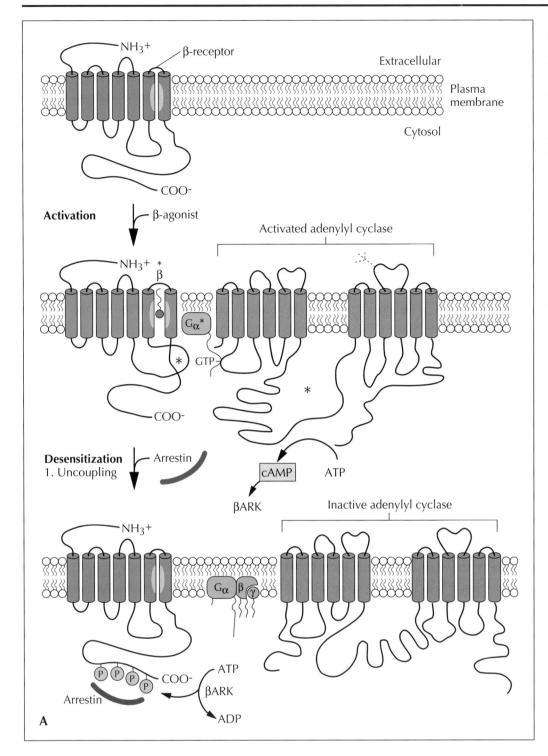

FIGURE 1-24. Mechanisms by which prolonged activation can desensitize (downregulate) β-adrenergic receptors [2]. **A,** Binding of a β-adrenergic agonist to its receptor (*activation*), which stimulates adenylyl cyclase to produce cyclic adenosine monophosphate (cAMP), can, when sustained, cause *desensitization*, which proceeds through three sequential steps. The first, *uncoupling*, is initiated when the cAMP produced by activated adenylyl cyclase stimulates a cAMP-dependent protein kinase called β-adrenergic receptor kinase (βARK), which phosphorylates the β-receptor. The coupling protein that activates βARK has recently been suggested to be $G_{\beta\gamma}$. The phosphorylated receptor (P) then binds arrestin, an inhibitor protein that prevents further interaction of the receptor with the G proteins. (*continued*)

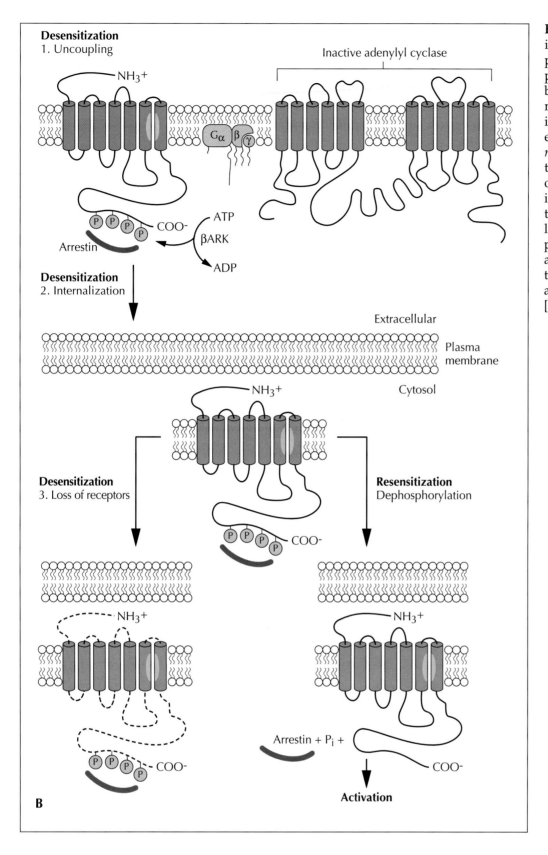

FIGURE 1-24. (*continued*) **B,** Uncoupling is followed by *internalization*, a reversible process that occurs when the phosphorylated receptor-arrestin complex becomes detached from the plasma membrane and moves into the cytosol. The internalized receptors can then undergo either of two further reactions. One, *loss of receptors*, continues receptor desensitization through irreversible proteolytic digestion of the internalized receptors. Alternatively, if the β-adrenergic stimulation ends before the internalized receptors are digested, the latter can be dephosphorylated by a phosphoprotein phosphatase, which causes arrestin to dissociate, allowing the receptor to return to the plasma membrane. ATP—adenosine triphosphate. (*Adapted from* Katz [2]; with permission.)

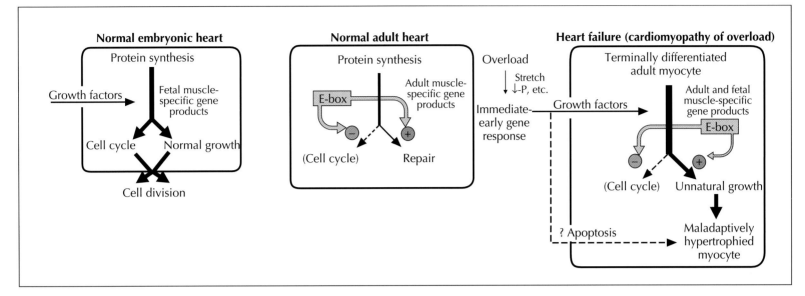

FIGURE 1-25. Differences in the overall growth patterns of proliferating myocytes of the embryonic heart, terminally differentiated myocytes of the adult heart, and maladaptively hypertrophied myocytes of the failing heart. In the embryonic heart, growth factors stimulate preferential synthesis of fetal protein isoforms, which, because it is matched to cell division, leads to the normal cell cycle. Withdrawal of the growth factors and binding of myogenic factors to the E-box in the terminally differentiated cells of the normal adult heart slows protein synthesis, inhibits the cell cycle, and favors the synthesis of adult muscle-specific gene products.

In the terminally differentiated cells of the normal adult heart, the slow rate of protein synthesis is appropriate for repair and renewal of cellular constituents. Overloading of the adult heart appears to initiate an unnatural growth response by activating an immediate-early gene response that renews growth factor stimulation, accelerates protein synthesis, and favors the expression of fetal muscle-specific gene products. In contrast to the embryonic heart, however, the cell cycle remains inhibited, so that the growth response of the overloaded adult cardiac myocytes is abnormal. Cell death in the overloaded heart, which probably plays an important role in the poor prognosis of patients with heart failure, may reflect, in part, the ability of some of the growth factors produced in the immediate-early gene response not only to stimulate protein synthesis, but also to cause programmed cell death (apoptosis). (*Adapted from* Katz [3]; with permission.)

REFERENCES

1. Katz AM: Molecular biology in cardiology: a paradigmatic shift. *J Mol Cell Cardiol* 1988, 20:355–366.

2. Katz AM: *Physiology of the Heart*, edn 2. New York: Raven Press; 1992.

3. Katz AM: The cardiomyopathy of overload: an unnatural growth response in the hypertrophied heart. *Ann Intern Med* 1994, 121:363–371.

4. Katz AM: Congestive heart failure: role of altered myocardial cellular control. *N Engl J Med* 1975, 293:1184–1191.

5. McNutt NA, Fawcett DW: Myocardial ultrastructure. In *The Mammalian Myocardium.* Edited by Langer GA, Brady AJ. New York: Wiley; 1974:1–49.

6. Herzberg O, James MNG: Structure of calcium regulatory protein troponin C at 28Å resolution. *Nature* 1985, 313:653–659.

7. Small JV, Fürst DO, Thornell L-E: The cytoskeletal lattice of muscle cells. *Eur J Biochem* 1992, 208:559–572.

8. Moncman CL, Wang K, Nebulette A: A 107 kD nebulin-like protein in cardiac muscle. *Cell Motil Cytoskeleton* 1995, 32:205–225.

9. Small JF, Fürst DO, Thornrell L-E: The cytoskeletal lattice of muscle cells. *Eur J Biochem* 1992, 208:559–572.

10. Fleischer S, Inui M: Biochemistry and biophysics of excitation-contraction coupling. *Ann Rev Biophys Biomol Chem* 1989, 18:333–364.

11. McDonald TF, Pelzer S, Trautwein W, Pelzer D: Regulation and modulation of calcium channels in cardiac, skeletal, and smooth muscle cells. *Physiol Rev* 1994, 72:365–507.

12. Katz AM: Selectivity and toxicity of antiarrhythmic drugs: molecular interactions with ion channels. *Am J Med* 1998, 104:179–195.

13. Lester HA, Dascal N: Potassium channels: the response to vagus-stoff. *Nature* 1993, 364:758–759.

14. Lytton J, MacLennan DH: Sarcoplasmic reticulum. In *The Heart and Circulation*, edn 2. Edited by Fozzard H, Haber E, Katz A, *et al.* New York: Raven Press; 1991:1203–1222.

15. Nicoll DA, Longoni S, Phillipson KD: Molecular cloning and functional expression of the cardiac sarcolemmal Na$^+$-Ca^{2+} exchanger. *Science* 1990, 250:562–565.

16. Toyoshima C, Sasabe H, Stokes DL: Three-dimensional cryo-electron microscopy of the calcium ion pump in the sarcoplasmic reticulum membrane. *Nature* 1993, 362:469–471.

17. Katz AM: Is the failing heart an energy-starved organ? *J Cardiac Failure* 1996, 2:267–272.

18. Lefkowitz RJ: Thrombin receptor: variations on a theme. *Nature* 1991, 351:353–354.

19. Fleming JW, Wister P, Watanabe AM: Signal transduction by G proteins in cardiac tissue. *Circulation* 1992, 85:420–433.

MYOCARDIAL MECHANISMS AND NEUROHUMORAL REGULATION OF THE CIRCULATION

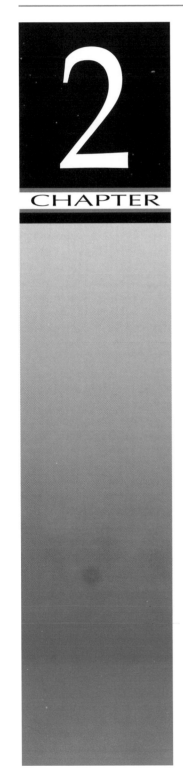

2

CHAPTER

Mark R. Starling

The principal function of the heart is to propel oxygenated blood to the peripheral tissues to meet their metabolic demands. The systemic arterial and venous systems provide the conduits. The interaction of the left ventricle (LV) with the arterial and venous systems is therefore integral to the satisfactory performance of this vital function. It is important to understand how the normal heart functions and how it interacts with the systemic arterial and venous systems to determine how it is affected by disturbances in the performance of this vital function that occur with various pathologic conditions. This chapter provides a physiologic framework for understanding normal cardiac contraction and relaxation and the interaction of the LV with the systemic arterial and venous systems by developing seven basic concepts. Taken together, these concepts can be used to provide insight into abnormal cardiac mechanisms in pathophysiologic conditions.

First, the mechanics of cardiac contraction are examined by analysis of muscle models; isometric contraction, the force-velocity relation, and the force-velocity-length relation; the concept of length-dependent activation; the ultrastructural basis for Starling's law of the heart, differences between cardiac and skeletal muscle; and the sarcomere length-ventricular performance relation. Second, these concepts are carried into the intact heart by examining the determinants of contraction through analysis of the cardiac cycle and of LV dynamic geometry and the complex control of the intact circulation. Third, the concept of LV preload is examined through an analysis of LV diastolic properties, including the concepts of the importance of the pericardium and ventricular interaction, the regulation of venous return, and the concepts of preload reserve and afterload mismatch.

Fourth, left ventricular contractility is analyzed using the time-varying elastance model to assess the effects of catecholamines and pharmacologic depressants on contractility and the interval-strength relationship. Fifth, LV afterload is defined and the contribution of arterial properties to afterload examined, as well as the effects of arterial impedance on LV contractility and ejection, and the concept of LV-arterial coupling. Sixth, an assessment of myocardial energetics, using the myocardial oxygen consumption/pressure-volume area relationship as an approach to evaluating the efficiency of work performed by the contractile element, is presented. Finally, neural control of contractility is examined, the concept of "accentuated antagonism" defined, and the effects of neural reflexes on contractility presented.

MECHANICS OF CARDIAC CONTRACTION

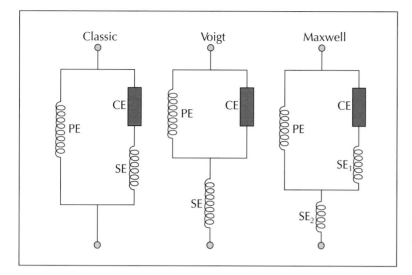

FIGURE 2-1. Muscle activity. Several muscle models have been proposed to describe muscle activity [1]. Each model is composed of three elements: first, a contractile element (CE), which is assumed to be freely distensible at rest but is capable of generating force and shortening with activation; second, one or two series elastic elements (SEs); and third, a parallel elastic element (PE). Whereas both the SE and PE are characterized by their length-tension curves, shortening of the CE is described by the relationship between force and velocity. During isometric contraction, the stimulated CE shortens, stretching the SE and thereby developing force in accordance with the stress-strain relationship of the SE. The rate of force development is therefore determined by the CE velocity and the stiffness of the SE. In the classic model, the passive length-tension curve defines the properties of the PE. In the Voigt and Maxwell models, both the PE and SE contribute to the passive length-tension curve.

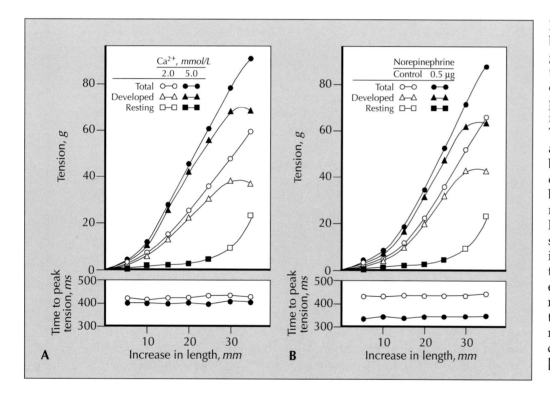

FIGURE 2-2. Tension. The relationship between developed and total tension generated at different muscle lengths at two calcium concentrations (A) and under control and enhanced contractile conditions produced by norepinephrine (B) in an isolated cat papillary muscle are illustrated. The resting length-tension curves are not altered by changes in contractile conditions, but with an increase in calcium concentration (A), there is an increase in both developed and total tension at each muscle length. In addition, at each muscle length the time to peak tension is shortened, demonstrating that an increase in tension development occurs in a shorter time, consistent with enhanced contractile element velocity. This is also true when norepinephrine is added (B), and the time to peak tension is achieved even more rapidly than with an increase in calcium concentration. (Adapted from Sonnenblick [2]; with permission.)

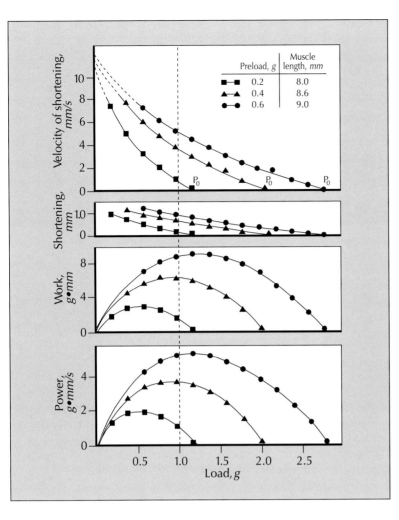

FIGURE 2-3. Preload. The effects of increasing preload, *ie* , initial muscle length, on the force-velocity and force-shortening relationship and on work and power are shown to demonstrate several concepts. First, with an increase in preload there is an increase in P_0 (isometric pressure), indicating an increase in isometric tension development consistent with the Frank-Starling mechanism. This is further illustrated for isotonic shortening by examining the effects of increasing preload on shortening and shortening velocity at the *dashed line*, representing a fixed afterload of 1.0 g. With increasing preload, there is an increase in both the extent and velocity of shortening at a fixed afterload. Second, extrapolation of the force-velocity relationship to V_{max} reveals that it is similar at all levels of preload, illustrating that preload has little or no effect on contractile element velocity. Finally, for any preload at which shortening occurs, both work and power increase as a function of increasing preload. *Work* is defined as the product of load (T) and the change in muscle length (work=T·Δl), and *power* is defined as the product of load and the rate of change in length (power=T·dl/dt). Note that at zero load both work and power are zero, and with an isometric contraction, both work and power are zero. Maximal work and power occur at an intermediate load. (*Adapted from* Sonnenblick [2]; with permission.)

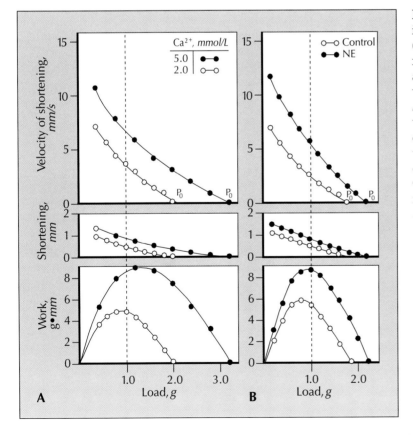

FIGURE 2-4. Force-velocity relationship. In contrast to the effects of initial muscle length, the effects of calcium and norepinephrine (NE) on the force-velocity relationship in an isolated cat papillary muscle are different [2,3]. With an increase in calcium (**A**) or administration of norepinephrine (**B**), there is an increase in the velocity of shortening for each afterload, as shown by the *dashed line,* for a load of 1.0 g. Isometric pressure, P_0, increased as it did with an increase in preload. However, in contrast to the effects of changes in preload alone, extrapolation of the force-velocity relationship to zero load indicates there is an increase in V_{max} consistent with an increase in contractile element (CE) velocity. Consistent with enhanced CE velocity in the isolated cat papillary muscle, there is an increase in shortening and an increase in work at each afterload. (*Adapted from* Sonnenblick [2]; with permission.)

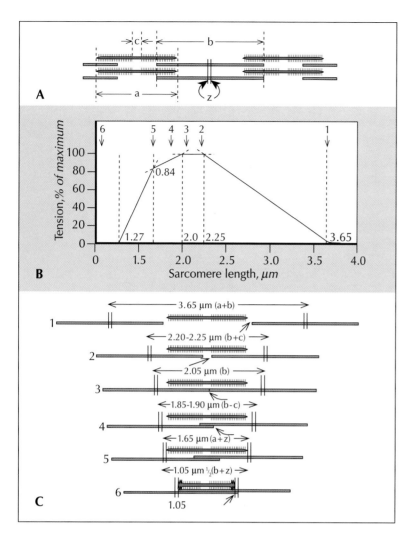

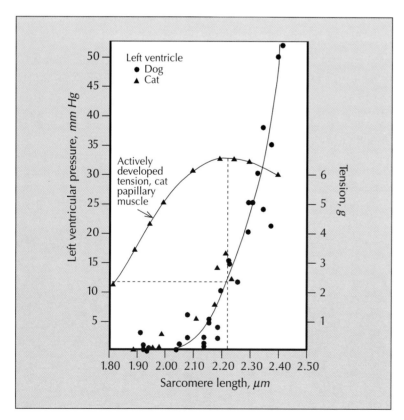

FIGURE 2-5. The Frank Starling Phenomenon. The capacity of the left ventricle to vary the force of contraction on a beat-to-beat basis is a function of preload, which reflects sarcomere length, and constitutes one of the major principles of cardiac function. It is generally referred to as the *Frank-Starling phenomenon*. This fundamental property of the heart is based on the myocardial length-tension relationship in which the force of contraction or extent of shortening is dependent on the initial muscle length. This, in turn, is dependent on the ultrastructural disposition of the thick and thin myofilaments of sarcomeres. The relationship between myofilament disposition and tension development in skeletal muscle is illustrated [4–6].

A, The myofilaments of the sarcomere are drawn to scale, where the thin filaments are 1.0 µm and the thick filaments are 1.6 µm in length. **B,** The relationship between tension developed at specific sarcomere lengths in a single skeletal muscle fiber as a percent of the maximal tension. The numbers shown across the *top* denote the specific break-points in the curve corresponding to the sarcomere lengths depicted in the diagram at the *bottom*. Note that there is no overlap of the myofilaments at 3.65 µm to the far right of the tension curve. **C,** Optimal overlap of the myofilaments occurs at sarcomere lengths between 2.0 µm and 2.25 µm. As the sarcomere length falls below 2.0 µm, the thick and thin filaments begin to overlap to various extents. At approximately 1.25 µm, no tension is developed, because the thick and thin filaments are completely overlapped and compressed below the length of the thick filaments. The overlapping below 2.0 µm interferes with the formation of cross-bridges and therefore may alter the ability of the thick and thin filaments to bind calcium, reduce the sensitivity of the overlapping thick and thin filaments to calcium, or generate significant internal loads that impede shortening of the sarcomere. a—thick filament length; b—thin filament length; c—central region on thick filament without cross-bridges; z—Z-line attachments of thin filaments. (*Adapted from* Gordon and coworkers [6]; with permission.)

FIGURE 2-6. The relationship between midwall sarcomere length and filling pressure from the left ventricle (LV) of both dog and cat. When the LV is empty the sarcomere length averages 1.9 µm, but as the LV fills the sarcomere length increases. At a filling pressure of 12 mm Hg, the sarcomere length reaches approximately 2.2 µm. As illustrated in Figure 2-5, this is the optimal sarcomere length for force generation. Note that because of the stiffness of the passive elastic (PE) element, further distention of the LV causes a sharp increase in filling pressures as the PE element attempts to resist overextension of the sarcomere and prevent disengagement of the myofilaments. Remember also that as preload is increased into these ranges, the series elastic (SE) element becomes important and may contribute to the resistance to disengagement of the myofilaments.

The relationship between tension development in the cat papillary muscle over the same range of sarcomere lengths has been superimposed on the resting length-tension relationship. This confirms the information from Figure 2-5 demonstrating that the optimal sarcomere length for maximal tension development is approximately 2.2 µm. *Dashed lines* indicate that the apex of the active length-tension relationship occurs at the optimal filling pressure of 12 mm Hg when sarcomere length approximates 2.25 µm. (*Adapted from* Spotnitz and coworkers [7]; with permission.)

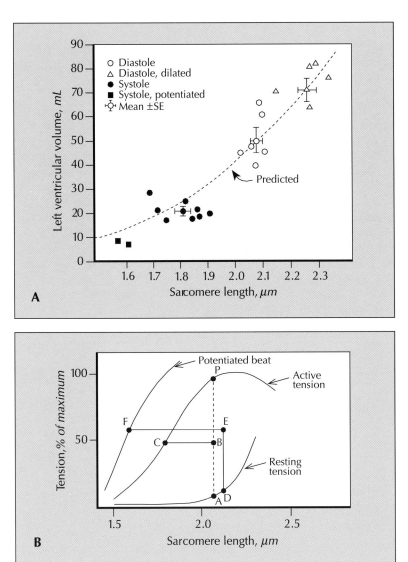

A

B

FIGURE 2-7. Ultrastructure-function relation. **A,** The relationship between left ventricular volume and midwall sarcomere length at end-diastole (*open circles*) and end-systole (*closed circles*) from an intact ejecting heart fixed *in situ* [8]. The *open triangles* indicate the end-diastolic volume and sarcomere length after dilatation of the chamber, and the *closed squares* indicate potentiated end-systolic left ventricular volumes and sarcomere lengths.

B, The data from *panel A* have been used to construct the length-tension relationship [9]. The resting length-tension relationship and two active length-tension relationships are constructed. At 2.1 μm on the passive length-tension curve (A), indicating the end-diastolic sarcomere length, the maximal pressure (tension) generated under isometric conditions is represented by P. If isotonic shortening is allowed to occur in the ejecting heart at B, sarcomere length decreases to approximately 1.8 μm, which is indicated on the active length-tension curve at point C. On a potentiated beat, end-diastolic sarcomere length would increase along the passive length-tension curve to point D. Pressure (tension) would rise to point E, and ejection would occur at the potentiated end-systolic sarcomere length of 1.6 μm (F), defining a new active length-tension curve that is shifted to the left and has a steeper slope.

Thus, it can be extrapolated that in an actively ejecting normal heart, a sarcomere length change of approximately 13% would equate to an ejection fraction of approximately 50%. With a potentiated beat, the change in sarcomere length would increase to 21%, which would produce an ejection fraction of approximately 75%. (Part A *adapted from* Sonnenblick and coworkers [8]; part B *adapted from* Ross and coworkers [9]; with permission.)

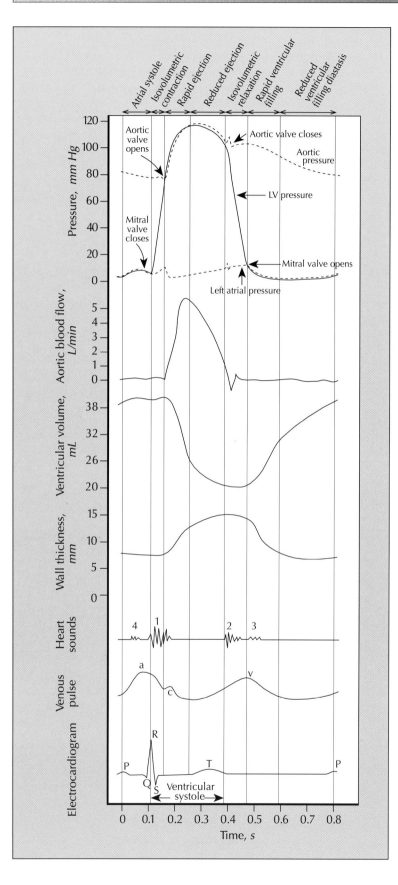

FIGURE 2-8. The events of the cardiac cycle. From *top* to *bottom*, aortic, left ventricular (LV), and left atrial pressure signals are shown, followed by the aortic flow signal, LV volume curve, LV wall thickness curve, heart sounds, the venous pulse, and the electrocardiogram. With electrical activation there is an abrupt increase in isovolumic LV pressure, followed by rapid ejection and sustained pressure elevation. Reduced ejection follows until closure of the aortic valve, achievement of zero flow, minimal volume, and maximal LV wall thickness occur, at which time diastolic events are initiated. The initial diastolic event, active LV pressure decline followed by rapid filling, manifests as a rapid increase in LV volume and thinning of the LV wall, followed by diastasis. Diastole is completed with atrial contraction. (*Adapted from* Berne and Levy [10]; with permission.)

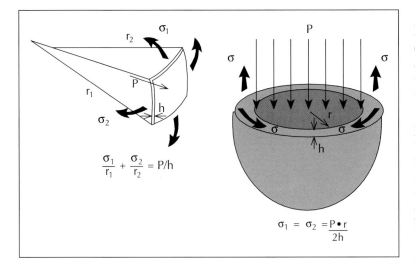

$$\frac{\sigma_1}{r_1} + \frac{\sigma_2}{r_2} = P/h$$

$$\sigma_1 = \sigma_2 = \frac{P \cdot r}{2h}$$

FIGURE 2-9. The heart compared with isolated muscle. In comparing the heart with isolated muscle, the heart's volume and pressure can be related to muscle length and tension [11]. In more complex formulations, the average circumferential wall stress (force per unit of cross-sectional area of wall) is related directly to the product of intraventricular pressure and radius, and inversely to wall thickness. In its simplest version, Laplace's law for a spherical ventricle is $\sigma = P \cdot r/2h$, where r is the left ventricular (LV) radius at the endocardial surface, P is intraventricular pressure, and h is LV wall thickness.

As illustrated here in its general form for a thin-walled sphere, the law relates the various stresses to the internal pressure, P, by the equation: $\sigma/r_1 + \sigma/r_2 = P/h$, where σ_1 and σ_2 represent stresses acting on the surface perpendicular to each other, r_1 and r_2 represent the radii of curvature of the surface, and h represents the wall thickness.

However, the LV is not a thin sphere, but rather is more appropriately represented by an ellipsoid of revolution, which is thick-walled, where σ_1 and σ_2 are not equal. Therefore, two different stresses, meridional stress acting perpendicular to the short axis and circumferential stress acting perpendicular to the long axis and in the direction of the midwall circumferential fibers, can be expressed by equations $Pb/2h (1-h/2b)^2$ and $Pb/h [1-h/2b-b^2/2a^2]$, respectively [12].

In the calculation of meridional and circumferential stress (σ_m and σ_c, respectively), a and b represent the midwall semi-major and semi-minor axes, respectively. Thus, not only do the calculations of meridional and circumferential stress vary but they may vary in a nonlinear fashion with changes in LV geometry. In the ejecting LV, the extent and rate of shortening are analogous to the extent and velocity of shortening of isolated muscle. LV pressure during ejection is therefore closely related to afterload, although geometric factors must be considered in calculating wall forces in the heart. (*Adapted from* Badke and O'Rourke [11]; with permission.)

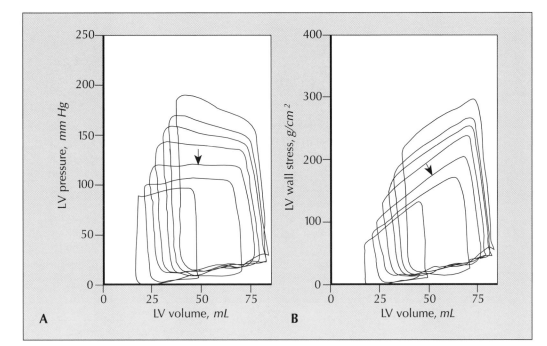

A

B

FIGURE 2-10. Left ventricular (LV) pressure-volume (**A**) and stress-volume (**B**) loops generated over a wide range of loading conditions produced by the infusion of intravenous angiotensin to increase LV pressure, or inferior vena caval obstruction to decrease LV pressure, are illustrated. The *arrows* indicate the control pressure-volume and stress-volume loops [5,13]. At end-systole the points from each pressure-volume or stress-volume loop are linear over this operating range of pressures and volumes, indicating little effect of volume and end-systolic pressure on these relationships. The configuration of the stress-volume loops clearly differs from the pressure-volume loops when LV wall thickness and geometry are included in the calculation. Nevertheless, both relationships show linearity at end-systole. The diastolic pressure-volume and stress-volume relations both appear to be curvilinear over this range of loading conditions. Consequently, both pressure-volume and stress-volume relations provide the basis for assessing both LV systolic (contractile) and diastolic function in the intact heart. (*Adapted from* Ross [13]; with permission.)

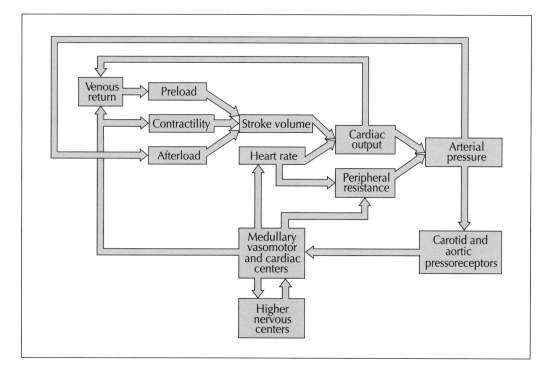

FIGURE 2-11. The various interactions controlling the intact circulation. The interaction of preload, contractility, and afterload in producing stroke volume is complex. Stroke volume combined with heart rate determines cardiac output, which, in turn, when combined with peripheral vascular resistance, determines arterial pressure for tissue perfusion. The characteristics of the arterial system also contribute to afterload on the heart. The interaction of these components with carotid and aortic arch baroreceptors provides a feedback mechanism to higher medullary and vasomotor cardiac centers and to higher levels in the central nervous system, to effect a modulating influence on heart rate, peripheral vascular resistance, venous return, and contractility [14]. Heart rate changes may also influence contractility. Cardiac output and peripheral vascular resistance can modulate venous return. This complex interaction is intrinsically fine-tuned to regulate beat-to-beat changes and thereby adapt the system in response to demand. (*Adapted from* Badke and O'Rourke [11]; with permission.)

PRELOAD

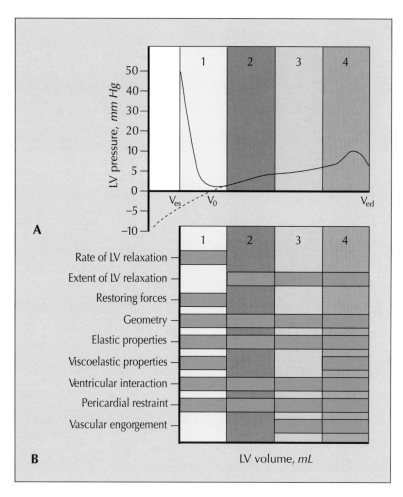

FIGURE 2-12. Left ventricular (LV) diastolic properties. **A,** LV diastole has four phases that include active relaxation during the period of isovolumic pressure decline (phase 1), rapid LV filling (phase 2), passive LV filling (phase 3), and the atrial contribution to LV filling (phase 4). LV relaxation begins at end-systolic volume (V_{es}) and is completed at end-diastolic volume (V_{ed}). V_0 represents the unstressed diastolic volume of the LV. **B,** The complex interaction of several factors can affect LV diastolic properties and include the rate of LV relaxation, the extent of LV relaxation, restoring forces of the LV, geometry of the LV, the elastic properties of the LV wall, the viscoelastic properties of the LV wall, right and left ventricular interaction, pericardial restraint, and vascular engorgement [15,16].

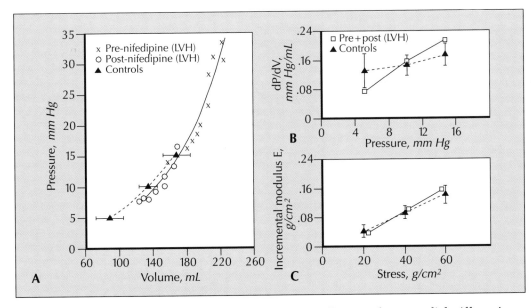

an exponential relationship between LV pressure and volume (**A**). When LV chamber stiffness is plotted against pressure, the relationship is linearized, and there is a distinct difference between the control subjects and patients with LVH, demonstrated by an increased slope in the LVH subjects consistent with increased stiffness of the LV chamber (**B**). In contrast, when myocardial stiffness is plotted against stress, there is no difference in the slope values between the control subjects and patients with LVH, indicating that the elastic stiffness of the muscle has not been affected by the hypertrophy process despite a significant change in the elastic stiffness of the LV chamber (**C**).

Therefore, LV chamber stiffness and myocardial stiffness can be used to differentiate the contribution of changes in myocardial properties to altered distensibility of the LV chamber. (*Adapted from* Mirsky [17].)

FIGURE 2-13. The use of left ventricular (LV) chamber stiffness and myocardial stiffness in differentiating the impact of pathologic processes (in this case, hypertrophy) on diastolic properties of the LV.

The plots of LV pressure versus volume in control subjects and patients with LV hyper-trophy (LVH) before and after use of nifedipine are curvilinear, representing

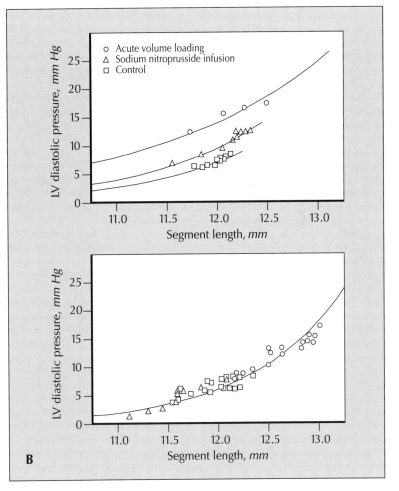

FIGURE 2-14. The pericardium has a substantial role in determining the left ventricular (LV) diastolic pressure-volume relationship. **A,** The canine pericardial pressure-volume relationship is uniquely bimodal [18]. The pericardial pressure-volume relationship was generated as right heart volume (RHV) was progressively increased from 0 to 50 mL. The pericardial pressure-volume relationships were little affected by right heart volumes. At low pericardial volumes, the pericardial pressure-volume relationship is quite flat, but it becomes extremely steep as pericardial volumes exceed approximately 225 mL. Therefore, the pericardial pressure-volume relationship has very little effect on LV diastolic properties at low pressures and volumes, but it has a substantial restraining effect at high pressures and volumes.

B, LV pressure-segment length relations in conscious, chronically instrumented dogs were analyzed during acute volume loading with (*top*) and without (*bottom*) an intact pericardium [19]. With acute volume loading they are superiorly displaced, and with sodium nitroprusside they are

inferiorly displaced toward the control level. In the same animal with the pericardium removed, these relationships are not shifted superiorly, but they remain on a continuum despite the same sequence of volume loading and sodium nitroprusside infusion. Therefore, with acute cardiac dilatation the pericardium contributes substantially to the increase in LV diastolic pressure because of shifts in the LV diastolic pressure-segment-length relationship. (*continued*)

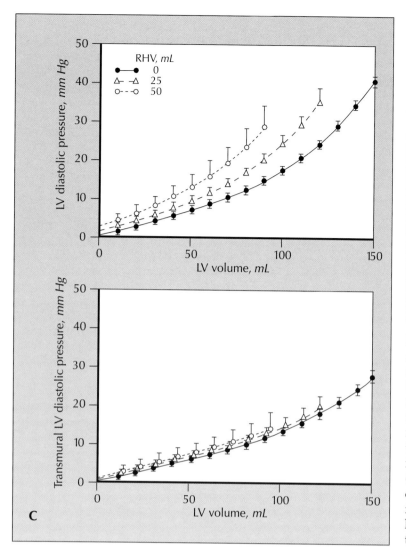

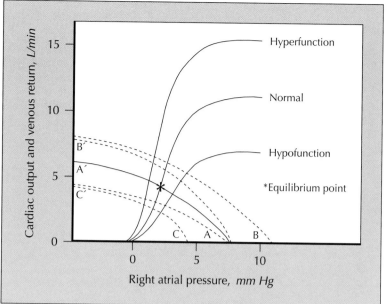

FIGURE 2-15. The regulation of venous return. The Y-axis represents cardiac output and venous return, and the X-axis represents right atrial pressure [20,21]. The *solid line* from A, on the X-axis, to A', on the Y-axis, indicates the resting venous return curve. At A, the right atrial pressure is high enough to provide no pressure gradient from the peripheral tissue to the heart, and therefore there is zero venous return. As right atrial pressure falls, the gradient from the peripheral tissues to the heart increases, and therefore venous return also increases. With superimposition of a normal cardiac output curve (normal), the crossing of the cardiac output and venous return curves is the equilibrium point at which venous return to the heart from the peripheral tissues is matched with cardiac output from the heart to the peripheral tissues. With hypofunctioning of the heart there is a shift in this equilibrium point to a higher right atrial pressure, thereby reducing venous return to the heart. With parallel upward displacement, the venous return curve operates from B to B'; with a parallel downward displacement, the venous return curve operates from C to C'.

These kinds of parallel displacements are consistent with changes in systemic venous pressure that may be attributable to changes in vasomotor tone, blood volume, interstitial fluid volume, intra-abdominal pressure, or muscle compression of the venous system. For example, with blood loss, the venous return curve shifts from the A-A' curve to the C-C' curve, and a lower equilibrium point is therefore achieved at a lower right atrial pressure and cardiac output. The opposite effect is seen with an increase in blood volume or vasomotor tone. For example, with an increase in catecholamine activity seen with exercise, the venous return curve shifts from the A-A' curve to the B-B' curve. With hyperfunction of the heart associated with enhanced catecholamine activity, as with exercise, there is a greater venous return at a lower right atrial pressure to maintain cardiac filling during the demand for high output.

A different pattern of venous return curves results from alterations in peripheral vascular resistance at the arteriolar level. With a decrease in peripheral vascular resistance, the venous return curve shifts to the A-B' curve, and with an increase in peripheral vascular resistance, the venous return curve shifts to the A-C' curve. These changes in the venous return curve result from dilatation or constriction, respectively, of the systemic arterioles. Therefore, there is dynamic equilibrium between cardiac output and venous return, which is finely regulated on a beat-to-beat basis and with changes in demand, such as exercise, to maintain cardiac output and tissue perfusion.

FIGURE 2-14. *(continued)* This kind of upward displacement of the diastolic pressure-segment length or volume relationship is indicative of the restraining effect of the pericardium. This phenomenon can also be observed with dilatation of chambers of one side of the heart. **C,** The effects of increasing RHVs on the LV pressure-volume relationship have been studied in postmortem canine hearts [18]. As RHVs are incrementally increased with the pericardium intact, LV pressures are also incrementally increased *(top).* Over a comparable range of LV volumes, there is an upward displacement of the LV pressure-volume relationship due to ventricular interaction. As a consequence, for comparable LV volumes, LV pressures are disproportionately elevated and provide an inaccurate determination of LV filling pressure. In contrast, if transmural LV pressure, which takes into account both the LV pressure and pericardial pressure, is used, there are no differences in transmural pressure across the full range of right and LV volumes *(bottom),* suggesting that transmural pressure represents a better measure of LV distending pressure. If right atrial pressure is substituted for pericardial pressure, then a simple approximation of transmural pressure can be calculated. (Parts A and C adapted from Hess and coworkers [18]; part B adapted from Shirato and coworkers [19]; with permission.)

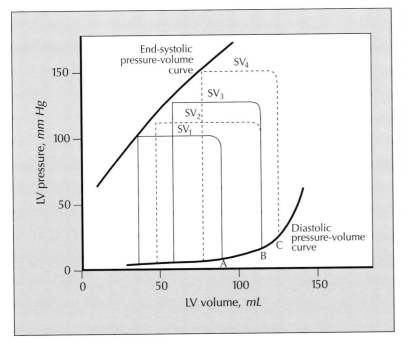

FIGURE 2-16. The concept of preload reserve and afterload mismatch. This concept has been proposed by Ross [22]. As illustrated in studies in normal conscious dogs by Lee *et al.* [23], this concept provides a possible explanation for the descending limb of the Starling curve. During acute angiotensin II infusions without volume loading, stroke volume (SV) was progressively reduced. This relationship between left ventricular (LV) stroke volume and

either end-diastolic pressure or volume was shifted upward and to the right when an angiotensin II infusion was combined with volume loading. The LV appeared to operate on a single diastolic and end-systolic pressure-volume relationship, suggesting no change in LV diastolic chamber elastance or contractility.

An attempt to graphically depict this relationship in an intact circulation that is allowed to freely adapt to alterations in LV pressure and volume is shown here, assuming a single diastolic and end-systolic pressure-volume relationship. Starting at point A and following the *lower solid line* at a constant contractile state, SV$_1$ is generated. With volume loading alone, movement up the diastolic pressure-volume curve to point B occurs, and the *lower dashed line* is followed generating SV$_2$, which is greater than SV$_1$, indicating the presence of preload reserve. Similarly, with pressure loading there is an increase in end-diastolic volume and pressure to point B along the diastolic pressure-volume curve; the *upper solid line* is followed generating SV$_3$, which is equal to SV$_1$. Therefore, despite an increase in LV pressure, stroke volume is maintained owing to preload reserve. In contrast, with a further increase in LV pressure following the *upper dashed line*, stroke volume is decreased, as shown by SV$_4$, due to an afterload mismatch. Preload reserve is exhausted at point C on the diastolic pressure-volume curve and is therefore insufficient to compensate for the increase in afterload. This is consistent with the observations of Lee *et al.* [23] in conscious animals, indicating that preload reserve is substantial in the normal heart and that it can compensate for increases in afterload on a beat-to-beat basis without changes in the passive diastolic pressure-volume relationship or contractility as long as venous return is adequate.

CONTRACTILITY

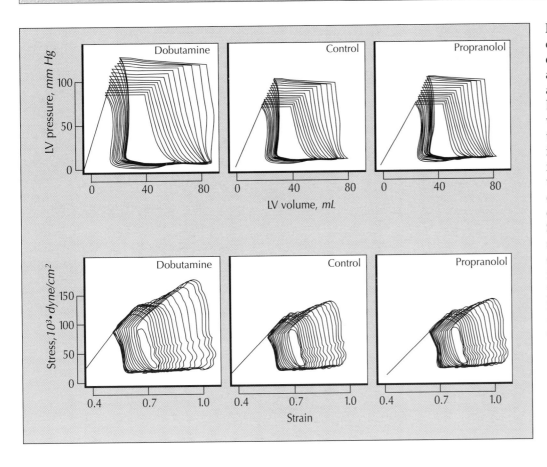

FIGURE 2-17. The effects of the β-agonist dobutamine and the β-antagonist propranolol on left ventricular (LV) contractility, as evaluated by both the pressure-volume and stress-strain relationships in the dog. By examining representative LV pressure-volume (*top*) and stress-strain (*bottom*) relationships, it is apparent that dobutamine increased the slope of the pressure-volume relation with very little change in the volume-axis intercept, and propranolol decreased the slope with no significant change in the volume-axis intercept. Similar observations were seen with the stress-strain relation. The slope of the LV end-systolic pressure-volume relationship is unique to the inotropic state. Both the LV pressure-segment length and stress-strain relationships provide similar information. (*Adapted from* Kaseda and coworkers [24]; with permission.)

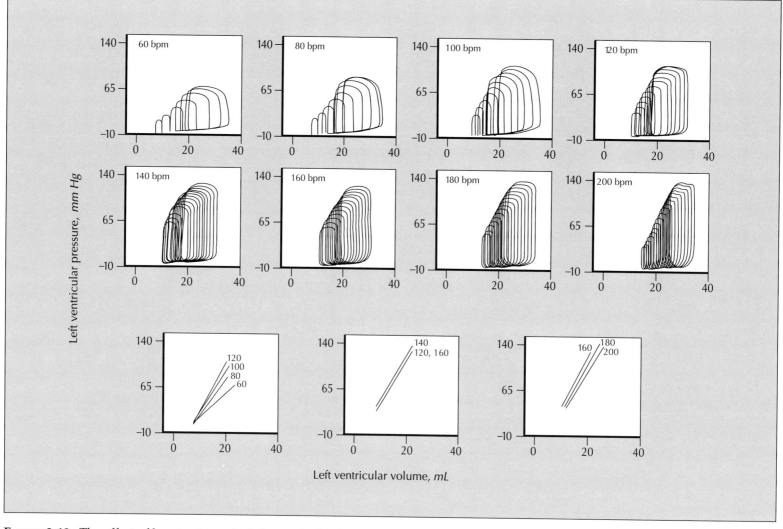

FIGURE 2-18. The effect of heart rate on the left ventricular (LV) end-systolic pressure-volume relationship (E_{es}) is shown from isolated, ejecting canine LV preparations to illustrate the interval-strength relationship [25]. Over a heart rate range from 60 to 120 bpm, the slope of the E_{es} increased significantly from 3.5 to 5.3 mm Hg/mL (*lower left*). There was very little change in the average E_{es} above 120 bpm. Over the same heart rate range there is very little change in the volume-axis intercept, V_0. These changes are consistent with a positive inotropic effect such as that observed with catecholamines [26]. The interval-strength relationship in the isolated heart preparation is therefore similar to the interval-strength relationship documented in isolated muscle [2] or other canine preparations [27–30], which is indicative of the heart rate–dependence of contractility. (*Adapted from* Maughan and coworkers [25]; with permission.)

AFTERLOAD

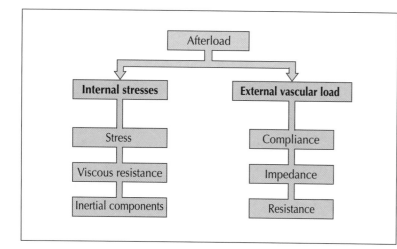

FIGURE 2-19. Afterload. The afterload against which the myocardium must work is composed of internal stresses, resistance, and inertial components. The external vascular load is composed of compliance, impedance, and resistance characteristics of the arterial vasculature. The components of stress, left ventricular (LV) pressure, mass, and geometry have been described. The viscous drag and inertial forces that must be overcome to generate blood movement are minor and are usually ignored. However, the characteristics of vascular load and their effects on LV ejection and contractility cannot be ignored because they contribute to the internal forces that the myocardium must carry during each contraction.

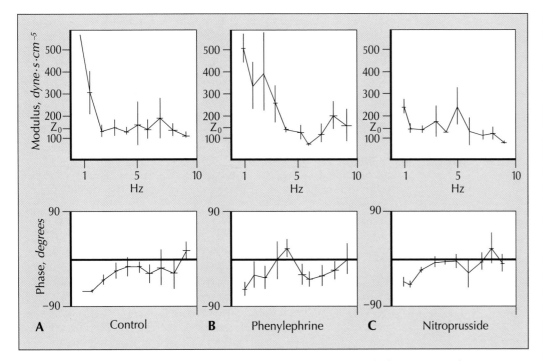

FIGURE 2-20. The average systemic arterial impedance moduli and phase spectra from normotensive baboons under control conditions and during phenylephrine and nitroprusside infusions are illustrated [31]. The *impedance* concept is an effort to present a quantitative description of the opposition to blood flow presented by the arterial vasculature [32]. Impedance should not be equated with *afterload*, which is a term that has been developed to describe the opposition to muscle shortening. Nevertheless, impedance can contribute to afterload through its influence on pressure, loading sequence, and geometry. Both resistance and compliance are properties of the arterial vasculature that contribute to, but are not equivalent to, total vascular impedance or opposition to blood flow.

Two specific terms, *input impedance* and *characteristic impedance*, have been used to differentiate the total opposition to blood flow: input impedance, if there were no wave reflections in the system; characteristic impedance, the average of impedance moduli over the second to tenth harmonics as frequencies (Hz), which are indicative of wave reflections in the system.

A, Under control hemodynamic conditions, the input impedance falls from a high value at zero frequency (mean aortic pressure divided by a mean flow or vascular resistance) to a minimum and then oscilates around a mean characteristic impedance (Z_0) of approximately 140 dynes•s•cm^{-5}. The impedance phase is negative over this range, indicating that flow is leading pressure.

B, When phenylephrine is administered, the moduli for characteristic impedance rise to an average Z_0 of approximately 225 dynes•s•cm^{-5}, indicating increased wave reflections in the system. Oscillations in phase initially begin as negative, indicating that flow leads pressure, then becomes positive as pressure leads flow, and then return to negative.

C, Nitroprusside decreases these oscillations and characteristic impedance moduli. Similar observations have been reported in normal human systemic arterial vasculature [33,34]. It has also been demonstrated that heart rate and respiratory variation do not affect these quantitative measures of the systemic arterial vasculature [34]. (*Adapted from* Latham and coworkers [32]; with permission.)

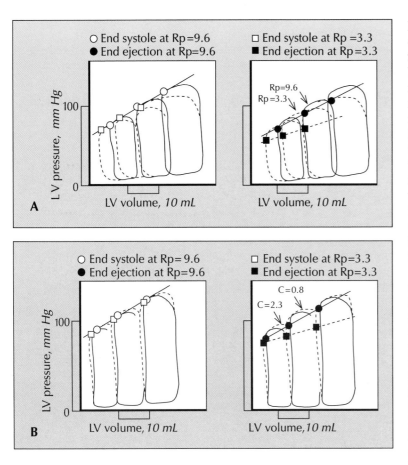

FIGURE 2-21. The effects of alterations in vascular characteristics on both left ventricular (LV) end-systole and end-ejection. **A,** Systemic arterial resistance (Rp) was independently altered, and LV pressure-volume loops were generated over this range of resistance values. Whereas the LV end-systolic pressure-volume relationship (*left*), was not affected by these changes in arterial resistance, the LV end-ejection pressure-volume relationship (*right*) was greatly affected. At a higher resistance level, indicated by the *solid pressure-volume loops*, end-ejection appeared to be similar to end-systole (*left*). However, at reduced arterial resistance, indicated by the *dashed pressure-volume loops*, end-ejection (*right*) was substantially dissociated from end-systole (*left*). This indicates that independent changes in arterial resistance that exceed the expected variation in the normal vasculature *in situ* have little impact on the time of end-systole and this contractile index, but they have substantial effects on ejection characteristics of the LV.

B, In the same preparation, independent changes in arterial compliance (C) over a sixfold range were used to generate a wide range of LV loads. The end-systolic pressure-volume relations were not affected by these large changes in arterial compliance (*left*). In contrast, reduced arterial compliance, represented by the *solid pressure-volume loops*, produced LV end-ejection pressure-volume relationships (*right*) that were similar to the LV end-systolic pressure-volume relationships (*left*). When arterial compliance was substantially improved, as indicated by the *dashed pressure-volume loops* (*right*), there was a substantial dissociation of end-ejection from end-systole. This demonstrates, once again, a significant impact of changes in arterial compliance on ejection characteristics of the LV but not the time of end-systole or this contractile index. (*Adapted from* Nishioka and coworkers [35]; with permission.)

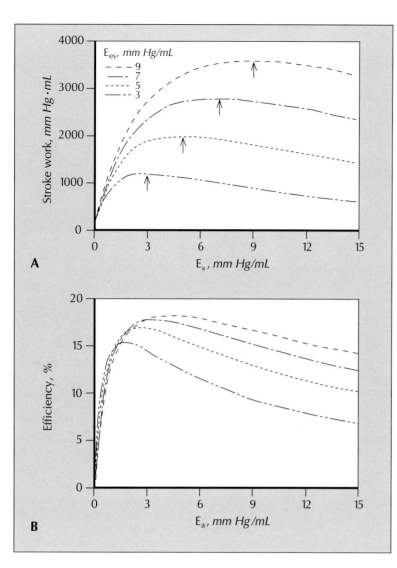

FIGURE 2-22. Interaction between the left ventricle (LV) and arterial system. A framework for analysis of the interaction between the LV and arterial system has been developed whereby LV pump function can be predicted and analyzed. Sunagawa *et al.* [36,37] developed a model of LV coupling that characterizes both the LV and arterial system by their end-systolic pressure-volume and end-systolic pressure-stroke volume relationships, respectively. The interaction of these two relationships can predict LV stroke volume. The final result of this analysis provides a formulation for predicting stroke volume at a known preload as a function of ventricular properties (chamber elastance [E_{es}], extrapolated volume-axis intercept, and ejection time) and arterial properties (modeled by the three-element Windkessel).

Using this model, Burkhoff and Sagawa [38] derived analytical expressions for LV stroke work (**A**) and mechanical efficiency (**B**) in terms of the LV contractile and arterial properties. As indicated here (*A*), when the LV contractile properties were quantitated in terms of LV E_{es} and arterial properties in terms of effective arterial elastance (E_a), these authors found that the model predicted maximal LV stroke work (*A*) when the LV and arterial elastances were equal, irrespective of the contractile state. In contrast, the E_a that resulted in the greatest efficiency (*B*) was less than that which provided maximal LV stroke work. In addition, with reduced LV contractile properties, as indicated by E_{es}, stroke work and myocardial efficiency were more sensitive to changes in arterial properties than in a heart with normal contractile properties. Although others have suggested that the LV and arterial systems are controlled to maximize LV output, this analytical model indicates that, under normal physiologic conditions, LV and arterial properties may be adjusted more toward maximal efficiency than maximal LV output, suggesting that the heart and circulation may have control mechanisms other than maximal output. (*Adapted from* Burkhoff and Sagawa [38].)

MYOCARDIAL ENERGETICS

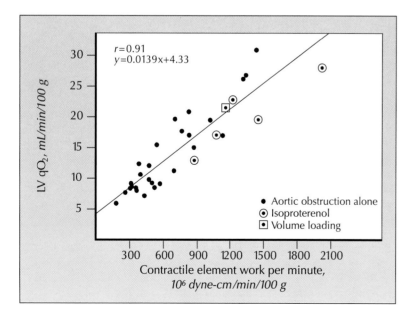

FIGURE 2-23. Formulation of muscle energetics. In 34 studies carried out in 23 dogs with various degrees of aortic obstruction, Britman and Levine [39] measured cardiac output, left ventricular (LV) and aortic pressures, heart rate, LV volume, coronary sinus blood flow, and coronary sinus oxygen extraction. They then compared LV oxygen consumption (LVqO_2) in mL/min/100 g of LV mass with contractile element work per minute in dynes•cm/min/100 g of LV weight. As shown here, over a wide range of loading conditions (volume loading) and contractile states (isoproterenol), contractile element work was the major determinant of myocardial oxygen requirements. They concluded that the ultimate formulation of muscle energetics must include consideration of the energy cost of resting cardiac muscle, excitation-contraction coupling, and isovolumic and ejecting work. (*Adapted from* Britman and Levine [39]; with permission.)

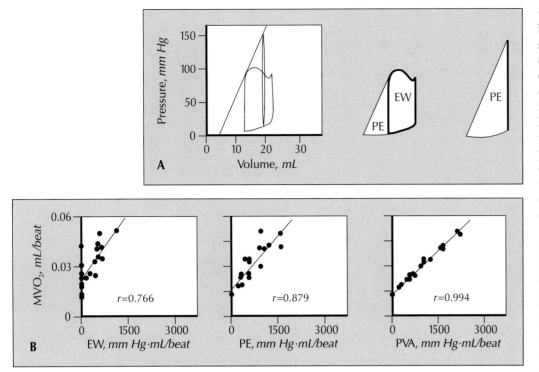

FIGURE 2-24. Suga *et al.* [40,41] took the muscle-energetics concept into the pressure-volume plane. They regressed myocardial oxygen consumption (MVO$_2$) against the pressure-volume area (PVA) from isolated canine left ventricular (LV) preparations. **A,** The PVA

was defined in isovolumic and ejecting beats as the area enclosed by the LV end-systolic pressure-volume relationship, the diastolic curve, and the systolic portion of each pressure-volume trajectory, which differed from the definition used in the initial studies of Monroe and French [42]. It had two components in the ejecting beat, the external work (EW) performed and the potential energy (PE) stored within the contractile element to perform external work [43], whereas in the isovolumic beat only PE was stored in the contractile element.

B, When MVO$_2$ was regressed against EW, PE, or the PVA, there was a highly linear relationship between MVO$_2$ and the PVA. This indicates that neither external nor potential energy alone is sufficient for predicting MVO$_2$, but the PVA, which is the simple sum of EW and PE and reflective of the total potential work that can be performed by the contractile element, can reliably predict MVO$_2$ in a given heart under a stable set of contractile conditions. (*Adapted from* Suga and coworkers [40]; with permission.)

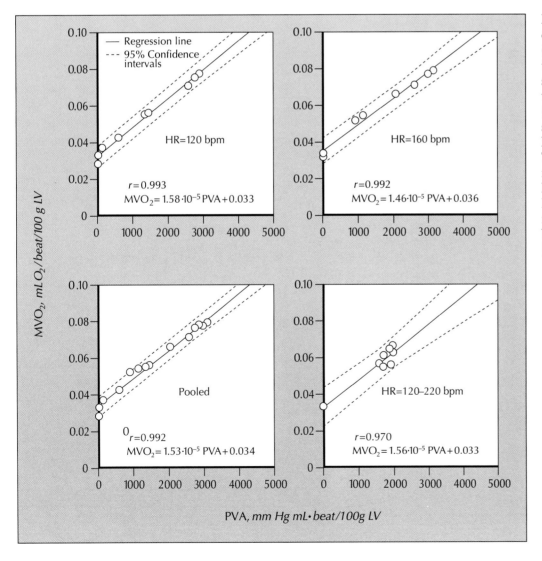

FIGURE 2-25. The effect of heart rate (HR) on the myocardial oxygen consumption (MVO$_2$)/ pressure-volume area (PVA) relationship. Because both MVO$_2$ and PVA are standardized to heart rate and 100 g of left ventricular (LV) mass, the pooled data (*bottom left*) are highly linear and do not show any significant variation whether the heart rate is 120, 160, or up to 220 bpm. These data indicate that the MVO$_2$/PVA relationship is essentially independent of heart rate when expressed in these terms. However, the importance of heart rate is reflected in the expression of MVO$_2$ per beat. (*Adapted from* Suga and coworkers [44]; with permission.)

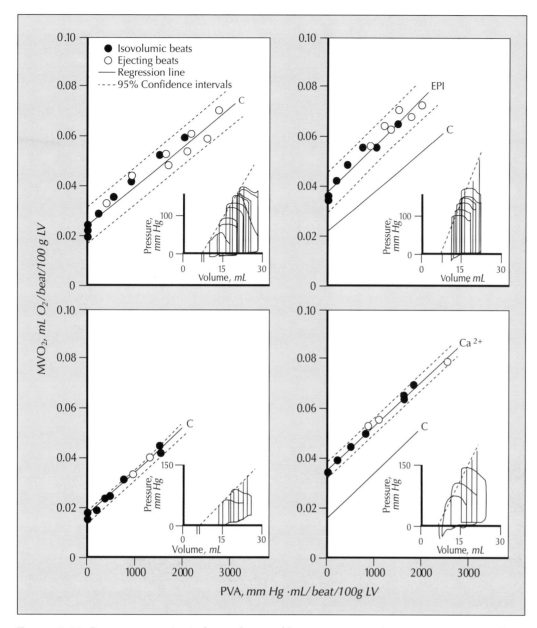

FIGURE 2-26. In contrast to its independence of heart rate, a positive inotropic agent has an important effect on the myocardial oxygen consumption (MVO_2)/pressure-volume area (PVA) relationship, as indicated here [45]. The same isolated canine left ventricular (LV) preparation was used to examine the relationship between MVO_2 and the PVA under control contractile conditions (C) and after either epinephrine (EPI) or calcium (Ca). These agents both increased the slope of the LV end-systolic pressure-volume relationship, a measure of LV contractility, by approximately 70%. The regression of MVO_2 on the PVA during the control and enhanced contractile states provided comparable slopes but an increase in the Y-axis intercepts with the enhanced contractile states. The reciprocal of the slope, which reflects contractile efficiency,

remained similar under the control and enhanced contractile conditions at approximately 30%. An increase in the Y-axis intercept reflects the increment in MVO_2 needed for excitation-contraction coupling, since basal metabolic rate should remain constant.

The incremental energy utilization for a given level of mechanical performance under the enhanced contractile state has been ascribed to the oxygen-wasting effect of inotropic agents. This oxygen-wasting effect has been related to the increased shortening velocity of the myocardium [46]. Others have ascribed the same effect to the augmented energetics for force-independent heat generation associated with calcium release and retrieval in the excitation-contraction coupling process [47].

The MVO_2/PVA relationship is unique in that it enables us to examine the mechanism for the augmented myocardial use of oxygen under enhanced contractile conditions. Because excitation-contraction coupling is known to require a large amount of energy at the sarcoplasmic reticulum and because both epinephrine and calcium augment calcium uptake by the sarcoplasmic reticulum, although by different mechanisms, the increase in MVO_2 needed during the enhanced contractile state probably results from the increase in energy utilization for excitation-contraction coupling produced by these positive inotropic agents. The constant efficiency observed in the MVO_2/PVA relationship indicates that the efficiency of energy conversion of the contractile machinery is constant over the wide range of loading conditions and contractile states employed in these studies. The independence of the slope, and therefore contractile efficiency from the contractile state, has not, however, been observed in all *in situ* hearts [48,49]. Therefore, the MVO_2/PVA relationship is a concept that can provide new and useful insights into myocardial energy utilization in the intact LV. (*Adapted from* Suga and coworkers [45]; with permission.)

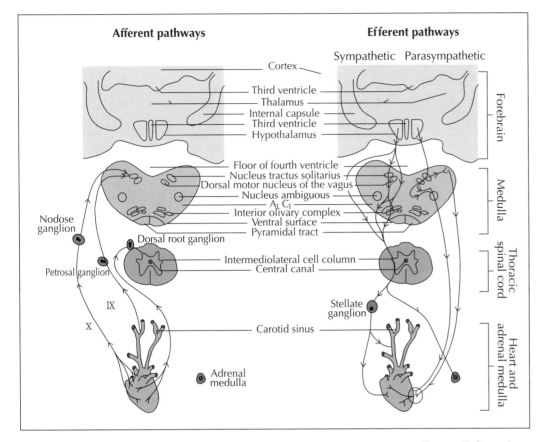

Afferent pathways

Efferent pathways

Sympathetic   Parasympathetic

FIGURE 2-27. The cardiovascular sympathetic and parasympathetic afferent (*left*) and efferent (*right*) pathways. The sympathetic and parasympathetic preganglionic cells represent the final common pathway of neural impulses to the cardiovascular system. They receive excitatory and inhibitory impulses predominantly from the medullary centers. These centers may operate independently and are capable of regulating cardiac contractility and heart rate, arterial pressure, and regional blood flow distribution. Under normal steady-state conditions, their activity is influenced by higher centers,

principally the cerebral cortex. Tonic excitatory medullary center activity is constantly influenced by inhibitory impulses from cardiovascular mechano- and chemoreceptors. An increase in activity in the carotid sinus and aortic nerves, as well as the vagal afferent fibers from the heart, reflexly reduces neural activity in the efferent sympathetic fibers and augments efferent vagal activity.

The sympathetic preganglionic neurons lie in the intermedial lateral horns of the spinal cord, leave the spinal cord, synapse with the postganglionic neurons in the chain of ganglia on each side of the spinal cord, and send peripheral sympathetic nerves to the heart and blood vessels. Some preganglionic sympathetic nerve fibers pass directly through these chains to the adrenal medulla. Whereas the postganglionic sympathetic nerves originating from the right stellate ganglion are distributed primarily to the sinus node and right atrium and control heart rate, those from the left stellate ganglion supply the left atrium and ventricle for control of contractile function. Terminal sympathetic innervation of the heart is a plexiform structure extending around the muscle cells in close apposition to them. The ventricular myocardium is only sparsely innervated by parasympathetic nerves. (*Adapted from* Corr and coworkers [50]; with permission.)

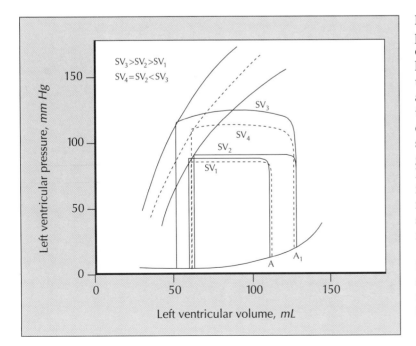

FIGURE 2-28. The interaction of the postganglionic sympathetic and parasympathetic neural fibers on myocardial contractility has been described as "accentuated antagonism" [51–53], which is illustrated here. Starting at point A and following the *solid lines* and *dashed lines* under the basal contractile state where sympathetic activity is low and parasympathetic restraint is dominant, heightened activity of the parasympathetic system (*dashed line*) does not significantly affect contractile function or depress stroke volume (SV_1). Heightened sympathetic neural activity, particularly from the left stellate ganglion, increases left atrial transfer function, thereby increasing left ventricular (LV) preload and moving on the passive diastolic filling curve from A to A_1, increasing stroke volume (SV_2). In addition, myocardial contractility is increased and pressure generation and shortening are improved, moving to a new LV pressure-volume relationship and enhancing stroke volume (SV_3).

During heightened sympathetic neural activity, an increase in parasympathetic neural activity becomes more apparent and decreases LV contractility, as indicated by a downward and rightward displacement of the LV pressure-volume relationship to the *dashed line*, with a reduction in stroke volumes (SV_4).

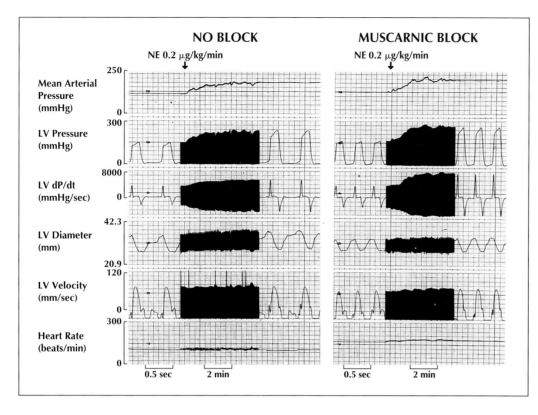

NO BLOCK

NE 0.2 μg/kg/min

MUSCARNIC BLOCK

NE 0.2 μg/kg/min

Mean Arterial Pressure (mmHg)

LV Pressure (mmHg)

LV dP/dt (mmHg/sec)

LV Diameter (mm)

LV Velocity (mm/sec)

Heart Rate (beats/min)

0.5 sec   2 min

0.5 sec   2 min

FIGURE 2-29. The steady-state effects of intravenous norepinephrine (NE) on mean arterial and left ventricular (LV) pressures, the rate of change of LV pressure (LV dP/dt), LV diameter and velocity of shortening, and heart rate before and after muscarinic blockade with atropine is shown from a conscious-dog preparation. After muscarinic blockade there is a greater increase in LV pressure, LV dP/dt, and LV shortening velocity with norepinephrine. The parasympathetic nervous system can therefore exert a tonic inhibitory influence on inotropic responses to peripherally administered sympathomimetic amines. The striking augmentation of the inotropic potential of sympathomimetic amines by muscarinic blockade is probably mediated through the vagal release of acetylcholine, which may inhibit the action of sympathomimetic amines at the β-adrenergic receptor at a postsynaptic site. (*Adapted from* Vatner and coworkers [54]; with permission.)

REFERENCES

1. Parmley WW, Sonnenblick EH: Series elasticity in heart muscle. *Circ Res* 1967, 20:112–123.

2. Sonnenblick EH: Force-velocity relations in mammalian heart muscle. *Am J Physiol* 1962, 202:931–939.

3. Burns JW, Covell JW, Ross J: Mechanics of isotonic left ventricular contractions. *Am J Physiol* 1973, 224:725–732.

4. Kentish JC, Wrzosek A: Changes in force and cytosolic Ca2+ concentration after length changes in isolated rat ventricular trabeculae. *J Physiol* 1998, 506:431–444.

5. Braunwald E, Sonnenblick EH, Ross J: Mechanisms of cardiac contraction and relaxation. In *Heart Disease: A Textbook of Cardiovascular Medicine*, ed 3. Edited by Braunwald E. Philadelphia: WB Saunders; 1988:383–425.

6. Gordon AM, Huxley AF, Julian FJ: The variation in isometric tension with sarcomere length in vertebrate muscle fibers. *J Physiol* 1966, 184:170–192.

7. Spotnitz HM, Sonnenblick EH, Spiro D: Relation of ultrastructure to function in the intact heart. Sarcomere structure relative to pressure-volume curves of intact left ventricles of dog and cat. *Circ Res* 1966, 18:49–66.

8. Sonnenblick EH, Ross J, Covell JW, *et al.*: The ultrastructure of the heart in systole and diastole. *Circ Res* 1967, 21:423–431.

9. Ross J Jr, Sonnenblick EH, Covell JW, *et al.*: Architecture of the heart in systole and diastole: technique of rapid fixation and analysis of left ventricular geometry. *Circ Res* 1967, 21:409–421.

10 Berne RM, Levy MN: *Cardiovascular Physiology*, edn 3. St Louis: CV Mosby; 1977.

11. Badke FR, O'Rourke RA: Cardiovascular physiology. In *Internal Medicine*, edn 1. Edited by Stein JH. Boston: Little, Brown and Co.; 1983:407–423.

12. Mirsky I: Left ventricular stresses in the intact human heart. *Biophys J* 1969, 9:189–208.

13. Ross J: Applications and limitations of end-systolic measures of ventricular performance. *Fed Proc* 1984, 43:2418–2422.

14. Potts JT, McKeown KP, Shoukas AA: Reduction in arterial compliance alters carotid baroreflex control of cardiac output in a model of hypertension. *Am J Physiol* 1998, 274(suppl H):1121–1131.

15. Glantz SA, Parmley WW: Factors which affect the diastolic pressure-volume curve. *Circ Res* 1978, 42:171–180.

16. Gilbert JC, Glantz SA: Determinants of left ventricular filling and of the diastolic pressure-volume relation. *Circ Res* 1989, 64:827–852.

17. Mirsky I: Assessment of diastolic function: suggested methods and future considerations. *Circulation* 1984, 69:836–841.

18. Hess OM, Bhargava V, Ross J, *et al.*: The role of the pericardium in interactions between the cardiac chambers. *Am Heart J* 1983, 106:1377–1383.

19. Shirato K, Shabetai R, Bhargava V, *et al.*: Alteration of the left ventricular diastolic pressure-segment length relation produced by the pericardium. *Circulation* 1978, 57:1191–1197.

20. Rothe CF: Physiology of venous return: an unappreciated boost to the heart. *Arch Intern Med* 1986, 146:977–982.

21. Guyton AC, Jones CE, Coleman TG: Graphical analysis of cardiac output regulation. In *Circulatory Physiology: Cardiac Output and its Regulation*, edn 2. Edited by Guyton AC, Jones CE, Lobwan TG. Philadelphia: WB Saunders; 1973:237–252.

22. Ross J: Afterload mismatch and preload reserve: a conceptual framework for the analysis of ventricular function. *Prog Cardiovasc Dis* 1976, 18:255–264.

23. Lee JD, Tajimi T, Ptritti J, *et al.*: Preload reserve and mechanisms of afterload mismatch in normal conscious dog. *Am J Physiol* 1986, 250:H464–H473.

24. Kaseda S, Tomoike H, Ogata I, *et al.*: End-systolic pressure-volume, pressure-length and stress-strain relations in canine hearts. *Am J Physiol* 1985, 249:H648–H654.

25. Maughan WL, Sunagawa K, Burkhoff D, *et al.*: Effect of heart rate on the canine end-systolic pressure-volume relationship. *Circulation* 1985, 72:654–659.

26. Suga H, Sagawa K: Instantaneous pressure-volume relationships and their ratio in the excised supported canine left ventricle. *Circ Res* 1974, 35:117–126.

27. Mitchell JH, Wallace AG, Skinner NS: Intrinsic effects of heart rate on left ventricular performance. *Am J Physiol* 1963, 205:41–48.

28. Covell JW, Ross J, Taylor R, *et al.*: Effects of increasing frequency of contraction on the force-velocity relation of left ventricle. *Cardiovasc Res* 1967, 1:2–8.

29. Higgins CB, Vatner SF, Franklin D, *et al.*: Extent of regulation of the heart's contractile state in the conscious dog by alteration in the frequency of contraction. *J Clin Invest* 1973, 52:1187–1194.

30. Klautz RJ, Baan J, Teitel DF: The effect of sarcoplasmic reticulum blockade on the force/frequency relationship and systolic contraction patterns in the newborn pig heart. *Eur J Physiol* 1997, 435:130–136.

31. Latham RD, Rubal BJ, Sipkema P, *et al.*: Ventricular/vascular coupling and regional arterial dynamics in the chronically hypertensive baboon: correlation with cardiovascular structural adaptation. *Circ Res* 1988, 63:798–811.

32. Finkelstein SM, Collins VR: Vascular hemodynamic impedance measurement. *Prog Cardiovasc Dis* 1982, 24:401–418.

33. Nichols WW, Conti CR, Walker WE, Milnor WR: Input impedance of the systemic circulation in man. *Circ Res* 1977, 40:451–458.

34. Murgo JP, Westerhof N, Giolma JP, *et al.*: Aortic input impedance in normal man: relationship to pressure wave forms. *Circulation* 1980, 62:105–116.

35. Nishioka O, Maruyama Y, Ashikawa K, *et al.*: Effects of changes in afterload impedance on left ventricular ejection in isolated canine hearts: dissociation of end ejection from end-systole. *Cardiovasc Res* 1987, 21:107–118.

36. Sunagawa K, Maughan WL, Burkhoff D, *et al.*: Left ventricular interaction with arterial load studied in isolated canine ventricle. *Am J Physiol* 1983, 245:H773–H780.

37. Sunagawa K, Maughan WL, Sagawa K: Optimal arterial resistance for the maximal stroke work studied in isolated canine left ventricle. *Circ Res* 1985, 56:586–595.

38. Burkhoff D, Sagawa K: Ventricular efficiency predicted by an analytical model. *Am J Physiol* 1986, 250:R1021–R1027.

39. Britman NA, Levine HJ: Contractile element work: a major determinant of myocardial oxygen consumption. *J Clin Invest* 1964, 43:1397–1408.

40. Suga H, Hayashi T, Shirahata M, *et al.*: Regression of cardiac oxygen consumption on ventricular pressure-volume area in dog. *Am J Physiol* 1981, 240:H320–H325.

41. Suga H, Yasumura Y, Nozawa T, *et al.*: Prospective prediction of O_2 consumption from pressure-volume area in dog hearts. *Am J Physiol* 1987, 252:H1258–H1264.

42. Monroe G, French GN: Left ventricular pressure-volume relationships and myocardial oxygen consumption in the isolated heart. *Circ Res* 1961, 9:362–374.

43. Suga H: External mechanical work from relaxing ventricle. *Am J Physiol* 1979, 236:H494–H497.

44. Suga H, Hisano R, Hirata S, *et al.*: Heart rate-independent energetics and systolic pressure-volume area in dog hearts. *Am J Physiol* 1983, 244:H206–H214.

45. Suga H, Hisano R, Goto Y, *et al.*: Effect of positive inotropic agents on the relation between oxygen consumption and systolic pressure-volume area in canine left ventricle. *Circ Res* 1983, 53:306–318.

46. Sonnenblick EH, Ross J, Covell JW, *et al.*: Velocity of contraction as a determinant of myocardial oxygen consumption. *Am J Physiol* 1965, 209:919–927.

47. Gibbs CL, Gibson WR: Isoprenaline, propranolol and the energy output of rabbit cardiac muscle. *Cardiovasc Res* 1972, 6:508–515.

48. Nozawa T, Yasumura Y, Futaki S, *et al.*: Relation between oxygen consumption and pressure-volume area of in situ dog heart. *Am J Physiol* 1987, 253:H31–H40.

49. Starling MR, Mancini GBJ, Montgomery DG, *et al.*: Relation between maximum time-varying elastance pressure-volume areas and myocardial oxygen consumption in dogs. *Circulation* 1991, 83:304–314.

50. Corr PB, Yamada KA, Witkowski FX: Mechanisms controlling cardiac autonomic function and their relation to arrythmogenesis. In *The Heart and Cardiovascular System*. Edited by Fozzard HA, Haber E, Jennings RB, *et al*. New York: Raven Press; 1986:1357–1371.

51. Levy MN, Martin PJ: Neural control of the heart. In *Physiology and Pathophysiology of the Heart*, edn. 1. Edited by Sperilakis N. Boston: Martinus Nijhoff Publishing; 1984:337–354.

52. Levy MN: Sympathetic-parasympathetic interactions in the heart. *Circ Res* 1971, 29:437–445.

53. DeGeest H, Levy MN, Zieske H, *et al.*: Depression of ventricular contractility by stimulation of the vagus nerves. *Circ Res* 1963, 17:222–235.

54. Vatner SF, Rutherford JD, Ochs HR: Baroreflex and vagal mechanisms modulating left ventricular contractile responses to sympathomimetic amines in conscious dogs. *Circ Res* 1979, 44:195–207.

Pathophysiology

THE ETIOLOGIC BASIS OF CONGESTIVE HEART FAILURE

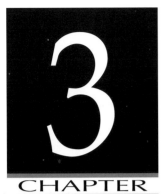

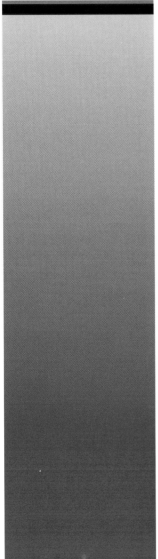

CHAPTER 3

Joshua M. Hare

Appropriate management of congestive heart failure requires recognition of the underlying etiologic basis. Currently, sequelae of ischemic heart disease are the most common causes of congestive heart failure in the United States. Mechanical causes of heart failure, which include coronary artery, valvular, and pericardial disease, must be diagnosed correctly in order to offer appropriate surgical therapy. Primary diseases of the myocardium, *ie*, cardiomyopathies, account for approximately 20% of cases of congestive heart failure [1]. Many systemic diseases, such as rheumatologic disorders, metabolic derangements, toxin exposures, and endocrinopathies, may affect cardiac function and present as a cardiomyopathy [2]. Although these secondary cardiomyopathies are rare, taken together they represent a significant proportion of new cases of dilated cardiomyopathy. As with mechanical causes, recognition of secondary cardiomyopathies is essential because treatment may result in the reversal of cardiac dysfunction.

Recent immunologic and molecular biologic studies are beginning to shed light on the etiologic basis of dilated cardiomyopathy. Among patients who present with new-onset dilated cardiomyopathy, approximately 10% have myocarditis [3,4]. Molecular biologic techniques have demonstrated that viral infection of the heart causing myocarditis can also lead to chronic dilated cardiomyopathy. In addition to coxsackie B virus, which is the most common cause of myocarditis, human immunodeficiency virus (HIV) represents a growing cause of myocarditis and dilated cardiomyopathy. Recent clinical and molecular biologic studies also have provided evidence that specific genetic defects may either directly cause or predispose to the development of dilated cardiomyopathy.

Despite the multiple different causes, left ventricular failure progresses by the common pathways of myocyte hypertrophy, fibrosis deposition, and left ventricular chamber enlargement. Abnormalities of function during systole, diastole, or both may contribute to diminished cardiovascular performance. In this chapter, a categorization of cardiomyopathic entities is presented. The causes of cardiomyopathy that are potentially reversible if appropriately diagnosed and treated are emphasized.

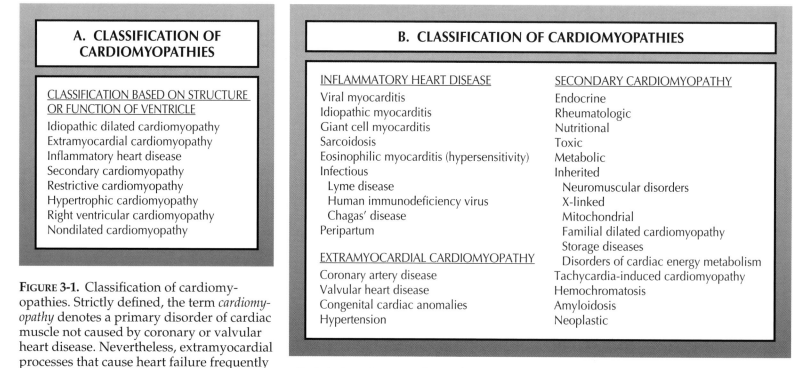

A. CLASSIFICATION OF CARDIOMYOPATHIES

CLASSIFICATION BASED ON STRUCTURE
OR FUNCTION OF VENTRICLE
Idiopathic dilated cardiomyopathy
Extramyocardial cardiomyopathy
Inflammatory heart disease
Secondary cardiomyopathy
Restrictive cardiomyopathy
Hypertrophic cardiomyopathy
Right ventricular cardiomyopathy
Nondilated cardiomyopathy

B. CLASSIFICATION OF CARDIOMYOPATHIES

INFLAMMATORY HEART DISEASE	SECONDARY CARDIOMYOPATHY
Viral myocarditis	Endocrine
Idiopathic myocarditis	Rheumatologic
Giant cell myocarditis	Nutritional
Sarcoidosis	Toxic
Eosinophilic myocarditis (hypersensitivity)	Metabolic
Infectious	Inherited
Lyme disease	Neuromuscular disorders
Human immunodeficiency virus	X-linked
Chagas' disease	Mitochondrial
Peripartum	Familial dilated cardiomyopathy
	Storage diseases
EXTRAMYOCARDIAL CARDIOMYOPATHY	Disorders of cardiac energy metabolism
Coronary artery disease	Tachycardia-induced cardiomyopathy
Valvular heart disease	Hemochromatosis
Congenital cardiac anomalies	Amyloidosis
Hypertension	Neoplastic

FIGURE 3-1. Classification of cardiomyopathies. Strictly defined, the term *cardiomyopathy* denotes a primary disorder of cardiac muscle not caused by coronary or valvular heart disease. Nevertheless, extramyocardial processes that cause heart failure frequently cause secondary changes in myocardial structure and function.

A, A general classification of cardiomyopathic processes based on observations in a large clinical series of patients followed over a 10-year period [2].

B, Subclassification of specific extramyocardial etiologies that can produce cardiomyopathy-like syndromes, inflammatory diseases of the heart, and specific second-ary conditions that can manifest as dilated cardiomyopathy. Although most secondary cardiomyopathies are described in the literature as case reports or small series, in aggregate they may account for up to 50% of new cases of dilated cardiomyopathy [2].

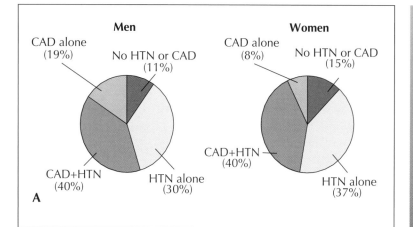

Men
CAD alone (19%)
No HTN or CAD (11%)
CAD+HTN (40%)
HTN alone (30%)

Women
CAD alone (8%)
No HTN or CAD (15%)
CAD+HTN (40%)
HTN alone (37%)

A

B. ETIOLOGIES OF CONGESTIVE HEART FAILURE

ETIOLOGY	PATIENTS, *n(%)*	NONISCHEMIC DISEASE WITH ETIOLOGY (%)
Ischemic	936(50.3)	
Nonischemic	925(49.7)	
No etiology provided	247(13.3)	
Etiology provided	678(36.4)	
Idiopathic	340(18.2)	(50.1)
Valvular	75(4.0)	(11.1)
Hypertensive	70(3.8)	(10.3)
Ethanol	34(1.8)	(5.0)
Viral	9(0.4)	(1.3)
Postpartum	8(0.4)	(1.2)
Amyloidosis	1(0.1)	(0.1)
Other/ unspecified	141(7.6)	(20.8)

FIGURE 3-2. The epidemiology of congestive heart failure in the United States. The Framingham Heart Study, which followed a cohort of 9405 Americans over a 40-year period, has provided valuable information regarding the etiologic basis of congestive heart failure in the United States [5]. **A,** Of 331 men and 321 women who developed heart failure, the majority had coronary artery disease (CAD) with or without hypertension (HTN), and approximately one third had HTN alone. At present, idiopathic dilated cardiomyopathy has replaced HTN as the second most important etiologic factor in the development of heart failure. CAD continues to be the most common risk factor for the development of heart failure in the United States.

B, Large treatment trials provide another valuable source of information about the causes of heart failure. Data are from a compilation of heart failure trials published between July 1989 and June 1990; categories are based on the presence or absence of significant ischemic heart disease [6]. In this analysis, 50% of cases were attributable to coronary disease; 18.2% of all patients and approximately 50% of those with nonischemic disease had idiopathic dilated cardiomyopathy. Less commonly, valvular heart disease, HTN, and excess alcohol consumption were identified as significant etiologic factors. (Part A *adapted from* Ho and coworkers [5]; part B *adapted from* Teerlink and coworkers [6].)

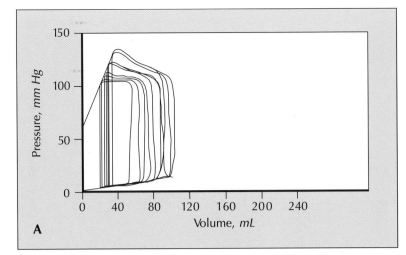

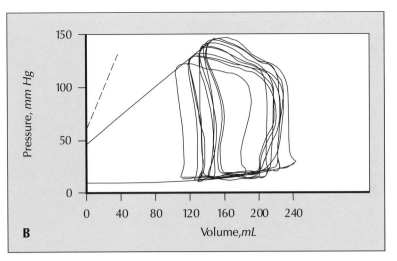

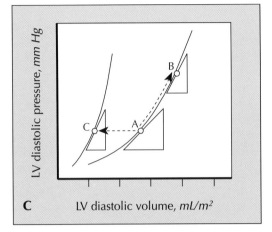

FIGURE 3-3. Systolic and diastolic heart failure. Abnormalities of ventricular function during systole, diastole, or both may produce congestive heart failure. Furthermore, the interaction of the heart with the circulation (*ie*, the loading conditions placed on the heart) is an important determinant of overall cardiovascular performance. Pressure-

volume diagrams can be used to characterize systolic dysfunction, altered diastolic compliance, and the influence of loading conditions on cardiac function.

A, A series of pressure-volume loops obtained from a patient with normal cardiac function. Each loop represents a cardiac cycle sampled during inflation of a balloon in the inferior vena cava to alter loading conditions. The slope of the end-systolic pressure-volume loop relationship (ESPVR, *solid line*) reflects end-systolic ventricular elastance, a relatively load-independent index of contractility. **B,** In dilated cardiomyopathy ventricular volumes are higher, and the ESPVR slope is reduced compared with normal (*dashed line*). Ventricular enlargement is a final common pathway in the heart with systolic impairment.

C, Diastolic dysfunction also may produce heart failure, either primarily or in conjunction with systolic failure. Myocardial ischemia, fibrosis, myocyte hypertrophy, elevated afterload, and pericardial constriction all may contribute to diastolic dysfunction [7]. The end-diastolic pressure-volume relationship (EDPVR) can be used to assess the passive properties of the ventricular chamber. The *operative volume stiffness* of the ventricle is defined as dP/dV (the slope of a tangent to the EDPVR), and the *compliance* of the ventricle is defined as the reciprocal of stiffness (*ie*, dV/dP). Alterations in diastolic function may occur because of increases in stiffness due to rises in chamber preload (A toward B) or actual shifts in the EDPVR (A toward C). Leftward shifts in the EDPVR can occur acutely with ischemia or chronically with fibrosis and hypertrophy. With such shifts, the EDPVR is steeper, and increments in volume produce an exaggerated rise in pressure. LV—left ventricular. (Parts A and B *courtesy of* David Kass, Baltimore, MD. Part C *adapted from* Gaasch and coworkers [8]; with permission.)

HEART FAILURE ASSOCIATED WITH CORONARY DISEASE

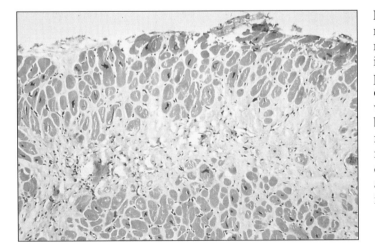

FIGURE 3-4. Histology of ischemic cardiomyopathy demonstrating replacement fibrosis. Myocyte hypertrophy occurs secondarily in response to increases in pressure or volume loads [9]. Fibrosis, the increased deposition of collagen, results from either repair of parenchymal myocyte injury (replacement fibrosis) or pathologic deposition in the interstitium. Histologic studies reveal that patients with ischemic cardiomyopathy display more replacement fibrosis but less myocyte hypertrophy than those with idiopathic cardiomyopathy. Depicted is a focus of replacement fibrosis in an endomyocardial biopsy sample obtained from a patient with ischemic cardiomyopathy. In one study, such foci were found to be 92% specific and 48% sensitive for a diagnosis of ischemic cardiomyopathy versus idiopathic dilated cardiomyopathy [10].

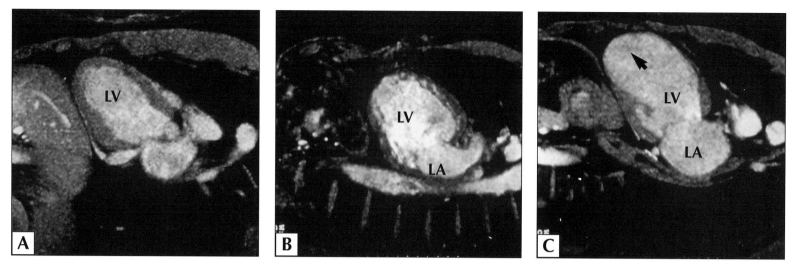

FIGURE 3-5. Magnetic resonance images depicting the normal left ventricle (LV; *panel A*), ischemic cardiomyopathy (*panel B*), and LV aneurysm (*panel C*). These images were obtained in the saggital view through the LV. Ischemic cardiomyopathy may develop months or years after a myocardial infarction due to remodeling of the ventricle, a process affecting both infarcted and viable (*ie,* noninfarcted) segments. Although the contractile abnormality is focal, particularly early in the process, progressive ventricular enlargement and eventual failure of noninfarcted myocardium can lead to a state that clinically resembles idiopathic dilated cardiomyopathy. The ventricle shown here (*panel B*) is diffusely enlarged and more spherical than the normal ventricle. LV aneurysms (*arrow*) are large segments of ventricular wall composed of fibrous tissue. These areas exhibit paradoxical systolic expansion, which impairs ventricular function despite preserved function of the viable myocardium, and may lead to heart failure following large myocardial infarcts. About one half of patients with moderate to large aneurysms experience symptoms of heart failure with or without angina pectoris, and in such patients aneurysm resection may lead to a significant improvement in global LV function [11]. LA—left atrium. (*Courtesy of* Joachim Gaa and Robert Edelman, Boston, MA.)

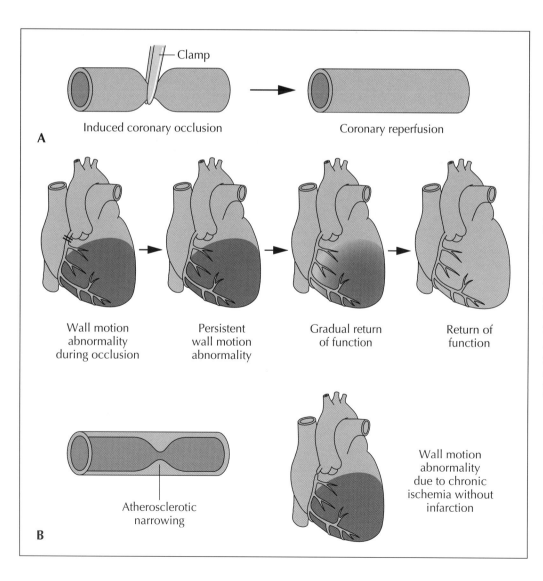

FIGURE 3-6. Stunned and hibernating myocardium. Both chronic myocardial ischemia and reperfusion of ischemic muscle may produce a reversible form of ventricular dysfunction. **A,** Stunned myocardium refers to left ventricular dysfunction after coronary reperfusion. Coronary occlusion, such as that occurring during acute myocardial infarction, may lead to regional dysfunction beyond the area of infarction. Despite restoration of flow, regional wall-motion abnormalities persist in these areas with viable myocytes. This process usually reverses over a period of several days after myocardial infarction. **B,** Hibernating myocardium results from chronic ischemia. Blood flow may be adequate to maintain myocyte viability, but may not be sufficient to support the full metabolic needs of normal contraction. After revascularization, myocardial function may significantly improve. (*Adapted from* Kloner and coworkers [12]; with permission.)

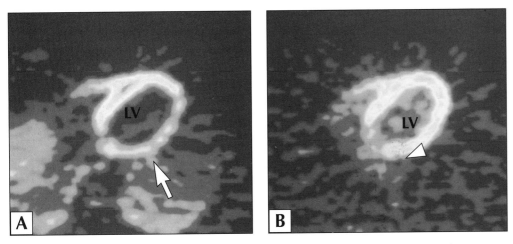

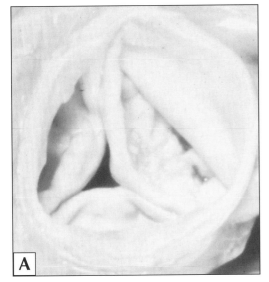 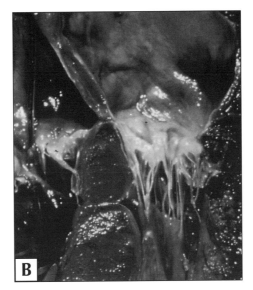

FIGURE 3-7. Positron emission tomogram demonstrating hibernating (viable but dysfunctional) myocardium in a patient with severe three-vessel CAD who presented with heart failure. In this technique, images are obtained after injection of isotopes that assess both myocardial perfusion and metabolic activity. In these images, active perfusion or metabolic activity appears yellow to red. **A,** A $[^{13}N]$-ammonia scan demonstrating a large anterolateral perfusion defect (*arrow*). **B,** The corresponding $[^{18}F]$-fluorodeoxyglucose image demonstrates that metabolic activity is preserved in this region (*arrowhead*). After coronary bypass surgery, the patient experienced a dramatic improvement in left ventricular function. Other imaging techniques valuable in the assessment of hibernating myocardium include thallium imaging and dobutamine stress echocardiography. These techniques can predict, with 80% or greater accuracy, if there will be significant improvement in left ventricular function with revascularization. Recently, detection of viable myocardium with ^{201}Tl scintigraphy has been shown to predict patient survival following coronary artery bypass surgery [13]. Therefore, patients may be considered as candidates for bypass surgery as an alternative to heart transplantation. (*Courtesy of* Henry Gewirtz, Boston, MA.) (*See* Color Plate.)

HEART FAILURE ASSOCIATED WITH VALVULAR LESIONS

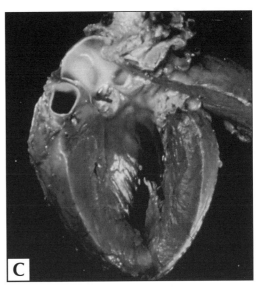

FIGURE 3-8. Heart failure associated with aortic valvular lesions. Heart failure represents a cardinal manifestation of both stenotic and regurgitant valvular heart disease. Aortic stenosis affects cardiac function by imposing progressively increasing systolic wall stress on the ventricle. Chronic aortic stenosis results in concentric left ventricular hypertrophy and fibrosis, and thereby increases wall thickness. The increase in wall thickness can initially restore wall stress to normal, but frequently heart failure ensues because of inadequate hypertrophy (afterload mismatch) or depression of myocardial contractility [14]. Heart failure may also reflect diastolic dysfunction due to increased diastolic stiffness. Heart failure in patients with aortic stenosis bodes a poor prognosis, with patients surviving only 1 to 1.5 years; however, it is generally responsive to valve replacement [15]. Aortic regurgitation imposes an excessive volume load on the ventricle. The rising end-diastolic volume increases diastolic wall stress and leads to eccentric hypertrophy of the left ventricle. The ventricle initially is capable of handling large volumes of regurgitant flow and generates an adequate forward flow without elevation of filling pressures. Heart failure usually ensues when end-diastolic volume continues to rise in the presence of a falling ejection fraction. The ratio of wall thickness to cavity diameter declines, wall tension increases, and further afterload mismatch occurs [14]. The end-systolic volume serves as a good index of prognosis: patients with volumes greater than 90 mL/m^2 generally have a poor operative mortality and fail to recover ventricular function. Ventricular dysfunction with exercise can be detected before the onset of symptoms and is an indication for surgery. Shown is a pathologic specimen from a patient in whom aortic stenosis (**A**) produced marked concentric ventricular hypertrophy (**B**). Also shown is a specimen from a patient with massive eccentric hypertrophy due to chronic aortic regurgitation secondary to healed bacterial endocarditis (**C**). Chronic aortic insufficiency produces the largest end-diastolic volumes of any heart condition, a condition termed *cor bovinum*. The weight of this specimen exceeded 1000 g. (*Courtesy of* Frederick J. Schoen, Boston, MA.)

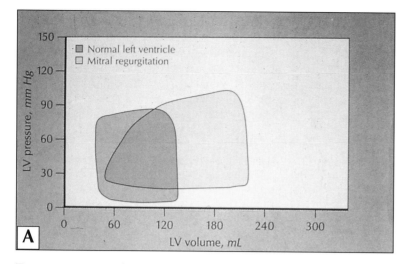

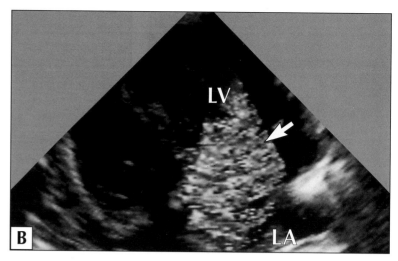

FIGURE 3-9. Heart failure associated with mitral regurgitation. When mitral regurgitation is acute, it may produce symptomatic pulmonary edema as well as pulmonary hypertension and right heart failure. Mitral regurgitation can also cause chronic left ventricular (LV) dysfunction, which, if left untreated, can lead to the development of dilated cardiomyopathy. Incompetence of the mitral valve reduces ventricular afterload and increases the velocity of contractile element shortening; thus, the LV ejection fraction may be normal despite significant LV dysfunction. **A,** Pressure-volume diagram typical of mitral regurgitation. Ventricu-lar volume decreases in early systole before opening of the aortic valve. After aortic valve closure, the ventricle continues to eject into the left atrium (LA), resulting in non-isovolumic relaxation. Contractility may be depressed in patients with mitral regur-

gitation as reflected by a diminished ratio of pressure to volume at the end-systolic point, an estimate of ventricular elastance (*see* Fig. 3-3). In chronic mitral regurgitation, the ventricle operates at a greater volume and, as with aortic regurgitation, ventricular size has proven to be predictive of impaired postoperative function. **B,** Echocardiogram with color Doppler depicting severe mitral regurgitation in a 70-year-old woman with a myxomatous mitral valve and a ruptured chordae. The Doppler jet demonstrates the systolic regurgitant flow-velocity from LV to LA (*arrow*). Ventricular enlargement has ensued with an LV enddiastolic dimension of 6.6 cm (normal range, 3.6 to 5.2 cm) and an LV end-systolic dimension of 4.2 cm (normal range, 2.3 to 3.9 cm). (Part A *adapted from* Kontos and coworkers [16]; with permission.) (*See* Color Plate for part B.)

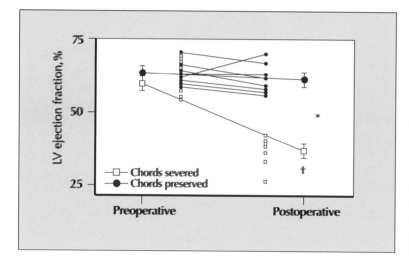

FIGURE 3-10. Paradoxically, dilated cardiomyopathy may appear to worsen after mitral valve replacement due to surgical transection of the subvalvular apparatus. Development of operative techniques for mitral repair and chordal preservation has largely eliminated this type of postoperative impairment of ventricular performance [17]. This graph shows the effect of chordal preservation on postoperative left ventricular (LV) ejection fraction. Patients received mitral valve replacement with or without preservation of the chordae tendineae. Only patients who had severance of their chordal structures experienced a decrease in ejection fraction with surgery (*asterisk*, $P<0.05$ between groups; *dagger*, $P<0.05$ before vs after mitral valve replacement). In this study, chordal preservation resulted in decreases in both diastolic and systolic volumes, as well as a decrease in end-systolic wall stress. In contrast, chordal transection led to an increase in both end-systolic volume and wall stress. (*Adapted from* Rozich and coworkers [17]; with permission.)

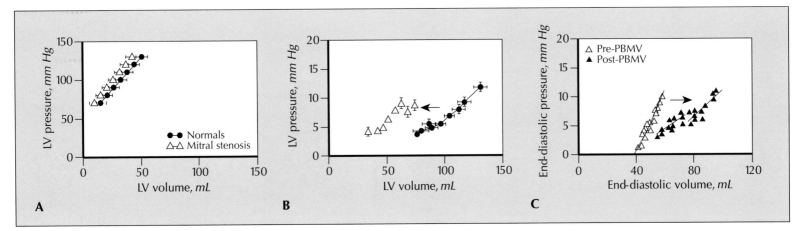

A **B** **C**

FIGURE 3-11. Diastolic dysfunction in mitral stenosis resulting primarily from the transvalvular gradient and subsequent pulmonary hypertension. Diminished cardiovascular performance has been associated with mitral stenosis. Liu *et al.* [18], using *in vivo* pressure-volume analysis, have demonstrated that cardiovascular impairment in mitral stenosis may be attributable, in part, to reduced diastolic compliance.

A, Comparison of the end-systolic pressure-volume relationship in normal subjects and patients with mitral stenosis. These relationships were very similar except for a small shift to lower volumes in the mitral stenosis group.

B, In contrast, the end-diastolic pressure-volume relationship (EDPVR) in patients with mitral stenosis demonstrates both a leftward shift to lower volumes and a slope increase indicative of reduced compliance.

C, The effect of percutaneous balloon mitral valvuloplasty (PBMV) on the EDPVR in mitral stenosis was used to assess the mechanism of this increase in diastolic stiffness. Immediately after valvuloplasty, the slope of the EDPVR indicated increased compliance, suggesting that the thickened, immobile valve apparatus exerted a mechanical constraining effect. The chamber compliance increased even further at 3 months of follow-up, approaching normal values. LV—left ventricular. (*Adapted from* Liu and coworkers [18]; with permission.)

IDIOPATHIC DILATED CARDIOMYOPATHY

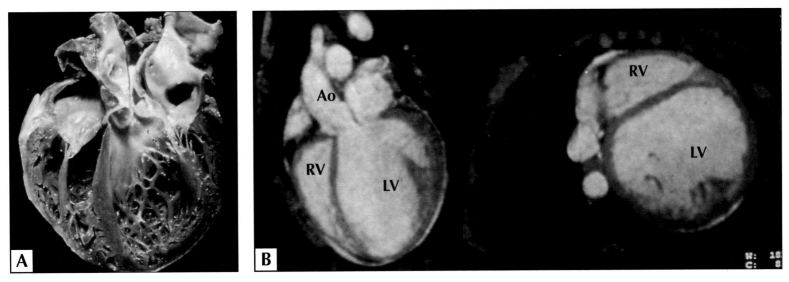

A **B**

Figure 3-12. Idiopathic dilated cardiomyopathy. Idiopathic dilated cardiomyopathy, a diagnosis of exclusion, is the second most common cause of heart failure in the United States, following ischemic heart disease (*see* Fig. 3-2B). Among patients who present with dilated cardiomyopathy, up to half have specific underlying etiologies, which in many cases are treatable. In addition, it is becoming apparent that many cases previously labeled "idiopathic" may actually reflect prior myocarditis or genetic disease.

A, Gross appearance of the heart in idiopathic dilated cardiomyopathy. This condition leads to four-chamber dilatation and

hypertrophy. In this example, focal anteroseptal apical wall thinning was a result of an infarct of embolic origin. The coronary arteries were free of obstructive narrowing.

B, Magnetic resonance images of dilated cardiomyopathy in four-chamber (*left*) and short-axis (*right*) views. This imaging technique provides an excellent *in vivo* assessment of cardiac structure and function. Ao—aorta; LV—left ventricle; RV—right ventricle. (Part A *courtesy of* Frederick J. Schoen, Boston, MA; part B *courtesy of* Joachim Gaa and Robert Edelman, Boston, MA.)

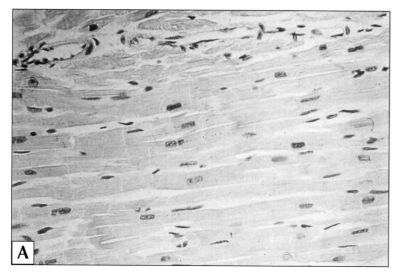

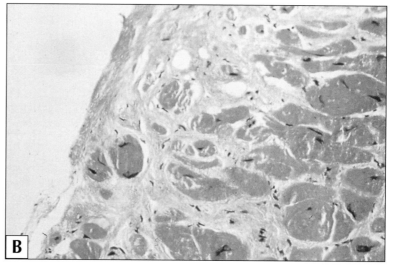

FIGURE 3-13. Pathology of idiopathic dilated cardiomyopathy. **A,** Histologic architecture of normal myocardium, demonstrating parallel alignment of uniformly sized myocytes without significant fibrosis. **B,** In contrast, the myocardium from a patient with idiopathic dilated cardiomyopathy demonstrates myocyte hypertrophy with variability in myocyte size and enlargement of nuclei. There is significant deposition of fibrotic tissue in the interstitium. (Part A *courtesy of* Evan Loh, Philadelphia, PA.)

INFLAMMATORY DISEASES OF THE MYOCARDIUM

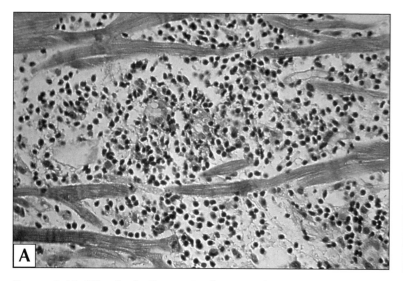

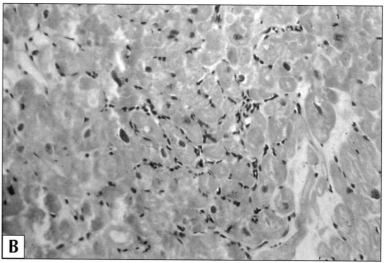

FIGURE 3-14. Histologic diagnosis of myocarditis. The Dallas Criteria [19] were formulated by a panel of cardiac pathologists, and have led to standardization of the histologic diagnosis of myocarditis by endomyocardial biopsy. **A,** As defined by the Dallas Criteria, a diagnosis of myocarditis requires the presence of both inflammatory infiltrates and evidence of myocardial necrosis.

B, Borderline myocarditis is defined as an inflammatory infiltrate without clear evidence of myocyte necrosis. These criteria were used as enrollment criteria in the Myocarditis Treatment Trial for the assessment of immunosuppressive therapy in patients with myocarditis. Interestingly, the degree of inflammation or the presence of myocyte necrosis does not necessarily indicate the presence of viral infection or provide prognosis [20].

As shown in Fig. 3-16C, enteroviral infection may cause severe ventricular dysfunction without inflammation. Furthermore, myocardial inflammation with or without myocyte necrosis may occur in nonviral disease processes (*see* Fig. 3-22). Despite the limitation of sampling error, endomyocardial biopsy remains the gold standard for the diagnosis of myocarditis [21]. It is hoped that the application of molecular and immunologic assays of myocardial tissue will enhance the clinical value of endomyocardial biopsy in the future. When endomyocardial biopsy is performed in centers that have experience with the technique, the incidence of major complications that require intervention or lead to patient death is less than 1% [22,23]. (*Courtesy of* H. Thomas Aretz for the Myocarditis Treatment Trial, Boston, MA.)

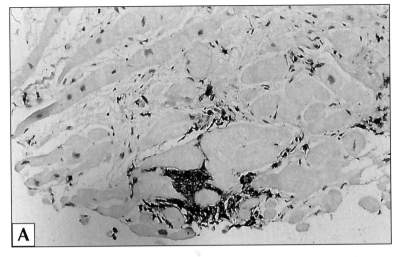

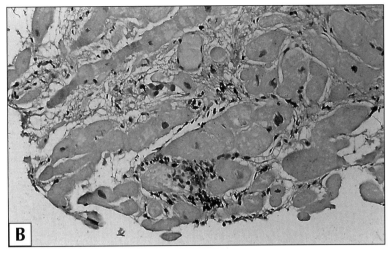

FIGURE 3-15. In addition to the Dallas criteria, immunohistochemical staining is valuable to characterize myocardial lymphocytic infiltration. Most human and animal myocarditis is characterized by infiltration with T cells that utilize the α-β T-cell receptor [24]. **A,** Immunohistochemical staining for CD3$^+$ T cells (general T-cell surface marker). **B,** CD8$^+$ T cells (cytotoxic/suppressor T cells) obtained from a patient with chronic active myocarditis. CD8$^+$

T cells are commonly detected in human myocarditis. Immunohistochemical staining has the potential to play a role in distinguishing autoimmune from viral myocarditis because the former may be characterized by T cells that contain the γ-δ T-cell receptor as opposed to α-β T cells [24]. Immunopositive cells stain *black*. (*Courtesy of* R. Hruban, Baltimore, MD.)

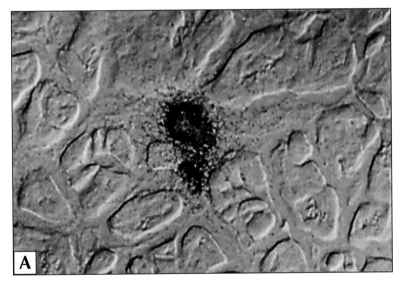

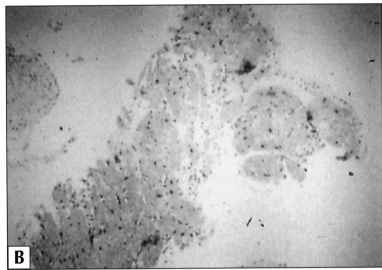

FIGURE 3-16. Viral myocarditis. Myocarditis accounts for approximately 10% of patients with new-onset congestive heart failure [3,25,26]. Enteroviruses of the Picornaviridae family have been implicated as the most common offending agents. Recent studies have implicated adenovirus as an additional myocarditis-causing virus that may affect pediatric patients more commonly than adults [27]. Molecular techniques such as polymerase chain reaction amplification [28] and *in situ* hybridization [29,30] have clearly demonstrated the presence of a viral genome in heart tissue from patients with acute myocarditis and in those with dilated cardiomyopathy, suggesting that viral myocarditis is a precursor to some cases of dilated cardiomyopathy.

A, Interference contrast microscopy (× 1000) demonstrating *in situ* hybridization of ^{35}S-labeled coxsackievirus B3 cDNA to the myocardium of a patient with an 8-year history of chronic dilated cardiomyopathy. The autoradiographic silver grains localize to distinct infected myocytes. Kandolf [30] has found enteroviral infection in 17% of 47 patients with idiopathic cardiomyopathy.

B, The typical pattern of enteroviral infection in an adult patient with recurrent myocarditis presenting with severe heart failure. The autoradiographic silver grains localize to individual myocytes. Mononuclear cellular infiltration lies adjacent to infected myocytes. (*continued*)

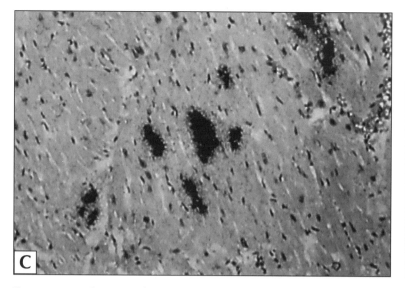

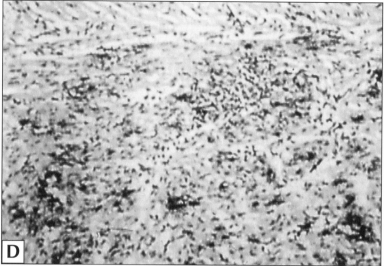

FIGURE 3-16. (*continued*) C, Early viral infection in a patient dying from fulminant heart failure. The high intensity of autoradiographic staining indicates a high copy number of replicating viral genomes. In this patient there is relatively little cellular inflammatory response, indicating that cardiac dysfunction may ensue from viral infection in the absence of inflammation.

D, Fulminant enteroviral infection with an inflammatory response in neonatal myocarditis. This section demonstrates extensive auto-radiographic staining, inflammatory infiltration, and progression of infection from inflamed to noninflamed areas, suggestive of cell-to-cell spread of the virus. (Part A *adapted from* Kandolf [29]; parts B to D *adapted from* Kandolf [30]; with permission.)

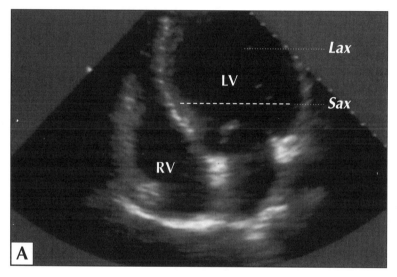

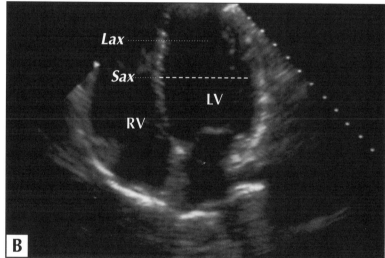

FIGURE 3-17. Ventricular chamber distortion in myocarditis. Myocarditis causes left ventricular enlargement and results in an increase in ventricular sphericity similar to that produced by postin-farction ventricular remodeling. Depicted are apical four-chamber echocardiograms from a patient with active myocarditis (**A**) and a

patient with a normal ventricle (**B**). In comparison with the normal ventricle, the ventricle affected by myocarditis is dilated and more spherical. The ventricular width at the short axis (Sax) has increased ralative to the length in the long axis (Lax). (*Courtesy of* Lisa Mendes for the Myocarditis Treatment Trial, Boston, MA.)

CLINICOPATHOLOGIC CLASSIFICATION OF MYOCARDITIS

	FULMINANT	ACUTE	CHRONIC ACTIVE	CHRONIC PERSISTENT
Left ventricular dysfunction	+++	++	++	-
Histology	Myo	Myo/BMyo	Myo/BMyo	Myo/BMyo
Response to immunosuppression	?	+/-	-	-
Natural history	Complete recovery or death	Incomplete recovery or DCM	DCM	Normal ventricular function

- —absent; ++—moderate; +++—severe.

FIGURE 3-18. A clinicopathologic classification of myocarditis. Lieberman *et al.* [3] have proposed a clinicopathologic description of myocarditis with four presentations that are analogous to those of viral hepatitis. This characterization was based on 35 of 348 patients who underwent endomyocardial biopsy for evaluation of cardiac dysfunction. *Fulminant myocarditis* manifested as acute, severe congestive heart failure with a clear-cut flu-like prodrome and severe histologic evidence of inflammation and myocyte necrosis, leading to either death or complete recovery. This presentation may be associated with progressive myocardial damage caused by ongoing viral infection.

Acute myocarditis was the most common presentation. Patients presented with minimally dilated hypokinetic ventricles with an indistinct onset of symptoms. Endomyocardial biopsy revealed either borderline (BMyo) or active (Myo) myocarditis. In this group, patients with BMyo responded to immunosuppressive therapy (prednisone and azathioprine) with improvement in ventricular function and regression of chamber dilatation [20]. Patients who did not respond to therapy developed end-stage dilated cardiomyopathy (DCM). *Chronic active myocarditis* presented in a manner similar to Myo. Patients experienced brief, dramatic but unsustained responses to immunosuppressive therapy and followed a slowly progressive course of deterioration to end-stage DCM. Initial histology revealed either BMyo or Myo and subsequent biopsies demonstrated the appearance of giant cells and extensive fibrosis. *Chronic persistent myocarditis* was characterized by ongoing myocardial inflammation in the absence of significant ventricular dysfunction. Patients had symptoms of palpitations or atypical chest pain. (*Adapted from* Lieberman and coworkers [3].)

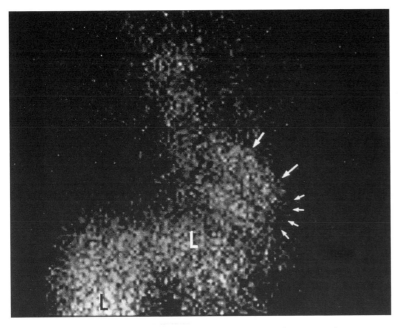

FIGURE 3-19. Nuclear imaging in the diagnosis of myocarditis. Antimyosin ^{111}In scintigraphy is a useful modality for the initial evaluation of patients with suspected myocarditis. This image depicts diffuse global uptake of radiolabeled antimyosin antibody by the left ventricle (*large arrows*) in an anterior planar image. The apical region has been relatively spared (*small arrows*). This patient presented with a syndrome masquerading as myocardial infarction with chest pain and elevations in creatine kinase MB isoenzymes. The left ventricle was dilated and hypocontractile. *L* denotes the normal hepatic activity of the labeled antibody. Compared with endomyocardial biopsy, antimyosin antibody imaging was 83% sensitive and 53% specific for the diagnosis of myocarditis [31]. (*From* Narula and coworkers [32]; with permission.)

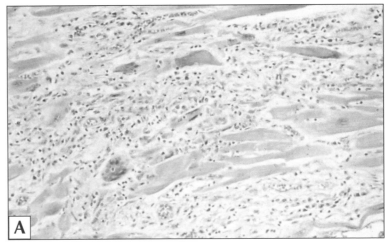

FIGURE 3-20. Giant-cell myocarditis and sarcoidosis. These are two rare inflammatory diseases of the myocardium distinguished by the presence of giant cells. **A,** Giant-cell myocarditis is characterized by lymphocytic infiltration, myocyte necrosis, and giant cells. Its course is slowly progressive yet insidious, and is often associated with ventricular arrhythmias or conduction system disease [3,33]. Giant-cell myocarditis has a very poor prognosis that may be improved by a cyclosporin-based immunosuppressive regimen or heart transplantation [34]. Rarely, giant-cell myocarditis may present as fulminant heart failure. (*continued*)

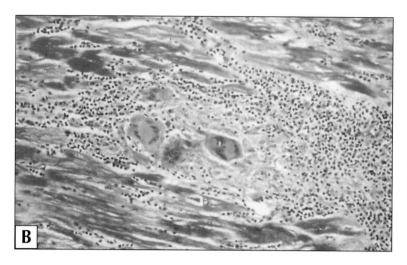

FIGURE 3-20. (*continued*) **B,** Section of left ventricular myocardium obtained at autopsy, demonstrating myocardial sarcoidosis. Myocardial sarcoidosis can be distinguished by the presence of true noncaseating granuloma within the myocardium. Approximately 5% of patients with sarcoidosis have clinically significant myocardial disease. However, involvement of the myocardium can be observed in 25% of autopsy cases [35]. The manifestations include cardiomyopathy, syncope, tachyarrhythmias, and sudden death. Patients may respond to corticosteroids and should be maintained on long-term, low-dose maintenance therapy [35]. (Part A *courtesy of* Frederick J. Schoen, Boston, MA; part B *courtesy of* Richard Mitchell, Boston, MA.)

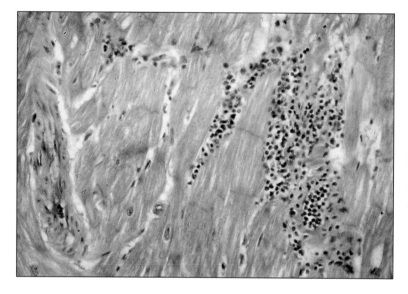

FIGURE 3-21. Hypersensitivity (eosinophilic) myocarditis. Some drugs, most commonly the sulfonamides, penicillins, and methyldopa, may cause an eosinophilic infiltration of the heart [36]. Typically, patients with hypersensitivity myocarditis present with the symptoms of an allergic drug reaction (*ie,* rash, fever, and eosinophilia) accompanied by cardiac symptoms, tachycardia, and electrocardiographic changes. Fulminant heart failure occurs rarely and is usually due to acute necrosis of the myocardium [37]. The presentation may also mimic myocardial infarction, with rises in creatine kinase MB fraction. Diagnosis can be achieved by endomyocardial biopsy, and management should include withdrawal of the offending medication and consideration of corticosteroid therapy. (*Courtesy of* Evan Loh, Philadelphia, PA.)

SPECIFIC CLINICAL CONDITIONS ASSOCIATED WITH A HISTOLOGIC DIAGNOSIS OF MYOCARDITIS IN 60 PATIENTS

CLINICAL CONDITION	PATIENTS, *n(%)*
Peripartum or postpartum	21(35)
Human immunodeficiency virus infection	17(28)
Chronic alcoholism	3(5)
Cocaine abuse	4(7)
Arrhythmias not associated with EF< 40%	4(7)
Familial cardiomyopathy	2(3)
Hyperthyroidism	2(3)
Systemic lupus erythematosus	2(3)
Sarcoidosis	2(3)
Restrictive cardiomyopathy	2(3)
Lyme disease	1(2)

FIGURE 3-22. The histologic prevalence of inflammatory heart disease in specific cardiomyopathies. Myocardial inflammation may play an important pathophysiologic role in several cardiomyopathic processes [38]. Midei *et al.* [39] have noted myocarditis in 78% of patients with peripartum cardiomyopathy. Furthermore, enteroviral RNA has been identified by the polymerase chain reaction in some patients with peripartum cardiomyopathy, indicating a viral etiology [28]. Myocarditis is also observed in patients who present primarily with arrhythmia or restrictive cardiomyopathy and in those with a history of drug exposure, endocrinopathy, or a familial predisposition to cardiomyopathy [38]. Myocarditis also plays a role in heart failure associated with rheumatologic illnesses, the prototype being systemic lupus erythematosus [40,41]. The most common cardiovascular manifestations of systemic lupus erythematosus include pericarditis (affecting 19% to 49% of patients) and Liebman-Sacks endocarditis. Approximately 10% of patients with systemic lupus erythematosus develop congestive heart failure, and 50% of these have myocarditis. Patients with systemic lupus erythematosus are also at increased risk for myocardial infarction on the basis of accelerated atherosclerosis or coronary arteritis, which may lead to the development of congestive heart failure. EF—ejection fraction. (*Adapted from* Herskowitz and coworkers [38].)

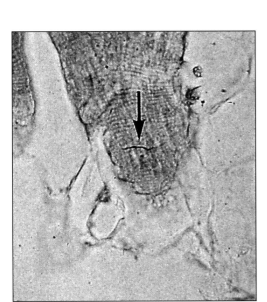

FIGURE 3-23. Detection of the spirochete *Borrelia burgdorferi* (*arrow*) in human myocardium (modified Steiner's silver stain). Lyme disease, a multisystem disorder caused by infection with *B. burgdorferi*, produces cardiac disease, notably arrhythmias and myocarditis, as a tertiary manifestation [42]. This infection is transmitted to humans from bites of ticks of the genus *Ixodes*. Here the spirochete is demonstrated in myocardium from a patient with a 4-year history of dilated cardiomyopathy and a serologic profile consistent with chronic Lyme disease. Despite therapy with ceftriaxone, the patient did not experience improvement in cardiac function. Bar=25 μm. (*From* Stanek and coworkers [42].)

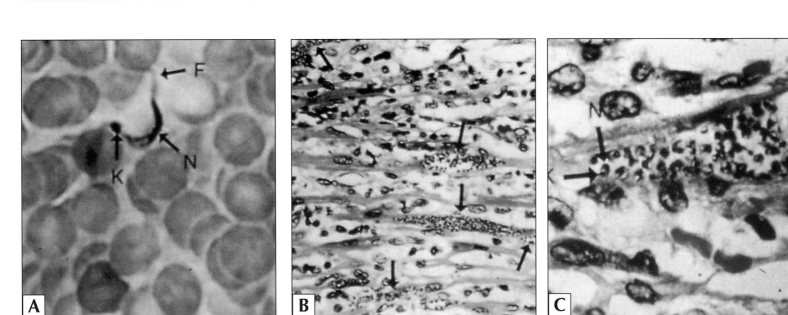

FIGURE 3-24. American trypanosomiasis (Chagas' disease). The most common infection of the heart worldwide is Chagas' disease, caused by the protozoan parasite *Trypanosoma cruzi*, which is spread by reduviid insects [43]. Infection with *T. cruzi* is endemic in Latin America and is now increasingly observed in the United States. Acute Chagas' disease is characterized by the systemic spread of the parasites to muscle, including myocardium. Two drugs, benznidazole and nifurtimox, shorten the acute phase of *T. cruzi* infection but achieve a cure in only 50% of patients. **A,** *T. cruzi* isolated from the blood of a patient with Chagas' disease. The trypomastigote is shown in mouse blood (Giemsa stain, × 2000). **B,** Histopathology of acute Chagas' myocarditis with a mononuclear infiltration. The *arrows* denote myocytes containing amastigote forms of the parasites (hematoxylin and eosin, × 360). **C,** High magni-fication of an infected myocyte (hematoxylin and eosin, × 900). F—flagellum; K—kinetoplast of amastigotes; N—nucleus. (*From* Kirchhoff [43]; with permission.)

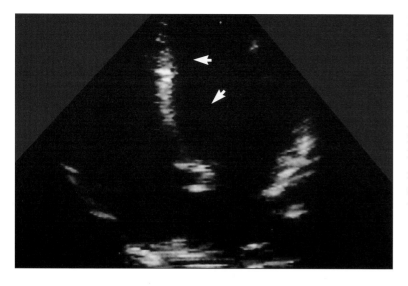

FIGURE 3-25. Chronic Chagas' disease. Patients chronically infected with *Trypanosoma cruzi* develop manifestations over a period of one to three decades [44]. Cardiac involvement is most common and manifests as biventricular enlargement, thinning of the ventricular walls, apical aneurysms (*arrows*), and mural thrombi. Clinically, patients experience heart failure, arrythmias, thromboembolic events, and sudden death. The prognosis of patients with Chagas' cardiomyopathy is worse than that of patients with idiopathic dilated cardiomyopathy [45].Cardiac transplantation has often been followed by recurrence of *T. cruzi* infection [43]. Depicted is a four-chamber echocardiogram showing two left ventricular apical aneurysms, which are characteristic of chronic Chagas' disease [44,45].

SECONDARY CAUSES OF CARDIOMYOPATHY

ENDOCRINE CAUSES

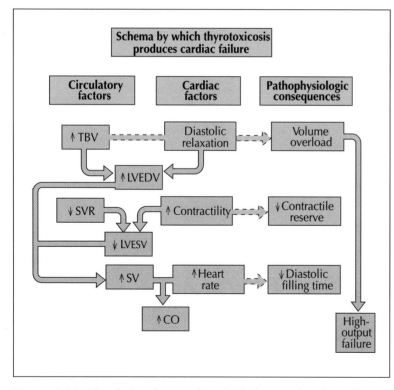

FIGURE 3-26. The chain of events by which thyrotoxicosis produces high-output cardiac failure. Excess circulating thyroxine influences both the vasculature and the heart, thereby affecting both cardiac

loading conditions and intrinsic cardiac function. Peripherally, thyrotoxicosis increases total blood volume (TBV), which increases preload, and decreases systemic vascular resistance (SVR), which decreases afterload. Thyroxine influences cardiac function by enhancing heart rate, increasing ventricular contractility, and lengthening diastolic relaxation. Therefore, baseline increases in cardiac performance associated with an increased volume load limit contractile reserve and may lead to heart failure and cardiac dilatation in about 6% of patients.

Risk factors for the development of congestive heart failure include age greater than 60 years and preexisting cardiac disease. A higher percentage of thyrotoxic patients also suffer from atrial fibrillation. Both congestive heart failure and atrial arrhythmias may respond favorably to treatment of hyperthyroidism.

Hypothyroidism also may produce dilated cardiomyopathy, which is reversible with therapy. Ladenson *et al.* [46] have recently reported a patient who experienced significant improvement in cardiac function during treatment for hypothyroidism. The clinical improvement was due to reversal of several molecular abnormalities associated with dilated cardiomyopathy (increased atrial natriuretic factor [ANF] and decreased α-myosin heavy chain and phospholamban). This case emphasizes that detection and treatment of thyroid, adrenal, and hypothalamic diseases in the patient with new-onset heart failure may lead to complete recovery of cardiac function. *Solid arrows* indicate direct effects; *dashed arrows* indicate potential consequences. CO—cardiac output; LVEDV—left ventricular end-diastolic volume; LVESV—left ventricular end-systolic volume; SV—stroke volume. (*Adapted from* Woeber [47]; with permission.)

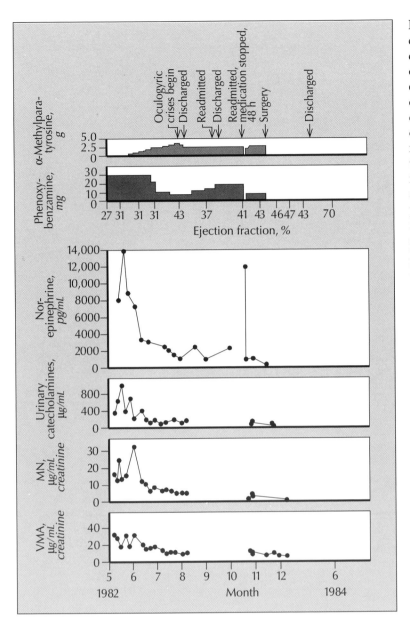

FIGURE 3-27. Reversal of dilated cardiomyopathy in pheochromo-cytoma. Several case reports document the development of dilated cardiomyopathy in patients with high levels of circulating cate-cholamines caused by pheochromocytoma [48–50]. A potential explanation for the pathophysiology of this lesion is that chronic adrenergic stimulation produces excessive activation of sarcolemmal calcium channels, increased cytosolic calcium, or accumulation of free radicals. Both increased calcium and free radicals may have toxic effects on the myocardium. Histologically, this lesion is characterized by myocyte vacuolization. Illustrated is the clinical course of a 12-year-old girl with pheochromocytoma and biventricular heart failure (initial ejection fraction, 27%). The patient was treated with α-methylparatyrosine and phenoxyben-zamine before surgical resection of the tumor. Six months after surgery she had recovered normal ventricular size and function. MN—metanephrine; VMA—vanillylmandelic acid. (*Adapted from* Imperato-McGinley and coworkers [49]; with permission.)

RHEUMATOLOGIC CAUSES

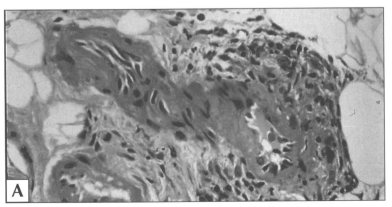

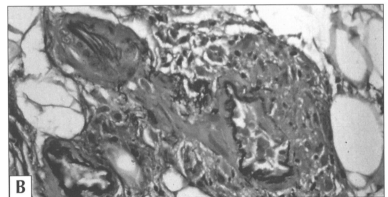

FIGURE 3-28. Necrotizing angiitis of a small intramural coronary artery in a patient with polyarteritis nodosa. Polyarteritis is a rare condition (incidence 6.3 in 100,00) that primarily affects the arteries of the kidney, peripheral nerves, skin, and abdominal viscera. Inflammation of the small branches of the coronary arteries represents a rare cause of cardiac microvascular disease and may produce myocardial infarction (often silent) and congestive heart failure. Depicted are sections of a right ventricular endomyocar-dial biopsy specimen from a patient with polyarteritis nodosa, chest pain, an inferoposterior thallium perfusion abnormality, and normal epicardial coronary arteries.

A, A small intramural artery is surrounded with fibrinoid degen-eration and cellular infiltration (hematoxylin and eosin, × 132). **B,** There is patchy destruction of the internal elastic membrane (elastica-van Gieson stain, × 132). (*From* Sugihara and coworkers [51]; with permission.)

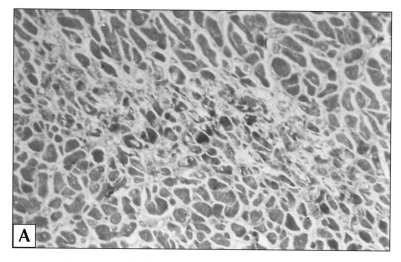

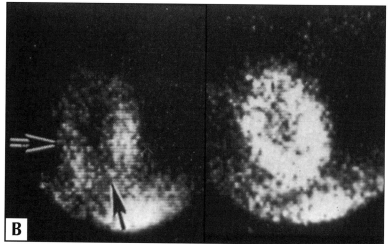

FIGURE 3-29. Myocardial involvement in systemic sclerosis. Micro-vascular vasoconstrictor abnormalities leading to myocardial fibrosis and left ventricular dysfunction are the hallmarks of scleroderma heart disease. The extent of myocardial fibrosis and contraction band necrosis predict the degree of left ventricular dysfunction [52].

A, Microinfarction with coagulation necrosis in the myocardium of a patient with systemic sclerosis (modified Masson's trichrome). The pathophysiology of the ischemic lesions appears to be microvascular disease similar to that observed in Raynaud's phenomenon [53]. Cardiac ischemia can be elicited by exposing patients with scleroderma to peripheral cold and detected as reversible thallium defects or transient segmental wall-motion abnormalities by echocardiography [53]. Kahan *et al.* [54] also have described impaired coronary flow reserve in response to dipyridamole in patients with systemic sclerosis.

B, Thallium scintigrams obtained from a patient with scleroderma obtained immediately after immersion of the patient's hand in ice water for 2 minutes (*left*) and after 3 hours of redistribution (*right*). Images were obtained in the 40° left anterior oblique view and demonstrate a septal and inferoapical perfusion defect (*arrows*) that completely resolved with redistribution. (Part A *courtesy of* Richard Mitchell, Boston, MA. Part B *from* Alexander and coworkers [53]; with permission.)

TOXIC AND METABOLIC CAUSES

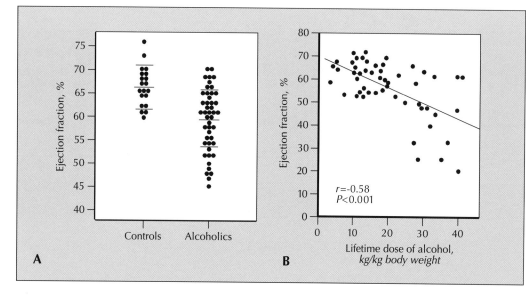

FIGURE 3-30. The toxic effects of alcohol consumption on cardiac function. Alcohol consumption has been implicated as an etiologic factor in approximately 5% of patients with nonischemic cardiomyopathy (*see* Fig. 3-2*B*). Urbano-Marquez *et al.* [55] have shown that fully one third of chronic alcoholics have cardiac dysfunction and that ethanol produces dose-related cardiac toxicity. **A,** Comparison of ejection fractions obtained by radionuclide ventriculography in 20 control subjects and 46 asymptomatic alcoholics in an outpatient rehabilitation program. The mean ejection fraction was 67% in the control subjects versus 59% in the alcoholic patients ($P<0.001$; SD depicted by *dashed lines*).

B, Correlation between total lifetime consumption of ethanol and left ventricular (LV) ejection fraction in 52 patients with alcoholism. In these patients, total lifetime consumption of alcohol was also positively correlated with LV mass (data not shown). Both relationships suggest a dose-related response to injury. Histologically, patients with alcoholic cardiomyopathy have changes indistinguishable from those of idiopathic cardiomyopathy, with interstitial and replacement fibrosis and myocyte hypertrophy. Alcoholics with early mild cardiac dysfunction may experience significant normalization in cardiac function if they abstain from alcohol consumption. (*Adapted from* Urbano-Marquez and coworkers [55].)

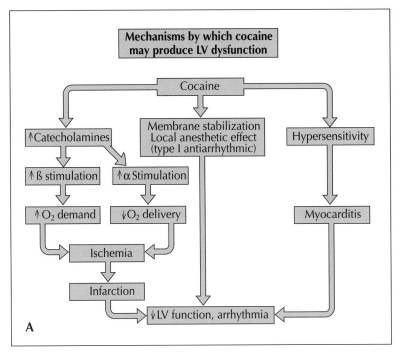

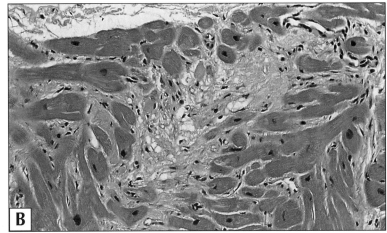

FIGURE 3-31. Schematic description of the potential mechanisms by which cocaine may produce cardiotoxicity and left ventricular (LV) dysfunction [56]. Cocaine, by inhibiting presynaptic reuptake of catecholamines, leads to increased β- and α-adrenergic stimulation. The former leads to increased heart rate and contractility and therefore to increased myocardial oxygen consumption. Increased α-adrenergic stimulation, on the other hand, causes rises in blood pressure and coronary vasoconstriction, thereby decreasing

oxygen delivery to the myocardium. The imbalance contributes to ischemia and possibly myocardial infarction. A second mechanism, that of decreased sodium transport leading to membrane stabilization or local anesthesia (a type I antiarrhythmic effect), may produce a negative inotropic effect that exceeds the positive inotropic effect of β-adrenergic stimulation. A third potential mechanism of LV dysfunction is that of hypersensitivity and myocarditis (*see* Fig. 3-22). Arrhythmias, QT and QRS prolongation, and sudden death occur due to LV dysfunction as well as to the direct type Ia effects of cocaine on the membrane. **B,** Histologic section obtained from a patient with dilated cardiomyopathy and chronic cocaine abuse. The section reveals replacement fibrosis, which may be a consequence of ischemia and microinfarction. (Part A *adapted from* Kloner and coworkers [56]; with permission. Part B *courtesy of* R. Hruban, Baltimore, MD.)

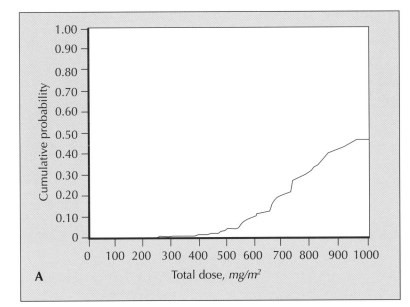

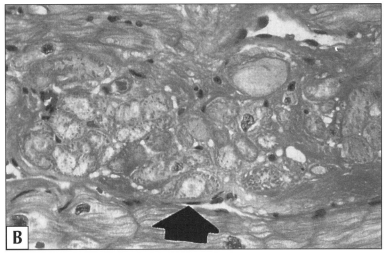

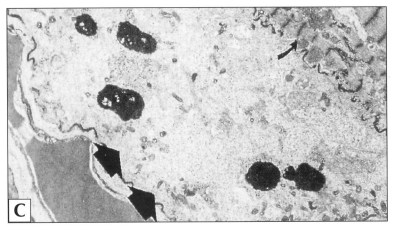

FIGURE 3-32. Anthracycline cardiomyopathy. Survivors of childhood malignancy represent one of the largest new groups of patients at risk for premature cardiovascular disease: 15% of patients in a pediatric cardiomyopathy registry had been treated for malignancy [57]. The anthracyclines doxorubicin and daunorubicin, widely used as chemotherapeutic agents, produce dose-related cardiotoxicity. It is likely that doxorubicin treatment impairs myocardial growth and leads to inadequate myocardial development. **A,** The cumulative probability of developing doxorubicin-induced congestive heart failure as a reflection of total cumulative dose in 3941 patients, 88 of whom experienced heart failure. **B,** Histologic changes characteristic of adriamycin cardiotoxicity. Light microscopic section showing characteristic myofibril loss and vacuolar degeneration (*arrow*). Hematoxylin and eosin, × 400. **C,** Electron microscopic image demonstrating extensive loss of myofilaments (*large arrows*). Normal, unaffected myocytes are also seen (*small arrows*). Original magnification, × 2800. (Parts B and C *from* Shan and coworkers [58]; with permission.)

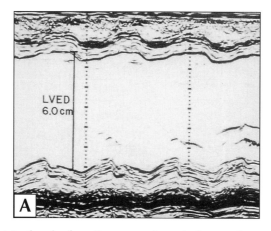 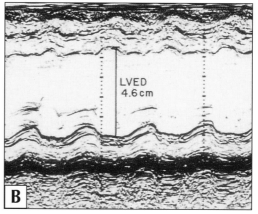

FIGURE 3-33. Left ventricular dysfunction secondary to hypocalcemia. M-mode echocardiograms from a patient with hypocalcemia before (**A**) and after (**B**) calcium repletion. Calcium exerts a fundamental regulatory role on cardiac contraction. Experimentally, the level of extracellular ionized calcium can be shown to correlate with the contractile state of the heart. Clinically, patients with persistent hypocalcemia may develop a reversible dilated cardiomyopathy. Shown is the echocardiogram of a patient with chronic renal insufficiency, previous subtotal parathyroidectomy, and persistent hypocalcemia. Chronic repletion of calcium with intravenous ionized calcium led to significant improvement of hemodynamics and partial resolution of cardiac dilatation over a 6-month period. LVED—left ventricular end-diastolic dimension. (*From* Feldman and coworkers [59]; with permission.)

INHERITED CAUSES

MYOCARDIAL DISEASE IN THE MAJOR HEREDOFAMILIAL NEUROMYOPATHIC DISORDERS

DISORDER	GENETICS	CARDIOMYOPATHY	CONDUCTION SYSTEM ARRHYTHMIA
Progressive muscular dystrophy			
Duchenne dystrophy; early-onset, rapidly progressive	X-linked	DCM	+
Becker dystrophy; late-onset, slowly progressive	X-linked	DCM	+
Limb-girdle dystrophy of Erb	Variable	-	-
Facioscapulohumeral (Landouzy-Dejerine)	AD	-	+
Emery-Dreifuss muscular dystrophy	X-linked	AP, DCM	+
Myotonic dystrophy (Steinert's disease)	AD	DCM	+
Friedreich's ataxia	AR	HCM, DCM	-
Kearns-Sayre syndrome	Mitochondrial	DCM	+

- —absent; + —present.

FIGURE 3-34. Myocardial disease in the major heredofamilial neuromyopathic disorders [60]. Shown are the major heredofamilial neuromyopathic disorders and their mode of inheritance. Also shown are the types of cardiomyopathic processes associated with these disorders, and whether arrhythmias or conduction system disease contribute to cardiovascular morbidity. AD—autosomal dominant; AP—atrial paralysis; AR—autosomal recessive; DCM—dilated cardiomyopathy; HCM—hypertrophic cardiomyopathy.

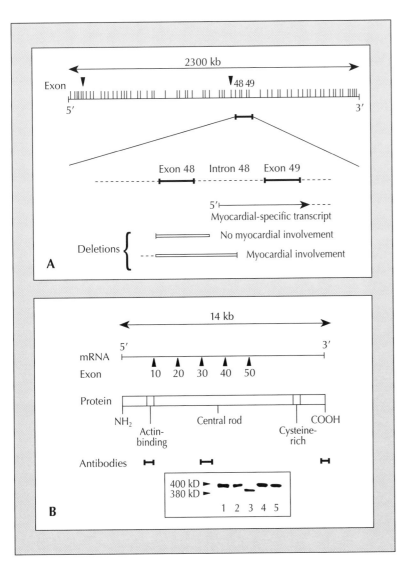

FIGURE 3-35. Neuromuscular disorders associated with cardiomy-opathy and mutations in the dystrophin gene. The dystrophin gene, spanning more than 2.3 million base pairs, is the largest mammalian gene. It codes for a cytoskeletal protein found in both striated and cardiac myocytes. Mutations of this gene cause both Duchenne and Becker muscular dystrophy. The former is associated with the complete absence of dystrophin, which results from an out-of-frame intragenic deletion producing a stop codon in the downstream sequence. In contrast, Becker muscular dystrophy results from an in-frame deletion in which only a part of the coding sequence is absent. Cardiac involvement has been noted in more than 80% of patients with Duchenne dystrophy and in approximately 50% of patients with Becker dystrophy.

A, The dystrophin gene: exons are indicated by *vertical bars* and *arrowheads* mark the sites where deletion breakpoints occur most often in Duchenne and Becker dystrophy. Melacini *et al.* [61] have described an association between cardiac involvement and intragenic deletions that include exons 48 and 49 in patients with Becker dystrophy. The finding that patients with deletions only in exon 48 have no cardiac involvement has led to the hypothesis that a myocardium-specific transcript exists whose 5' end is located within intron 48. Deletion of this sequence could be crucial in the development of cardiomyopathy in patients with muscular dystrophy.

B, The 14-kilobase (kb) dystrophin mRNA with exon numbers indicated and its corresponding protein product. Several domains of the protein are indicated: NH_2 (amino-terminal) domain, actin-binding domain, central-rod domain, cysteine-rich domain, and COOH (carboxy-terminal) domain. Using antibodies to various locations of the protein (*inset*), Western blotting can be used to demonstrate the abnormal lower molecular weight protein (lane 3,380 kD) in a patient with Becker muscular dystrophy compared to the normal 400-kD dystrophin protein in lanes 1, 2, 4, and 5. (*Adapted from* Melacini and coworkers [61]; with permission.)

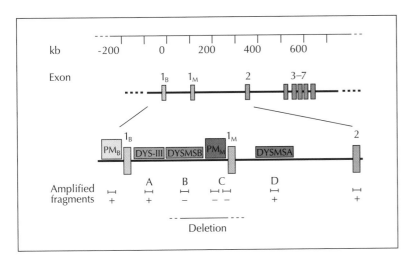

FIGURE 3-36. Dystrophin mutations in X-linked cardiomyopathies. Genetics may play a significant role in the etiology of idiopathic dilated cardiomyopathy (DCM) in the absence of neuromyopathic findings [62]. In 1987, Berko and Swift [63] reported a large kindred in which a progressive cardiomyopathy observed in teenage boys was inherited as an X-linked trait. Because both Duchenne and Becker muscular dystrophy have an X-linked pattern of inheritance, the intriguing possibility was raised that X-linked DCM was due to similar genetic abnormalities. Two studies in 1993 have now confirmed the association of X-linked DCM with mutations in the dystrophin gene [64] or its promoter region [65]. This figure shows the 5' end of the dystrophin gene. Muntoni *et al.* [65] used the polymerase chain reaction (PCR) to detect the presence of three polymorphic microsatellite loci (DYS-III, DYSMSB, and DYSMSA) in a kindred of patients with X-linked DCM. The *bars* beneath these regions indicate the fragments subject to PCR analysis. The letters *A, B, C,* and *D* above the bars correspond to the regions for which the PCR amplification was performed. The *plus* and *minus* signs indicate the presence or absence of the region in affected individuals, respectively. The approximate extent of the deletion is indicated at the bottom of the figure. These data indicate that X-linked cardiomyopathy is associated with a deletion of the muscle promoter and the first exon of the dystrophin gene, and imply that expression of dystrophin must be driven by the brain promoter (PM_B). PM_M—muscle promoter; 1_B—first brain exon; 1_M—first muscle exon. (*Adapted from* Muntoni and coworkers [65]; with permission.)

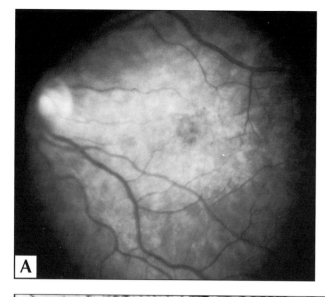

FIGURE 3-37. The Kearns-Sayre syndrome and mitochondrial cardiomyopathies. Dilated cardiomyopathy (DCM) is rarely associated with mitochondrial skeletal myopathies [66]. Kearns-Sayre syndrome is a rare mitochondrial myopathy characterized by ptosis, chronic progressive external ophthalmoplegia, abnormal retinal pigmentation, and conduction system abnormalities. Fewer than 20% of patients have cardiac involvement manifesting either as conduction system disease or cardiomyopathy. The genetics of mitochondrial cardiomyopathies have recently been elucidated; both mutations and deletions in the mitochondrial DNA have been associated with DCM [67,68]. **A,** The typical "salt and pepper" retinal pigmentation of Kearns-Sayre syndrome. **B,** Electron microscopic sections of normal and abnormal cardiac mitochondria from patients with Kearns-Sayre syndrome. *Panel I* demonstrates the appearance of normal mitochondria with closely packed cristae and granules. *Panels II* to *IV* depict mitochondrial abnormalities, with huge mitochondria with concentric cristae (*panel II*), enlarged mitochondria with transverse cristae (*panel III*), and small vacuolized mitochondria (*panel IV*). These abnormalities were found in seven of nine patients with Kearns-Sayre syndrome, demonstrating that a mitochondrial cardiomyopathy is part of this condition. (Part A *courtesy of* Tatsuo Hirose and Paul Arrigg. Part B *from* Schwartzkopff and coworkers [69]; with permission.)

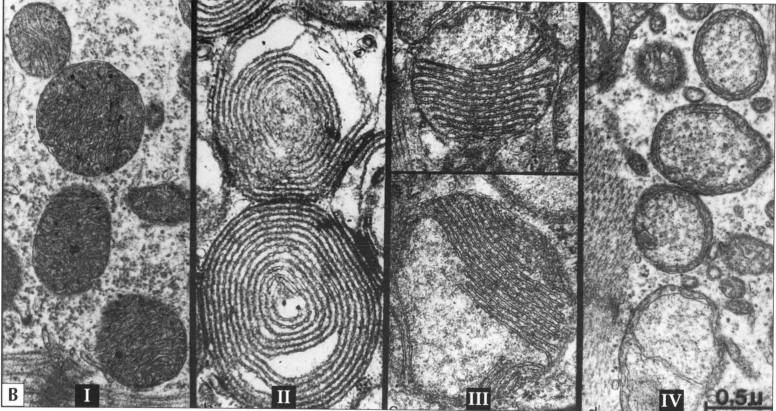

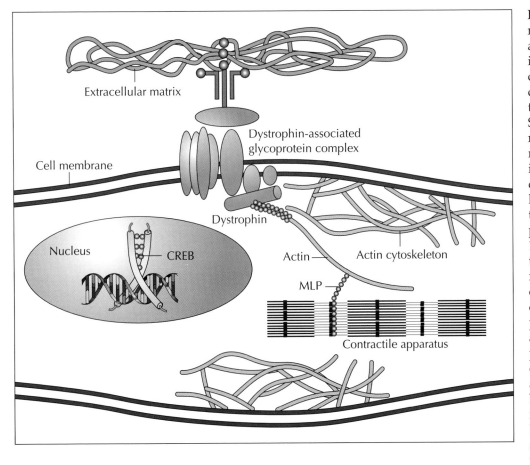

FIGURE 3-38. The genetics of dilated cardio-myopathy. Familial inheritance, usually with autosomal dominant transmission, has been implicated in 20% to 30% of cases of dilated cardiomyopathy [70]. Implicated genes encode cellular structural proteins, nuclear transcription factors, and as-yet unidentified products. Structural proteins that are involved in organizing the contractile apparatus of cardiac myocytes and maintaining their structural integrity have been implicated in dilated cardiomyopathy. The actin cytoskeleton is linked to the extracellular matrix by dystrophin and the dystrophin-associated glycoprotein complex. The muscle LIM (Lin-11, Isl-1, and Mec-3) protein, MLP, is thought to link the actin cytoskeleton to the contractile apparatus. Mutations in dystrophin, other members of the dystrophin-associated glycoprotein complex, and MLP have been shown to produce dilated cardiomyopathy in humans and mice. Nuclear transcription factors, gene products involved in controlling expression of other cardiac myocyte genes, such as cyclic adenosine monophosphate response element binding protein (CREB) have been implicated in experimental, murine cardiomyopathy. Linkage studies have identified gene loci, with as yet unidentified gene-products, associated with familial dilated cardiomyopathy [70]. (*Adapted from* Leiden [71]; with permission.)

INFILTRATIVE/RESTRICTIVE CARDIOMYOPATHIES

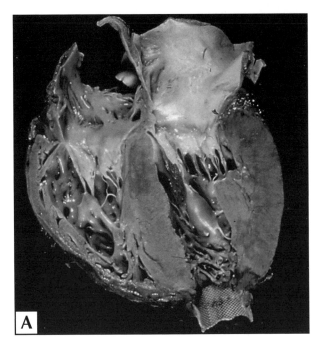

FIGURE 3-39. Myocardial iron deposition from hemochromatosis. Hemochromatosis is an inherited HLA-linked disorder of iron metabolism that results in iron deposition within parenchymal cells of the heart, liver, pancreas, synovium, and various endocrine glands, including the thyroid, parathyroid, and anterior pituitary. Infiltration of the heart produces a classic dilated cardiomyopathy. Early diagnosis is essential, as periodic venesection can prevent or reduce iron deposition. Iron depletion from the heart may not reverse cardiac dysfunction after a certain threshold of myocyte damage has been reached [72]. Iron loading from repeated blood transfusions can also produce iron deposition in parenchymal disease; patients with anemias associated with erythroid marrow hyperplasia and ineffective erythropoiesis are predisposed to iron deposition with transfusion.

A, The heart of a patient with hemochromatosis, demonstrating four-chamber hypertrophy and dilatation (heart weight, 500 g). The patient had received left and right ventricular assist devices for advanced heart failure. Shown is the left ventricular apical insertion site of a left ventricular assist device. (*continued*)

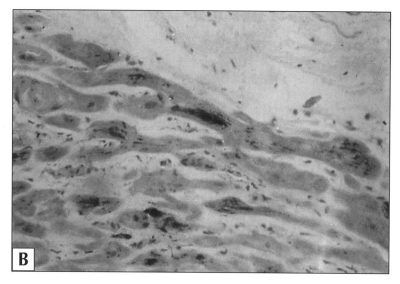

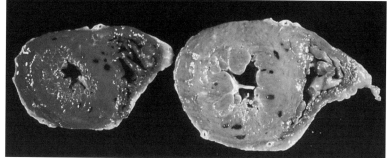

FIGURE 3-40. Neoplastic infiltration of the heart with metastatic melanoma. Tumor invasion of the heart is a rare cause of congestive heart failure. Flipse *et al.* [73] reported on a series of seven patients over a 7-year period in whom malignant neoplasms of the heart were diagnosed during life by endomyocardial biopsy. The important differential diagnosis to be considered in patients with known neoplasia is that of cardiac toxicity induced by treatment with anthracycline-based chemotherapy (*see* Fig. 3-32) or mediastinal radiation. (*Courtesy of* Richard Mitchell, Boston, MA.)

FIGURE 3-39. (*continued*) **B,** Microscopic section of myocardium from a patient with hemochromatosis, stained for iron with Prussian blue. The extensive hemosiderin deposits within the myocytes stain blue. (Part A *courtesy of* Richard Mitchell, Boston, MA; part B *courtesy of* Ralph Hruben, Baltimore, MD.) (*See* Color Plate for part B.)

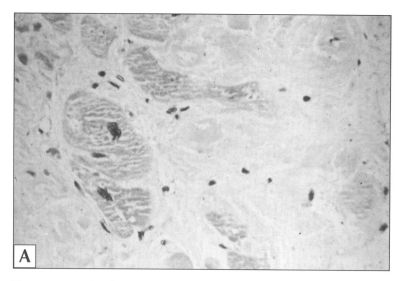

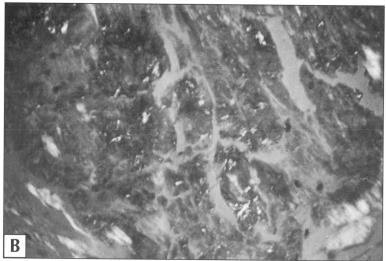

FIGURE 3-41. Cardiac amyloidosis. Amyloidosis is a condition in which tissue atrophy and necrosis result from deposition of insoluble protein fibrils. Although different proteins have the potential to deposit as amyloid, their common feature is the ability to form a specific molecular configuration, that of the β sheet. Cardiac amyloidosis may develop from the deposition of 1) proteins of immunologic origin, usually variable (κ or λ) immunoglobulin light chains, also known as Bence-Jones proteins (associated with multiple myeloma and primary amyloidosis); 2) abnormal transthyretin protein (familial amyloidosis); or 3) pre-albumin (senile cardiac amyloidosis). Amyloid deposition may result in either dilated, restrictive, or hypertrophic-like cardiomyopathy.

Survival of patients with familial amyloidosis is significantly better than that of patients with light chain amyloidosis, which warrants distinguishing these two etiologies by identifying the abnormal protein with immunohistochemistry or electrophoresis in the heart, bone-marrow, serum, or urine [74]. Digitalis, calcium channel blockers, and β-blocking drugs are contraindicated in amyloidosis. **A,** Histologic section from myocardium of a patient with senile amyloidosis, revealing scattered viable myocytes surrounded by a pale, hazy material, which represents the amyloid deposition (hematoxylin and eosin). **B,** Amyloid can be histologically identified by a characteristic green birefringence when viewed under polarized light (Sirius red). (*See* Color Plate for part B.)

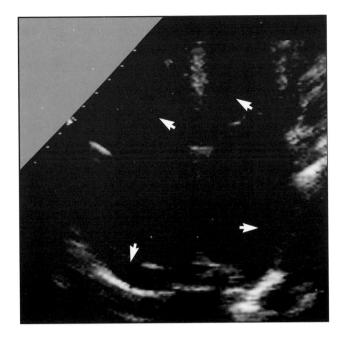

FIGURE 3-42. Echocardiographic features of restrictive cardiomyopathy. Apical four-chamber echocardiogram obtained from an 82-year-old man with progressive right heart failure. The notable features include thickened ventricular walls (*lower arrows*) with normal cavity sizes. There is biatrial enlargement (*upper arrows*), which develops to compensate for the restriction to filling. At cardiac catheterization the patient had equalization of the right atrial, right ventricular diastolic, pulmonary diastolic, and pulmonary arterial wedge pressures. Endomyocardial biopsy revealed cardiac amyloidosis.

HYPERTROPHIC CARDIOMYOPATHY

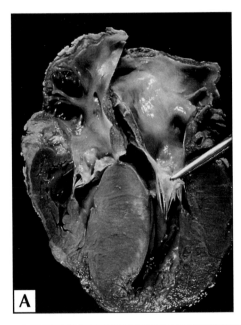

FIGURE 3-43. Hypertrophic cardiomyopathy. Familial hypertrophic cardiomyopathy is inherited as an autosomal-dominant trait. It causes hypertrophy of the ventricular walls in association with myofiber disarray. The genetic etiology of this condition has been linked to mutations in the cardiac β-myosin heavy chain gene [75]. The two most important clinical manifestations of hypertrophic cardiomyopathy are heart failure and sudden death. The development of heart failure is a consequence of increased chamber stiffness and diastolic dysfunction.

A, Gross appearance of hypertrophic cardiomyopathy. Although several different distributions of left ventricular hypertrophy exist, the most common is that of asymmetric septal hypertrophy. A characteristic fibrous plaque can be seen at the base of the septum in proximity to the anterior mitral leaflet, which probably results from systolic contact between the mitral valve and the septum. This interaction manifests on echocardiography as systolic anterior motion. **B,** Myocardial histology in hypertrophic cardiomyopathy. The characteristic appearance is that of bizarre and disordered myocardial architecture (hematoxylin and eosin). **C,** Myocardial fibrosis in hypertrophic cardiomyopathy (Masson's trichrome). (*Courtesy of* Frederick J. Schoen, Boston, MA.) (*See* Color Plate for parts B and C.)

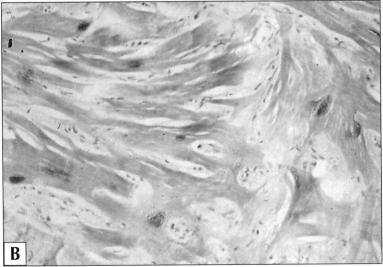

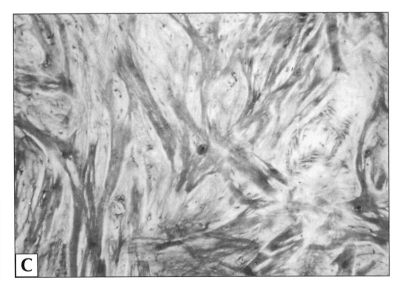

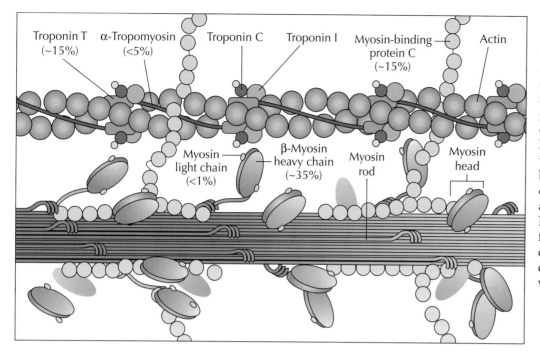

FIGURE 3-44. The genetics of hypertrophic cardiomyopathy. Hypertrophic cardiomyopathy may be caused by mutations affecting components of the myocardial contractile apparatus, thereby impairing myosin-actin interactions responsible for the generation of force. Mutations in four genes encoding proteins of the cardiac sarcomere have been implicated as causing hypertrophic cardiomyopathy. Mutations have been found in the genes for β-myosin heavy chain; cardiac troponin T, α-tropomyosin; and myosin-binding protein C genes. Percentages represent the estimated frequency with which a mutation on the corresponding gene causes hypertrophic cardiomyopathy. (*Adapted from* Spirito [75]; with permission.)

RIGHT VENTRICULAR CARDIOMYOPATHY

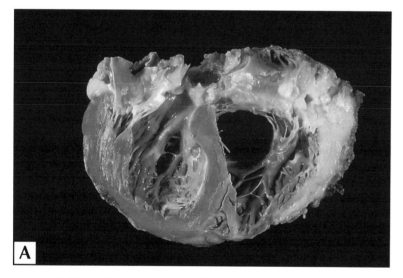

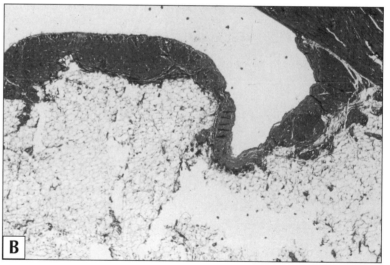

FIGURE 3-45. Arrhythmogenic right ventricular dysplasia. Arrhythmogenic right ventricular dysplasia is an isolated right ventricular cardiomyopathy characterized by extensive fibrotic and adipose infiltration of the right ventricular free wall. Approximately one third of patients have an autosomal dominant inheritance. Clinically there is a male predominance, symptoms of palpitations and syncope, a risk of sudden death often associated with ventricular fibrillation, and right ventricular dyskinesis. **A,** Explanted heart of a patient with right ventricular dysplasia. The right ventricle is markedly dilated, infiltrated with adipose tissue, and has a very thin rim of myocardial tissue. **B,** Histologic section through the right ventricular apex, showing regions of fibrosis, adipose infiltration, and myocardial thinning (Mason's trichrome). (*Courtesy of* G. Winters, Boston, MA.) (*See* Color Plate for part B.)

REFERENCES

1. Manolio TA, Baughman KL, Rodeheffer R, *et al.*: Prevalence and etiology of idiopathic dilated cardiomyopathy (summary of a National Heart, Lung, and Blood Institute workshop). *Am J Cardiol* 1992, 69:1458–1466.

2. Kasper EK, Agema WRP, Hutchins GM, *et al.*: The causes of dilated cardiomyopathy: a clinicopathologic review of 673 consecutive patients. *J Am Coll Cardiol* 1994, 23:586–590.

3. Lieberman EB, Hutchins GM, Herskowitz A, *et al.*: Clinicopathologic description of myocarditis. *J Am Coll Cardiol* 1991, 18:1617–1626.

4. Hrobon P, Kuntz KM, Hare JM: Should endomyocardial biopsy be performed for detection of myocarditis? A decision analytic approach. *J Heart Lung Transplant* 1998, 17:479–486.

5. Ho KKL, Pinsky JL, Kannel WB, *et al.*: The epidemiology of heart failure: the Framingham Study. *J Am Coll Cardiol* 1993, 22 (suppl A):6–13.

6. Teerlink JR, Goldhaber SZ, Pfeffer MA: An overview of contemporary etiologies of congestive heart failure. *Am J Cardiol* 1991, 121:1852–1853.

7. Bonow RO, Udelson JE: Left ventricular diastolic dysfunction as a cause of congestive heart failure: mechanisms and management. *Ann Intern Med* 1992, 117:502–510.

8. Gaasch WH, Levine HJ, Quinones NM, *et al.*: Left ventricular compliance: mechanisms and clinical implications. *Am J Cardiol* 1976, 38:645–653.

9. Weber KT, Anversa P, Armstrong PW, *et al.*: Remodeling and reparation of the cardiovascular system. *J Am Coll Cardiol* 1992, 20:3–16.

10. Hare JM, Walford GD, Hruban RH, *et al.*: Ischemic cardiomyopathy: endomyocardial biopsy and ventriculographic evaluation of patients with congestive heart failure, dilated cardiomyopathy and coronary artery disease. *J Am Coll Cardiol* 1992, 20:1318–1325.

11. Mangschau A, Forfang K, Rootwelt K, *et al.*: Improvement in cardiac performance and exercise tolerance after left ventricular aneurysm surgery: a prospective study. *Thorac Cardiovasc Surg* 1988, 36:320–325.

12. Kloner RA, Przyklenk K, Patel B: Altered myocardial states: the stunned and hibernating myocardium. *Am J Med* 1989, 86(suppl 1A):14–22.

13. Pagley PR, Beller GA, Watson DD, *et al.*: Improved outcome after coronary bypass surgery patients with ischemic cardiomyopathy and residual myocardial viability. *Circulation* 1997, 96:793–800.

14. Ross J Jr: Afterload mismatch in aortic and mitral valve disease: implications for surgical therapy. *J Am Coll Cardiol* 1985, 5:811–826.

15. Morgan DJR, Hall RJC: Occult aortic stenosis as cause of intractable heart failure. *Br Med J* 1979, 1:784–787.

16. Kontos GJ Jr, Schaff HV, Gersh BJ, *et al.*: Left ventricular function in subacute and chronic mitral regurgitation: effect of function early postoperatively. *J Thorac Cardiovasc Surg* 1989, 98:163–169.

17. Rozich JD, Carabello BA, Usher BW, *et al.*: Mitral valve replacement with and without chordal preservation in patients with chronic mitral regurgitation: mechanisms for differences in postoperative ejection performance. *Circulation* 1992, 86:1718–1726.

18. Liu CP, Ting CT, Yang TM, *et al.*: Reduced left ventricular compliance in human mitral stenosis: role of reversible internal constraint. *Circulation* 1992, 85:1447–1456.

19. Aretz HT, Bellingham ME, Edwards WD, *et al.*: Myocarditis: a histopathologic definition and classification. *Am J Cardiovasc Pathol* 1986, 1:3–14.

20. Jones SR, Herskowitz A, Hutchins GM, *et al.*: Effects of immunosuppressive therapy in biopsy-proved myocarditis and borderline myocarditis on left ventricular function. *Am J Cardiol* 1991, 68:370–376.

21. Chow LH, Radio SJ, Sears TD, *et al.*: Insensitivity of right ventricular endomyocardial biopsy in the diagnosis of myocarditis. *J Am Coll Cardiol* 1989, 14:915–920.

22. Deckers JW, Hare JM, Baughman KL: Complications of transvenous right ventricular endomyocardial biopsy in adult cardiomyopathy patients: a seven year survey of 546 consecutive diagnostic procedures in a tertiary referral center. *J Am Coll Cardiol* 1992, 19:43–47.

23. Starling RC, VanFossen DB, Hammer DF, *et al.*: Morbidity of endomyocardial biopsy in cardiomyopathy. *Am J Cardiol* 1991, 68:133–136.

24. Eck M, Greiner A, Kandolf R, *et al.*: Active fulminant myocarditis characterized by T-lymphocytes expressing the gamma-delta T-cell receptor: a new disease entity? *Am J Surg Path* 1997, 21:1109–1112.

25. Mason JW, O'Connell JB, Herskowitz A, *et al.*: A clinical trial of immunosuppressive therapy for myocarditis. *N Engl J Med* 1995, 333:269–275.

26. Hare JM, Baughman KL: Myocarditis: current understanding of the etiology, pathophysiology, natural history and management of inflammatory diseases of the myocardium. *Cardiol Rev* 1994, 2:165–173.

27. Martin AB, Webber S, Fricker FJ, *et al.*: Acute myocarditis: rapid diagnosis by PCR in children. *Circulation* 1994, 90:330–339.

28. Jin O, Sole MJ, Butany JW, *et al.*: Detection of enterovirus RNA in myocardial biopsies from patients with myocarditis and cardiomyopathy using gene amplification by polymerase chain reaction. *Circulation* 1990, 82:8–16.

29. Kandolf R: The impact of recombinant DNA technology on the study of enterovirus heart disease. In *Coxsackieviruses—A General Update*. Edited by Bendinelli M, Friedman H. New York: Plenum Publishing; 1988:293–318.

30. Kandolf R: Molecular biology of viral heart disease. *Herz* 1993, 18:238–244.

31. Dec GW, Palacios I, Yasuda T, *et al.*: Antimyosin antibody cardiac imaging: its role in the diagnosis of myocarditis. *J Am Coll Cardiol* 1990, 16:97–104.

32. Narula J, Khaw BA, Dec GW, *et al.*: Recognition of acute myocarditis masquerading as acute myocardial infarction. *N Engl J Med* 1993, 328:100–104.

33. Davidoff R, Palacios I, Southern J, *et al.*: Giant cell versus lymphocytic myocarditis: a comparison of their clinical features and long-term outcomes. *Circulation* 1991, 83:953–961.

34. Cooper LT, Berry GJ, Shabetai R: Idiopathic giant-cell myocarditis: natural history and treatment. *N Engl J Med* 1997, 336:1861–1866.

35. Johns CJ, Paz H, Kasper EK, *et al.*: Myocardial sarcoidosis: course and management. *Sarcoidosis* 1992, 9(suppl 1):231–236.

36. Kounis NG, Zavras GM, Soufras GD, *et al.*: Hypersensitivity myocarditis. *Ann Allergy* 1989, 62:71–73.

37. Getz MA, Subramanian R, Logemann T, *et al.*: Acute necrotizing eosinophilic myocarditis as a manifestation of severe hypersensitivity myocarditis: antemortem diagnosis and successful treatment. *Ann Intern Med* 1991, 115:201–202.

38. Herskowitz A, Campbell S, Deckers J, *et al.*: Demographic features and prevalence of idiopathic myocarditis in patients undergoing endomyocardial biopsy. *Am J Cardiol* 1993, 71:982–986.

39. Midei MG, DeMent SH, Feldman AM, *et al.*: Peripartum myocarditis and cardiomyopathy. *Circulation* 1990, 81:922–928.

40. Stevens MB: Lupus carditis. *N Engl J Med* 1988, 319:861–862.

41. Doherty HE, Siegel RJ: Cardiovascular manifestations of systemic lupus erythematosus. *Am Heart J* 1985, 110:1257–1265.

42. Stanek G, Klein J, Bittner R, *et al.*: Isolation of *Borrelia burgdorferi* from the myocardium of a patient with longstanding cardiomyopathy. *N Engl J Med* 1990, 322:249–252.

43. Kirchhoff LV: American trypanosomiasis (Chagas' disease): a tropical disease now in the United States. *N Engl J Med* 1993, 329:639–644.

44. Morris SA, Tanowitz HB, Wittner M, *et al.*: Pathophysiologic insights into the cardiomyopathy of Chagas' disease. *Circulation* 1990, 82:1900–1909.

45. Bestetti RB, Muccillo G: Clinical course of Chagas' heart disease: a comparison with dilated cardiomyopathy. *Int J Cardiol* 1997, 60:187–193.

46. Ladenson PW, Sherman SI, Baughman KL, *et al.*: Reversible alterations in myocardial gene expression in a young man with dilated cardiomyopathy and hypothyroidism. *Proc Natl Acad Sci U S A* 1992, 89:5251–5255.

47. Woeber KA: Thyrotoxicosis and the heart. *N Engl J Med* 1992, 327:94–98.

48. Lam JB, Shub C, Sheps SG: Reversible dilatation of hypertrophied left ventricle in pheochromocytoma: serial two-dimensional echocardiographic observations. *Am Heart J* 1985, 109:613–615.

49. Imperato-McGinley J, Gautier T, Ehlers K, *et al.*: Reversibility of catecholamine-induced dilated cardiomyopathy in a child with pheochromocytoma. *N Engl J Med* 1987, 316:793–797.

50. Case 15-1988: Case records of the Massachusetts General Hospital. *N Engl J Med* 1988, 318:970–998.

51. Sugihara N, Genda A, Shimizu M, *et al.*: Intramural coronary angiitis of periarteritis nodosa proved by endomyocardial biopsy. *Am Heart J* 1990, 119:1414–1416.

52. Follansbee WP, Miller TR, Curtiss EI, *et al.*: A controlled clinico-pathologic study of myocardial fibrosis in systemic sclerosis (scleroderma). *J Rheumatol* 1990, 17:656–662.

53. Alexander EL, Firestein GS, Weiss JL, *et al.*: Reversible cold-induced abnormalities in myocardial perfusion and function in systemic sclerosis. *Ann Intern Med* 1986, 105:661–668.

54. Kahan A, Nitenberg A, Foult JM, *et al.*: Decreased coronary reserve in primary scleroderma myocardial disease. *Arthritis Rheum* 1985, 28:637–646.

55. Urbano-Marquez A, Estruch R, Navarro-Lopez F, *et al.*: The effects of alcoholism on skeletal and cardiac muscle. *N Engl J Med* 1989, 320:409–415.

56. Kloner RA, Hale S, Alker K, *et al.*: The effects of acute and chronic cocaine use on the heart. *Circulation* 1992, 408:407–419.

57. Lipshultz SE, Sallan SE: Cardiovascular abnormalities in long-term survivors of childhood malignancy. *J Clin Oncol* 1993, 11:1199–1203.

58. Shan K, Lincoff AM, Young JB: Anthracycline-induced cardiotoxicity. *Ann Intern Med* 1996, 125:47–58.

59. Feldman AM, Fivush B, Zahka K, *et al.*: Congestive cardiomyopathy in patients on continuous ambulatory peritoneal dialysis. *Am J Kidney Dis* 1988, 11:76–79.

60. Perloff JK: Neurologic disorders and heart disease. In *Heart Disease, A Textbook of Cardiovascular Medicine*, edn 5. Edited by Braunwald E. Philadelphia: WB Saunders; 1997:1865–1886.

61. Melacini P, Fanin M, Danieli GA, *et al.*: Cardiac involvement in Becker muscular dystrophy. *J Am Coll Cardiol* 1993, 22:1927–1934.

62. Michels VV, Moll PP, Miller FA, *et al.*: The frequency of familial dilated cardiomyopathy in a series of patients with idiopathic dilated czardiomyopathy. *N Engl J Med* 1992, 326:77–82.

63. Berko BA, Swift M: X-linked dilated cardiomyopathy. *N Engl J Med* 1987, 316:1186–1191.

64. Towbin JA, Hejtmancik JF, Brink P, *et al.*: X-linked dilated cardio-myopathy: molecular evidence of linkage to the Duchenne muscular dystrophy (dystrophin) gene at the Xp21 locus. *Circulation* 1993, 87:1854–1865.

65. Muntoni F, Cau M, Ganua A, *et al.*: Deletion of the dystrophin muscle-promoter region associated with X-linked dilated cardiomyopathy. *N Engl J Med* 1993, 329:921–925.

66. Channer KS, Channer JL, Campbell MJ, *et al.*: Cardiomyopathy in the Kearns-Sayre syndrome. *Br Heart J* 1988, 59:486–490.

67. Zeviani M, Gellara C, Antozzi C, *et al.*: Maternally inherited myopathy and cardiomyopathy: association with mutation in mitochondrial DNA tRNA $^{Leu(UUR)}$. *Lancet* 1991, 338:143–147.

68. Suomalainen A, Paetau A, Leinonen H, *et al.*: Inherited idiopathic dilated cardiomyopathy with multiple deletions of mitochondrial DNA. *Lancet* 1992, 340:1319–1320.

69. Schwartzkopff B, Frenzel H, Breithardt G, *et al.*: Ultrastructural findings in endomyocardial biopsy of patients with Kearns-Sayre syndrome. *J Am Coll Cardiol* 1988, 12:1522–1528.

70. Bowles KR, Gajarski R, Porter P, *et al.*: Gene mapping of familial autosomal dominant dilated cardiomyopathy to chromosome 10q21-23. *J Clin Invest* 1996 98:1355–60.

71. Leiden, JM: The genetics of dilated cardiomyopathy: emerging clues to the puzzle. *N Engl J Med* 1997, 337:1080–81.

72. Westra WH, Hruban RH, Baughman KL, *et al.*: Progressive hemo-chromatotic cardiomyopathy despite reversal of iron deposition after liver transplantation. *Am J Clin Pathol* 1993, 99:39–44.

73. Flipse TR, Tazelaar HD, Holmes DR Jr: Diagnosis of malignant cardiac disease by endomyocardial biopsy. *Mayo Clin Proc* 1990, 65:1415–1422.

74. Dubrey SW, Cha K, Skinner, *et al.*: Familial and primary (AL) cardiac amyloidosis: echocardiographically similar diseases with distinctly different clinical outcomes. *Heart* 1997, 78:74–82.

75. Spirito P, Seidman CE, McKenna WJ, *et al.*: The management of hypertrophic cardiomyopathy. *N Engl J Med* 1997, 336:775.

MOLECULAR AND CELLULAR EVENTS IN MYOCARDIAL HYPERTROPHY AND FAILURE

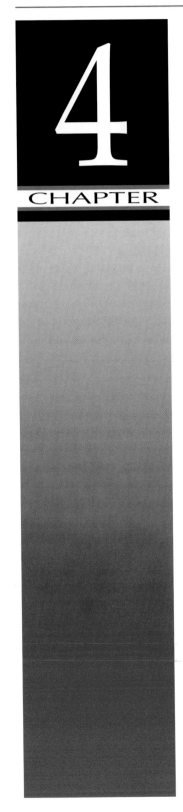

4

CHAPTER

Douglas B. Sawyer and Wilson S. Colucci

Whereas cardiac failure was once thought to be a static condition reflecting a damaged myocardium, it is now apparent that it reflects a dynamic process involving the continuous structural and functional reorganization, or remodeling, of the heart in response to environmental stresses and stimuli. The fundamental events that lead to cardiac remodeling occur at the molecular and cellular level in both the myocytes and the nonmyocyte cells of the heart. Observations made in failing human myocardium and in myocardium from animals with hypertrophy or failure suggest that there are multiple molecular and cellular alterations involving the excitation-contraction process, contractile and regulatory proteins, growth factors, and signaling pathways. A variety of stimuli that may be responsible for these alterations have been identified, including mechanical wall stresses, hormones, neurotransmitters, and peptide growth factors. Genetic manipulations in small animal models are refining our understanding of the stimuli and molecular events that lead to progression of heart failure. Although much remains to be learned about how these stimuli interact with signaling pathways to regulate the remodeling of the myocardium, it is now apparent that these events have an important impact on the clinical course of the patient and may offer new approaches to the prevention and treatment of myocardial failure.

As our understanding of the basic molecular and cellular biology of myocardial hypertrophy and failure advances, it is likely that additional new diagnostic and therapeutic approaches will emerge. For example, the ability to assess the "molecular status" of the myocardium may allow better tracking of disease progression, earlier detection of asymptomatic patients, improved prognostication, and the design of therapeutic regimens tailored at the molecular level. New classes of therapeutic agents will emerge. Drugs that block cytokine or growth factor receptors already exist, and these offer exciting prospects that may be evaluated in the near future. Finally, it is already reasonable to speculate that progress in our understanding of the regulation of cardiac gene expression will lead to the development of molecular therapies (*eg*, utilizing the transfer of genes or antisense oligonucleotides) aimed at preventing or reversing fundamental abnormalities that occur at the molecular and cellular level.

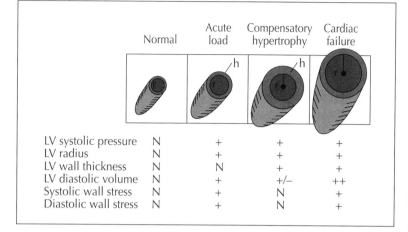

	Normal	Acute load	Compensatory hypertrophy	Cardiac failure
LV systolic pressure	N	+	+	+
LV radius	N	+	+	+
LV wall thickness	N	N	+	+
LV diastolic volume	N	+	+/–	++
Systolic wall stress	N	+	N	+
Diastolic wall stress	N	+	N	+

FIGURE 4-1. Hemodynamic overload is the most common stimulus for myocardial hypertrophy and remodeling. A frequent cause of hemodynamic overload is an increase (+) in left ventricular (LV) systolic pressure, as may occur in patients with hypertension or aortic stenosis. The normal (N) relationship between LV wall thickness (h) and chamber radius (r) is shown (*first panel*). An acute increase in systolic pressure causes an increase in systolic wall stress, which can be approximated by the equation $P \times r/h$, where *P* is LV systolic pressure. Diastolic wall stress is also increased when there is chamber dilatation or when diastolic pressure is elevated (*second panel*). If sufficient compensatory hypertrophy occurs, the increase in ventricular wall thickness may normalize the systolic and diastolic wall stresses (*third panel*). However, if additional chamber dilatation occurs or the increase in wall thickness is insufficient, systolic and diastolic wall stresses remain abnormally elevated. In this situation, further chamber dilatation may occur in association with hemodynamic failure (*fourth panel*). (*Adapted from* Swynghedauw and coworkers [1]; with permission.)

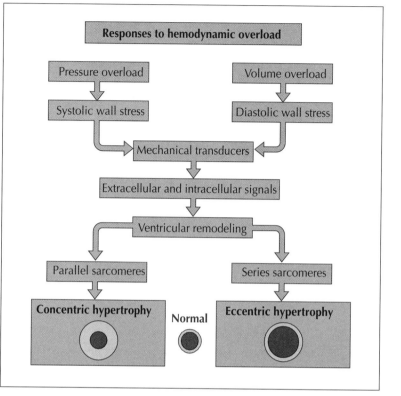

FIGURE 4-2. The morphologic characteristics of the response to a hemodynamic overload depend on the nature of the stimulus. With pressure overload, the increase in systolic wall stress leads to a parallel addition of sarcomeres and widening of cardiac myocytes. At the gross morphologic level there is concentric hypertrophy. Alternatively, if the hemodynamic stimulus consists primarily of an increase in ventricular volume (*eg*, due to regurgitant valvular disease), there is a series addition of sarcomeres and lengthening of cardiac myocytes. At the gross morphologic level there is eccentric hypertrophy.

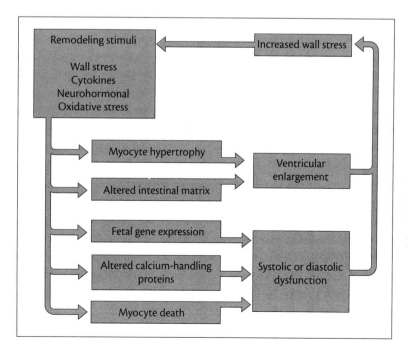

FIGURE 4-3. Remodeling stimuli. Chronic hemodynamic stimuli such as pressure and volume overload lead to ventricular remodeling through increases in myocardial wall stress, cytokines, signaling peptides, neuroendocrine signals, and perhaps, oxidative stress. The myocardium responds with adaptive as well as maladaptive changes. Myocyte hypertrophy and changes in interstitial matrix might at first normalize the wall stress but these occur at the expense of ventricular compliance. Re-expression of fetal contractile proteins and calcium handling proteins may contribute to impaired contraction and relaxation. Myocytes unable to adapt might be triggered to undergo programmed cell death (apoptosis). The net result of these changes is further impairment in pump function and increased wall stress, thus completing a vicious cycle that leads to further progression of the myocardial dysfunction.

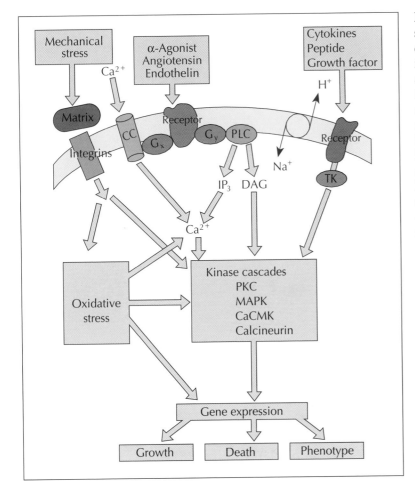

FIGURE 4-4. Signaling pathways in myocardial remodeling. Many signaling pathways have the potential to regulate the growth of cardiac cells acting through an increasingly complex network of intracellular signaling cascades. Agonists for α-adrenergic, angiotensin, and endothelin receptors couple to phospholipase C (PLC) and calcium influx channels (CC) by way of G-proteins (G_x and G_y). Activation of PLC results in the generation of two second messengers, inositol triphosphate (IP_3) and diacylglycerol (DAG). IP_3 causes the release of calcium from intracellular stores, and DAG activates protein kinase C (PKC). Changes in intracellular calcium stores can activate calcium-calmodulin–dependent kinases (Ca-CMK), as well as calcineurin, which can affect gene expression in multiple ways. PKC can affect gene expression directly or indirectly by its effects on Na^+-H^+ exchange (to regulate cellular pH) or by activating mitogen-activated protein kinase (MAPK) cascades.

Cytokines and peptide growth factors can be elaborated by various cells within the heart and may act in an autocrine or paracrine manner. These growth factors activate cellular receptors that usually possess tyrosine kinase (TK) activity and are coupled to a cascade of protein kinases (ras, Raf, MAPKK, MAPK). Mechanical deformation of cardiac myocytes through matrix-integrin interactions can lead to activation or modulation of several signaling pathways, at least in part through autocrine action of released agonists such as angiotensin. Both nitric oxide and oxidative stress may be induced after stimulation of signaling pathways and modulate the activity of kinase cascades and transcription factors leading to alterations in contractile phenotype, growth, and death in myocytes.

MYOCYTE HYPERTROPHY

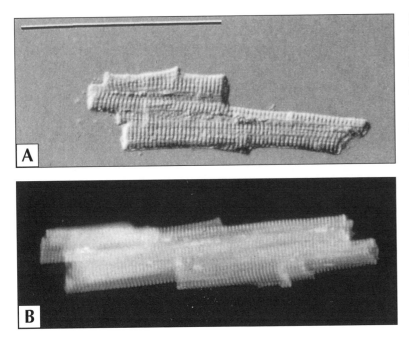

FIGURE 4-5. Isolated cardiac myocytes obtained from human left ventricular myocardium. **A,** Myocyte from a normal heart (*bar* = 100 μm). **B,** A hypertrophied myocyte from the left ventricle of a patient with ischemic cardiomyopathy, viewed at the same magnification as in *A*. This myocyte is longer and wider than the normal myocyte. The myocytes have been stained with rhodamine-phalloidin for visualization of the sarcomere structure. In the myocyte from the failing heart, there has been both series and parallel addition of sarcomeres, which are otherwise organized in a normal pattern. (*Adapted from* Gerdes and coworkers [2]; with permission.)

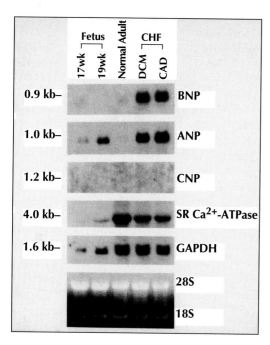

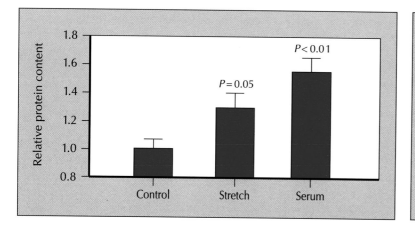

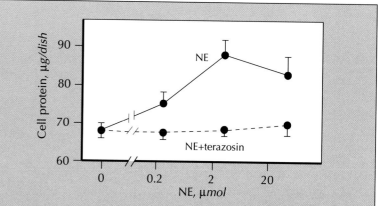

FIGURE 4-6. Although the sarcomeres in remodeled myocardium retain a normal gross morphologic appearance, the expression of several functionally important proteins is altered. Characteristics of the ventricular remodeling response to hemodynamic overload include reexpression of fetal genes that are not normally present in adult myocardium and reduced expression of several muscle-specific adult genes. Shown is a Northern blot illustrating mRNA levels for several proteins in human ventricular myocardium from a normal adult (*center lane*), fetal tissue (Fetus) and from two patients with heart failure (CHF), one due to dilated cardiomyopathy (DCM) and the other due to coronary artery disease (CAD).

Atrial natriuretic peptide (ANP) and brain natriuretic peptide (BNP), which are normally expressed in fetal tissue but are not present in normal adult ventricular tissue, are reexpressed in patients with heart failure. The quantity of cardiac sarcoplasmic reticulum Ca^{2+}-ATPase (Sr Ca^{2+}-ATPase), a protein important for excitation-contraction coupling and normally expressed in abundance in normal adult myocardium, is reduced in the myocardium from the patients with CHF. The amounts of glyceraldehyde-3-phosphate dehydrogenase (GAPDH) mRNA and ribosomal (28S and 18S) RNAs are shown as internal controls. CNP—C-type natriuretic peptide. (*Adapted from* Takahashi and coworkers [3]; with permission.)

FIGURE 4-7. An increase in the mechanical stresses on cardiac myocytes is a potential growth stimulus common to many forms of hypertrophy. To examine this mechanism experimentally, cardiac myocytes cultured from neonatal rat hearts were grown on a deformable membrane that could be stretched. Compared with control cells that were not stretched, cells that were stretched to increase their length by 20% for 48 hours showed an approximately 30% increase in cellular protein content, indicative of hypertrophy. Serum, which is rich in growth factors, was used for comparison purposes. Because under the conditions of these experiments no other cell types or extrinsic growth factors are present, these observations suggest that mechanical deformation of the myocyte can in itself cause hypertrophy. *P* values are versus control cells. (*Adapted from* Sadoshima and coworkers [4]; with permission.)

FIGURE 4-8. Another regulator of cell growth and differentiation is sympathetic innervation. Norepinephrine (NE), the primary sympathetic neurotransmitter, can affect the growth of cardiac myocytes. Neonatal rat cardiac myocytes in culture dishes were exposed to NE in various concentrations for 24 hours, after which cellular protein was measured. NE caused cellular hypertrophy (*ie*, increased protein), which was inhibited by terazosin, an α_1-selective antagonist. These findings indicate that the hypertrophic effect of NE is mediated by an α_1-adrenergic receptor located on the cardiac myocyte. (*Adapted from* Simpson and McGrath [5]; with permission.)

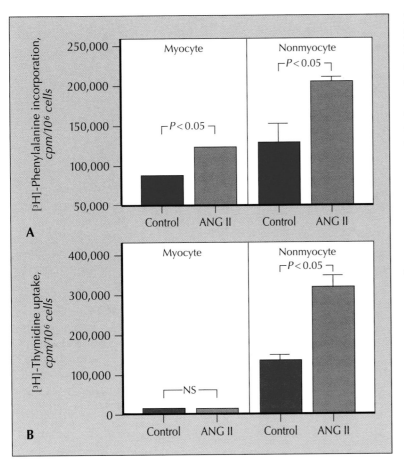

FIGURE 4-9. The levels of both circulating and tissue angiotensin are increased in many conditions associated with myocardial hypertrophy, and this peptide has therefore been implicated as a causative factor in myocardial hypertrophy. To examine whether angiotensin exerts direct effects on protein synthesis in cardiac cells, 10 nmol angiotensin (ANG II) was applied for 24 to 48 hours to either myocytes or nonmyocytes (the latter consisting primarily of fibroblasts) cultured from neonatal rat hearts. **A,** In both cardiac myocytes and nonmyocytes, angiotensin increased [³H]-phenylalanine incorporation, indicating a hypertrophic effect. **B,** Interestingly, angiotensin increased [³H]-thymidine incorporation, an index of DNA synthesis, only in the nonmyocytes. This observation suggests that, in addition to causing myocyte hypertrophy, angiotensin may play a role in the proliferation of fibroblasts and the development of interstitial fibrosis, important components of cardiac remodeling. NS—not significant. (*Adapted from* Sadoshima and Izumo [6]; with permission.)

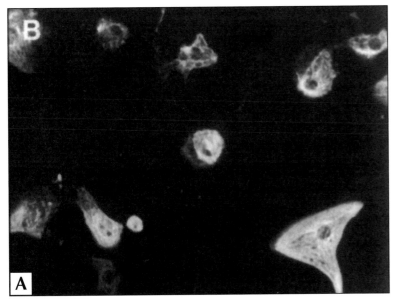

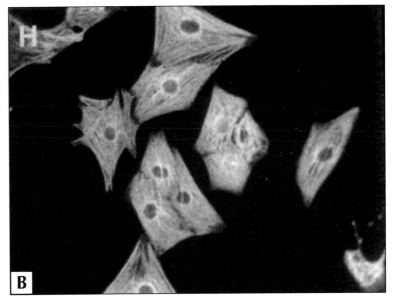

FIGURE 4-10. It has recently been appreciated that endothelin-1, a peptide produced primarily by endothelial cells, can have important effects on cardiac myocyte growth. Neonatal rat cardiac myocytes in culture were exposed to 10-nmol endothelin-1 for 48 hours. **A,** Immunofluorescence staining of myosin light chain–2 in control cells. **B,** Cells exposed to endothelin are increased in size and show increased expression of myosin light chain–2, which is organized into contractile units. Recent observations suggest that endothelin-1, which can be produced by a variety of cells in the myocardium, may play an autocrine or paracrine role in modulating the response to hypertrophic stimuli. (*From* Shubeita and coworkers [7]; with permission.)

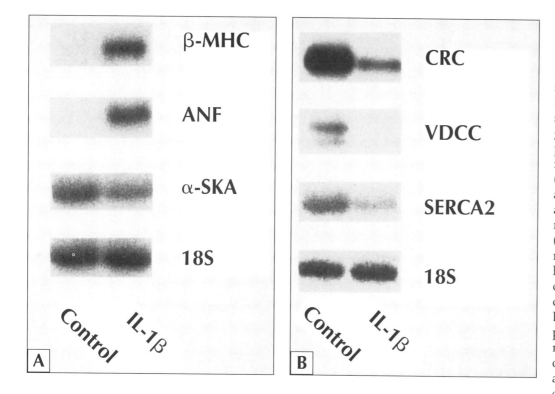

A

β-MHC

ANF

α-SKA

18S

Control   IL-1β

B

CRC

VDCC

SERCA2

18S

Control   IL-1β

FIGURE 4-11. Cytokines alter myocardial phenotype. Circulating or myocardial levels of cytokines including interleukin-1β, tumor necrosis-α and interleukin-6 are increased in some patients with heart failure. **A** and **B**, In isolated ventricular myocytes, Thaik *et al.* [8] showed that interleukin-1β induces cell growth, as evidenced by an increases in protein synthesis, the reexpression of the fetal genes for β-myosin heavy chain (β-MHC) and atrial natriuretic factor (ANF), and the decreased expression of several adult genes, including those for sarcoplasmic reticulum calcium adenosine triphosphatase (ATPase) (*ie, SERCA2*) and the calcium release channel (*ie, CRC*). Other investigators have shown that some inflammatory cytokines such as tumor necrosis factor–α can stimulate apoptosis in cardiac myocytes. Data such as these suggest that the local production of inflammatory cytokines in the myocardium in response to hemodynamic overload or inflammatory conditions can, among other things, regulate the growth and death of cardiomyocytes and may thus play an important role in the process of myocardial remodeling. (*From* Thaik and coworkers [8]; with permission.)

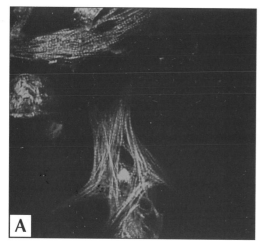

A

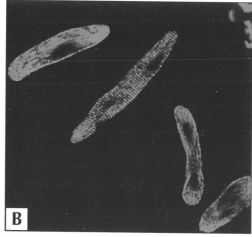

B

FIGURE 4-12. Peptide growth factors for heart failure. Some peptide growth factors may exert a survival effect on the myocardium. For example, neuregulins are a family of peptide growth factors that function in several organ systems, including the heart, to control normal tissue architecture. Mice genetically engineered to lack neuregulins or their receptors have growth arrest and die *in utero* with a poorly developed left ventricle. Neuregulins are expressed on nonmyocytes, including the microvascular endothelium of the heart in adulthood, and induce a growth response in isolated cardiac myocytes. Neuregulins also prevent the programmed cell death of isolated myocytes, suggesting that their stimulation may have survival value. **A,** Myocytes treated with neuregulin. **B,** Control myocytes. (*Courtesy of* R. Rogers and RA Kelly.)

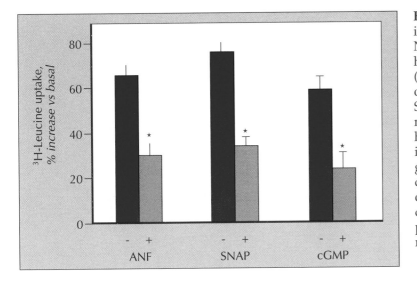

FIGURE 4-13. Counter-regulatory pathways. Myocyte hypertrophy is balanced in the cell by counter-regulatory pathways. Norepinephrine (NE) and adrenergic stimuli cause myocyte hypertrophy, as evidenced by an increased rate of protein synthesis (*see* Fig. 4-8), in this case tritiated leucine incorporation. The addition of atrial natriuretic factor (ANF), or the nitric oxide (NO) donor SNAP (S-nitroso-N-acetyl-D,L-penicillamine), inhibits the norepinephrine (NE)-induced increase in protein synthesis. Myocyte hypertrophy is associated with the reexpression of ANF. Thus, ANF in turn may act on the myocyte in an autocrine manner to limit the growth response. ANF increases intracellular levels of cGMP, and cGMP alone has similar effects. SNAP also increases myocyte levels of cGMP, suggesting that this pathway may play a role in the control of sympathetically stimulated myocyte hypertrophy by the parasympathetic system, which is known to regulate the activity of nitric oxide synthase. (*Adapted from* Calderone and coworkers [9].)

CALCIUM HANDLING

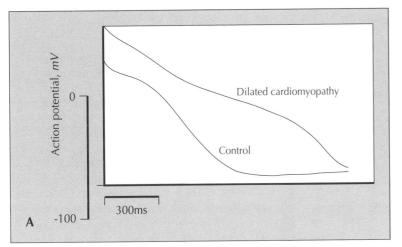

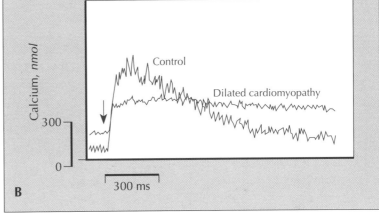

FIGURE 4-14. There is evidence that calcium handling is deranged in the myocardium of patients with end-stage heart failure.

A, The action potentials in single human cardiac myocytes obtained from patients with normal ventricular function (control) or dilated cardio-myopathy. The action potential is substantially prolonged in the cell from the patient with dilated cardiomyopathy.

B, The intracellular calcium transients in single cells, as assessed by the fura-2 technique. In the cell from a patient with dilated cardiomyopathy, the intracellular calcium fails to increase normally after stimulation and remains elevated for a prolonged time. Such abnormalities in calcium transients probably contribute to both systolic and diastolic ventricular dysfunction. (*Adapted from* Beuckelmann and coworkers [10]; with permission.)

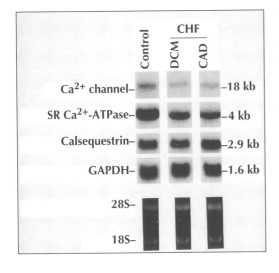

FIGURE 4-15. Abnormal calcium handling in failing myocardium appears to reflect altered expression of one or more important proteins. Shown is a Northern blot demonstrating typical decreases in the mRNA levels for both voltage-dependent Ca^{2+} channels and sarcoplasmic reticulum Ca^{2+}-ATPase (SR Ca^{2+}-ATPase) in myocardium from patients with idiopathic dilated cardiomyopathy (DCM) or ischemic cardiomyopathy (CAD). The mRNA level for calsequestrin, a protein that binds calcium within the sarcoplasmic reticulum, is normal in the myopathic myocardium. The levels of glyceraldehyde-3-phosphate dehydrogenase (GAPDH) and ribosomal RNA (18S and 28S) are shown as internal controls. kb—kilobases. (*Adapted from* Takahashi and coworkers [11]; with permission.)

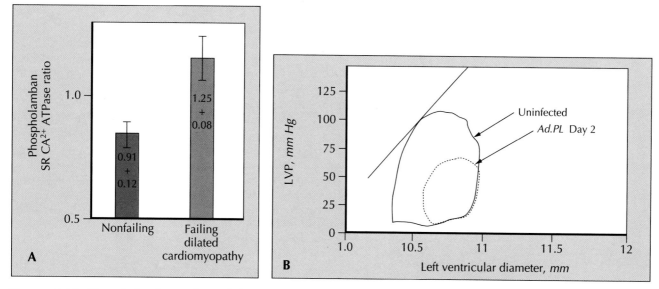

FIGURE 4-16. Pholpholamban in heart failure. Phospholamban regulates the activity of SERCA2 in the cardiac myocyte and thereby alters the cytosolic concentrations of calcium (Ca^{2+}). Whereas both phospholamban and SERCA2 expression are decreased in failing myocardium, phospholamban is not as reduced as SERCA2, so that the ratio of phospholamban to SERCA2 is increased (**A**). When the phospholamban/SERCA2 ratio was increased in rat heart by means of viral-mediated transfer of the phospholamban gene (Ad.PL), there was a downward shift in the left ventricular end-systolic pressure/volume relationship consistent with worsening systolic function (**B**). Thus, abnormal expression of calcium-regulating proteins could contribute to myocardial dysfunction in remodeled hearts. (Part A *adapted from* Hasenfuss and coworkers [12]; part B *adapted from* Hajjar and coworkers [13]; with permission.)

CALCIUM HOMEOSTASIS IN FAILING HUMAN MYOCARDIUM

INTRACELLULAR CALCIUM CONCENTRATION	CALCIUM-HANDLING PROTEINS (mRNA LEVELS)
Basal (diastolic) ↑	Voltage-dependent Ca^{2+} channels ↓
Peak (systolic) ↓	Na$^+$/Ca^{2+} exchanger ↑
Rate of fall ↓	SR Ca^{2+}-ATPase ↓
	Phospholamban ↓
	Phospholamban/SR Ca^{2+} ATPase ↑
	Ca^{2+} release channel ↓
	Calsequestrin ↔

FIGURE 4-17. The observed alterations in calcium handling and the levels of mRNA expression for several key calcium-handling proteins in myocardium from patients with cardiomyopathy. In failing myocardium there is elevation of the basal concentration of intracellular calcium and attenuation of the peak rise with depolarization. These functional abnormalities are associated with alterations in the mRNA levels for proteins involved in myocyte excitation-contraction coupling, suggesting that at least some of the functional abnormalities in failing myocardium are caused by alterations in gene expression. SR—sarcoplasmic reticulum.

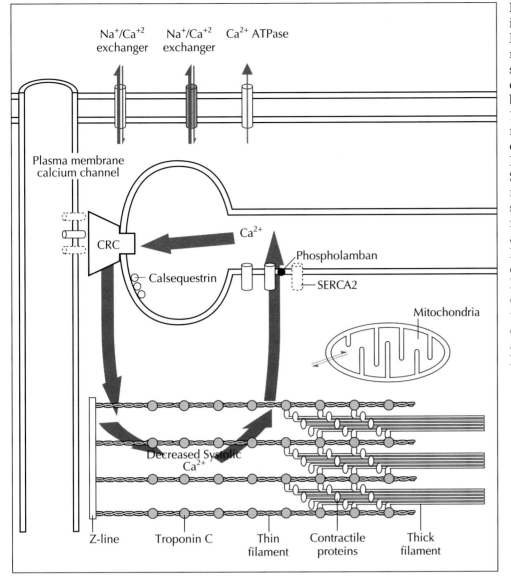

FIGURE 4-18. Myocyte contraction and relaxation in heart failure. As discussed in Chapter 1 (*see* Fig. 1-9), normal myocyte contraction and relaxation are dependent on the interaction of several calcium regulatory proteins. Changes in expression and activity of several of these have been observed in failing myocardium (*see* Fig. 4-17), as illustrated here. Increased expression is represented by *shaded* proteins. Decreased expression is represented by *dotted* proteins. Increases in the ratio of phospholamban to SERCA2 and the sodium/calcium exchanger reduces the amount of calcium in the sarcoplasmic reticulum that is available for release during systole, thereby diminishing the amplitude of the calcium transient, as shown in Figure 4-14. Decreases in the calcium release channel (CRC) and L-type calcium channels likewise diminish the calcium transient. As discussed in the next section, other alterations in the expression and calcium sensitivity of the contractile proteins may also contribute to the abnormal contractile phenotype of the failing heart. (*Adapted from* Katz [14]; with permission.)

CONTRACTILE ISOFORM EXPRESSION

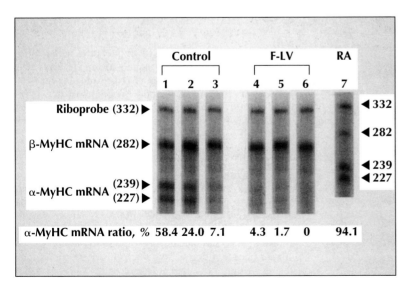

FIGURE 4-19. The myosin heavy chains (MHCs). The MHCs are the molecular motors of muscle that convert the calcium transients into muscle contraction. The α and β isoforms of MHC differ in their relative adenosine triphosphatase (ATPase) activity and velocity of shortening. Whereas α-MHC has relatively more ATPase activity and an increased velocity of shortening, β-MHC shortens more slowly and with greater economy of energy stores. The adult human heart has approximately 90% β-MHC and 10% α-MHC. In myocardium from patients with left ventricular failure (F-LV), Nakao *et al.* [15] have shown that there is decreased expression of α-MHC, which would be expected to result in a reduced velocity of shortening. (*From* Nakao and coworkers [15]; with permission.)

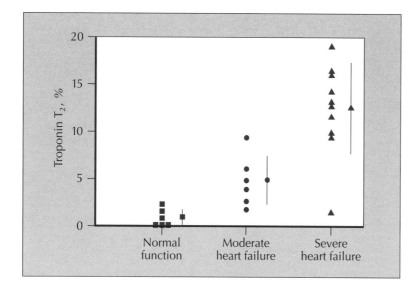

FIGURE 4-20. Altered troponin T in cardiomyopathy. There is evidence that the expression of troponin T, one of the proteins that regulates the interaction of actin and myosin, is altered in the myocardium of patients with cardiomyopathy. In myocardium from patients with normal ventricular function there is a single predominant isoform, referred to as *troponin T₁*. A second isoform, referred to as *troponin T₂*, accounts for only about 2% of the total troponin T. In contrast, in myocardium obtained from patients with moderate or severe heart failure, there is increased expression of the troponin T_2 isoform. Although the functional significance of the shift in troponin T isoforms is not known, this observation is important because it suggests that changes in regulatory elements of the contractile apparatus may contribute to functional abnormalities in the failing myocardium. (*Adapted from* Anderson and coworkers [16]; with permission.)

CELL DEATH

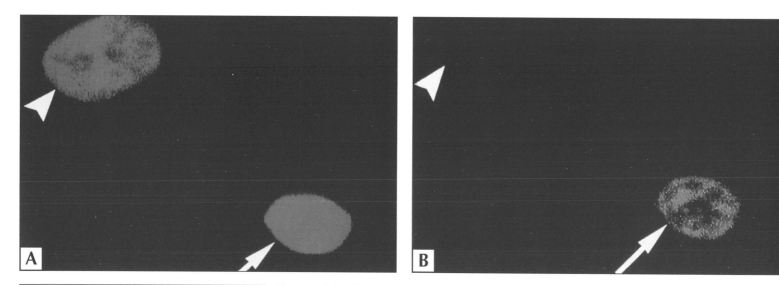

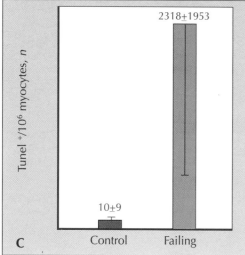

FIGURE 4-21. Loss of myocytes in heart failure. The slow loss of myocytes may contribute to the progressive decline in systolic function in heart failure. All cells have the ability to undergo programmed cell death, or apoptosis, in the presence of stimuli that activate the necessary signaling cascades. Cardiac apoptosis appears to play an important role in embryonic life as the heart "remodels" during development. Thus, apoptosis may be part of a fetal gene program. Apoptosis also occurs as a defense mechanism to rid an organ of infected or damaged cells without activation of inflammatory systems as would occur with necrosis. Olivetti *et al.* [17] demonstrated that apoptosis occurs in myocardium obtained from patients with heart failure by staining for fragmented DNA, a hallmark of the apoptotic process. **A**, Confocal microscopy of myocardial nuclei stained with propridium iodide. **B**, DNA fragments labeled with deoxyuridine triphosphate (Tunel) in apoptotic nucleus (*arrow*) but not normal nucleus (*arrowhead*). **C**, Counting of stained cells shows a large number of apoptotic cells (Tunel⁺) in failing, but not normal, myocardium. (Parts A and B *from* Olivetti and coworkers [17]; with permission. Part C *adapted from* Olivetti and coworkers [17].).

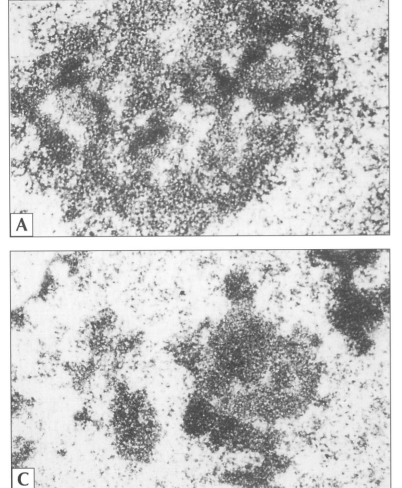

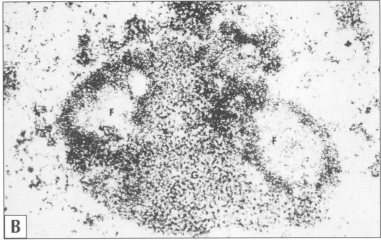

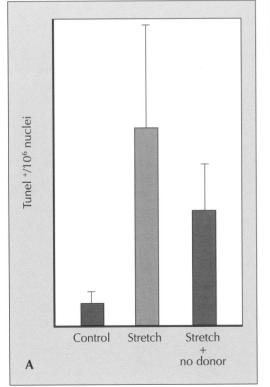

FIGURE 4-22. Electron micrographs of apoptotic cells show condensed chromatin due to the activity of specific endonucleases that cleave DNA between nucleosomes. Unverferth *et al.* [18] demonstrated this finding in the myocardium of patients 24 hours after a single dose of adriamycin, suggesting that myocyte apoptosis may play a role in the cardiotoxicity of anthracylines. **A**, Normal nucleus. **B**, Myocardial nucleus from a patient 4 hours after a single dose of adriamycin, showing some chromatin condensation. **C**, Nucleus from a patient 24 hours after adriamycin dose, showing chromatin condensation typical of apoptosis. (*From* Unverferth and coworkers [18]; with permission.)

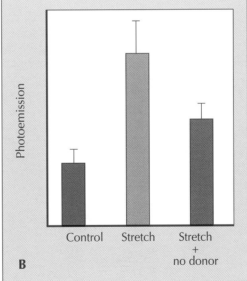

FIGURE 4-23. Increased mechanical stress on cardiac myocytes. This appears to be an important stimulus for myocardial remodeling. To determine whether mechanical stress can cause apoptosis, Cheng *et al.* [19] applied gentle mechanical strain to rat myocardium *in vitro*. The stretched myocardium exhibited an increase in the number of myocytes with DNA fragmentation characteristic of apoptosis (**A**). They further showed that mechanical stretch increased the production of reactive oxygen (*eg*, superoxide anion), and that the addition of a nitric oxide donor that can reduce the availability of superoxide anion reduced the extent of stretch-induced apoptosis (**B**) as detected using the Tunel method. Other studies have suggested that the release of angiotensin from the myocardium in response to mechanical stretch may be a signal for apoptosis and that stretch-mediated apoptosis can be inhibited by the angiotensin receptor antagonist losartan. (*Adapted from* Cheng and coworkers [19]; with permission.)

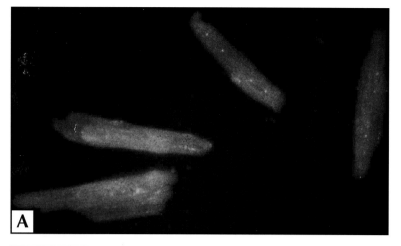

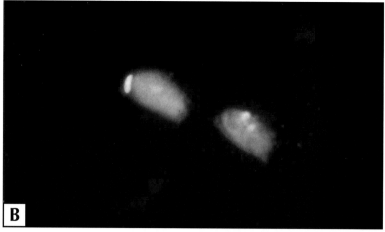

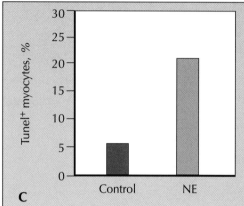

A

B

C

FIGURE 4-24. Other neurohormonal systems, including the sympathetic nervous system, have been implicated in the induction of apoptosis. Communal *et al.* [20] have shown that norepinephrine (NE) can stimulate apoptosis in isolated rat ventricular myocytes as demonstrated here by an increase in the number of cells staining positive for fragmented DNA using the Tunel method. **A,** Control myocytes. **B,** Apoptotic myocytes after 24 hours' treatment with 10 μm NE. **C,** The percent of apoptotic cells increases approximately four-fold. This effect is mediated by β-adrenergic receptors since it is blocked by the β-adrenergic antagonist propranolol but not the α-adrenergic antagonist prazosin. These observations suggest that increased sympathetic tone could contribute to progressive myocyte loss and provide a possible mechanism by which β-adrenergic antagonists might exert beneficial effects in patients with heart failure. (Parts A and B *from* Communal and coworkers [20]; with permission. Part C *adapted from* Communal and coworkers [20].)

EXTRACELLULAR MATRIX

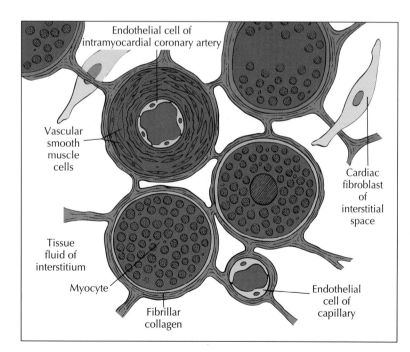

FIGURE 4-25. Although myocytes are the major components of the heart on the basis of mass, they represent only a minority of the cells on the basis of number. Nonmyocyte cellular contituents of the myocardium include fibroblasts, smooth muscle cells, and endothelial cells. Myocytes and nonmyocytes are interconnected by a complex of connective tissue and extracellular matrix. Components of the extracellular matrix include collagens, proteoglycans, glycoproteins (such as fibronectin), several peptide growth factors, and proteases (such as plasminogen activators). There is increasing appreciation that by regulating the nature and quantity of the extracellular matrix, nonmyocytes in the heart play an important role in determining the response of the myocardium to pathologic stimuli, such as hemodynamic overload. (*Adapted from* Weber and Brilla [21]; with permission.)

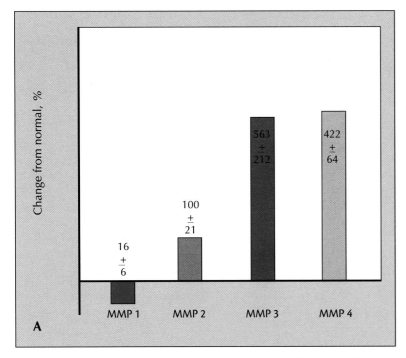

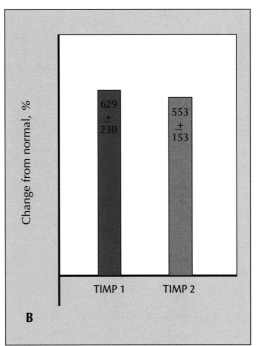

FIGURE 4-26. Metalloproteinases (MMPs) in remodeling of the extracellular matrix. The extracellular matrix that mechanically couples the myocytes must also "remodel" as the ventricle dilates. The extracellular matrix of the heart is constantly being broken down and reformed. This occurs in part through the activity of a group of enzymes called *MMPs* that degrade the extracellular matrix. **A,** The expression of at least two MMPs, MMP 3 and MMP 9, is increased in myocardium obtained from patients with heart failure. **B,** At the same time there appears to be increased expression of counter-regulatory inhibitors of MMPs referred to as *tissue inhibitors of metalloproteinase* (TIMP). Although the structural and functional consequences of these changes in matrix regulatory proteins is not yet known, it is possible that they play a role in myocardial remodeling by facilitating slippage of myocytes and thereby leading to chamber dilation. (*Adapted from* Thomas and coworkers [22].)

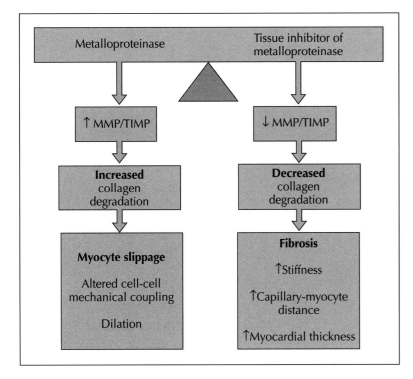

FIGURE 4-27. The balance between metalloproteinase (MMP) and tissue inhibitors of metalloproteinase (TIMP) activity. This balance determines the rate of matrix degradation and turnover. Increased MMP activity theoretically favors myocyte slippage, with reduced myocyte-to-myocyte mechanical coupling and dilation. Increased TIMP activity results in a net decrease in MMP activity and therefore theoretically favors matrix deposition. This perhaps leads to interstitial fibrosis, which may lead to increased stiffness and impaired supply of nutrients to myocytes because of an increased capillary-to-myocyte distance.

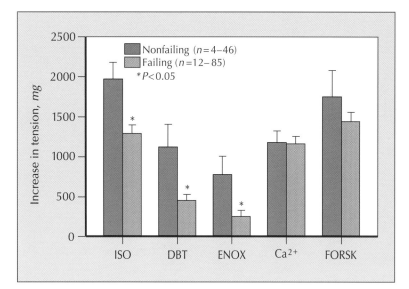

FIGURE 4-28. A characteristic physiologic abnormality in patients with heart failure is a reduction in the inotropic and chronotropic responses to exercise and other types of sympathetic stimulation. The responsiveness of trabeculae from normal hearts and hearts with end-stage failure was examined by determining the development of contractile tension in response to several agonists. By this approach, it was shown that although the contractile response to calcium (Ca^{2+}) is preserved in failing myocardium, the contractile responses to the β-adrenergic agonists isoproterenol (ISO) and dobutamine (DBT) are significantly reduced, as is the response to enoximone (ENOX), a phosphodiesterase inhibitor that is dependent on the availability of cAMP. In contrast, forskolin (FORSK), a substance that directly activates adenylate cyclase, thereby bypassing the β-adrenergic receptor, elicited a normal response in failing myocardium. These observations suggest that in heart failure, reduced adrenergic responsiveness of the myocardium is relatively specific for the β-adrenergic receptor pathway. (*Adapted from* Bristow [23]; with permission.)

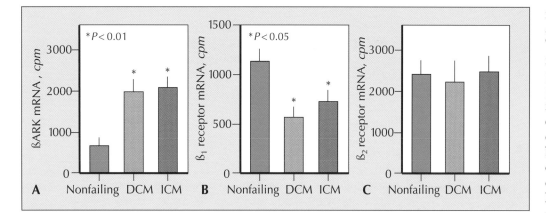

reduced (**B**). The level of mRNA for β_2-adrenergic receptors is unchanged (**C**). These data provide the molecular basis for the observation that the number of β_1-adrenergic receptors, but not of β_2-adrenergic receptors, is reduced in failing myocardium. The increased expression of βARK may explain the observation that the responsiveness to both β_1- and β_2-adrenergic agonists is often depressed out of proportion to the decrease in receptor number. Failing hearts include those with dilated cardiomyopathy (DCM) and ischemic cardiomyopathy (ICM). (*Adapted from* Ungerer and coworkers [24]; with permission.)

FIGURE 4-29. In myocardium from patients with end-stage heart failure, compared with control tissue from patients without failure, the level of β-adrenergic receptor kinase (βARK) mRNA is increased (**A**) and the level of β_1-adrenergic receptor mRNA is

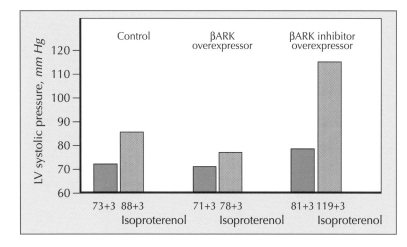

FIGURE 4-30. The functional importance of the increased expression of β-adrenergic receptor kinase (βARK) in failing myocardium. In transgenic mice with overexpression of βARK, there is a decreased ionotropic response to administration of the beta-adrenergic agonist isoproterenol. Conversely, in mice with overexpression of the βARK inhibitor has the opposite effect is seen with augmentation of the inotropic response to isoproterenol. LV—left ventricle. (*Adapted from* Koch and coworkers [25]; with permission.)

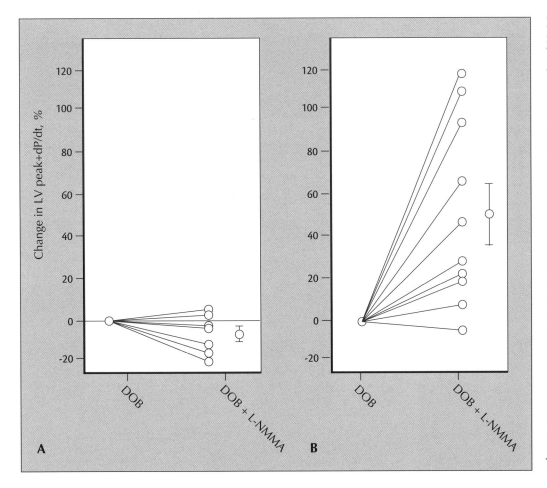

FIGURE 4-31. Evidence for modulation of myocardial β-adrenergic responsiveness beyond the level of the receptor. *In vitro* experiments have shown that nitric oxide (NO) can blunt the inotropic response to β-adrenergic stimulation. NO synthase (NOS) activity is increased in myocardium obtained from patients with heart failure due to the expression of the inducible form of NO synthase (NOS2), perhaps in response to inflammatory cytokines. To examine whether increased NO might have functional consequences *in vivo*, the NOS inhibitor L-N-monomethylarginine (L-NMMA) was infused into the left main coronary artery of patients at the time of catheterization, and the left ventricular (LV) contractile response to dobutamine was measured. In patients with normal LV function (**A**), L-NMMA had no effect on basal or dobutamine-stimulated contractility. However, in patients with LV systolic failure (**B**), L-NMMA infusion increased the inotropic response to dobutamine. This observation suggests that increased NOS activity is of functional importance in the failing heart by contributing to β-adrenergic hyporesponsiveness, a common feature in heart failure. (*Adaped from* Hare and coworkers [26]; with permission.)

RENIN-ANGIOTENSIN SYSTEM, ENDOTHELIN, AND INFLAMMATORY CYTOKINES

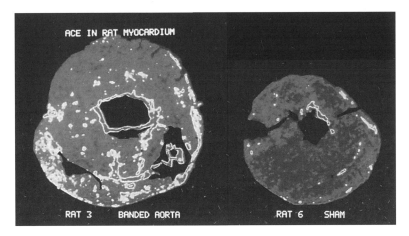

FIGURE 4-32. In rats with left ventricular hypertrophy caused by aortic banding, the expression of angiotensin-converting enzyme (ACE) activity is increased. To demonstrate this, ventricular tissue was sectioned, labeled with an isotopically tagged ACE inhibitor, and exposed to radiographic film. The autoradiographs were digitized and visualized such that the color scale represents the relative ACE density. In rats with hypertrophy (*left*) compared with sham-treated (SHAM) animals (*right*), there is increased ACE expression. These and other similar observations suggest that upregulation of the tissue renin-angiotensin system contributes to the ventricular remodeling that occurs with hemodynamic stress. (*Adapted from* Schunkert and coworkers [27]; with permission.) (*See* Color Plate.)

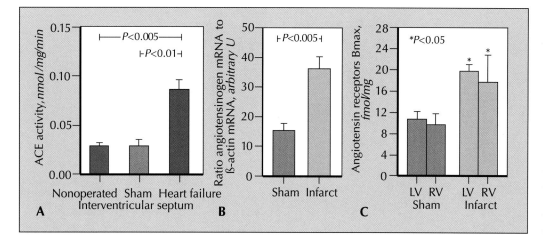

FIGURE 4-33. There is upregulation of several components of the renin-angiotensin system (RAS) in the noninfarcted myocardium of rats after myocardial infarction. There are significant increases in ACE activity (**A**), the level of angiotensinogen mRNA (**B**), and the density of angiotensin-II receptors (**C**). The increase in angiotensin-II receptor density suggests that in addition to increased activity of the tissue RAS, the responsiveness of the tissue to angiotensin may be increased. LV—left ventricle; RV—right ventricle. (Part A *adapted from* Hirsch and coworkers [28]; part B *from* Lindpaintner and coworkers [29]; and part C *from* Meggs and coworkers [30]; with permission.)

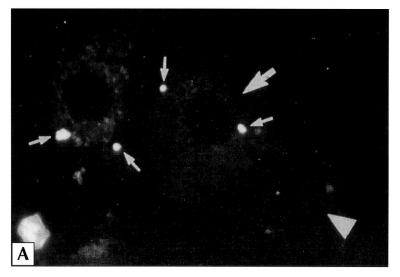

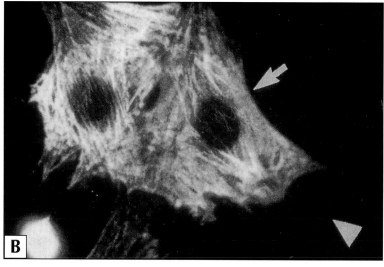

FIGURE 4-34. The cardiac myocyte may be a source of tissue angiotensin II. **A**, Fluorescence staining of a rat ventricular myocyte with an antibody directed against angiotensin II is shown. The focal areas of staining (*small arrows*) within the cell indicate the presence of angiotensin II. **B**, The same cell (note location of *large arrow*) stains avidly with an antisarcomeric myosin antibody, indicating that it is a myocyte. The *arrowhead* indicates a nonmyocyte. Stretching of

cultured neonatal rat cardiac myocytes on a silicone membrane induced the expression of fetal genes and increased protein synthesis, and these effects were blocked by the angiotensin-receptor antagonist losartan. These observations suggest that angiotensin II released from cardiac myocytes plays an autocrine role in regulating the cardiac myocyte growth response to hemodynamic overload. (*Adapted from* Sadoshima and coworkers [31]; with permission.)

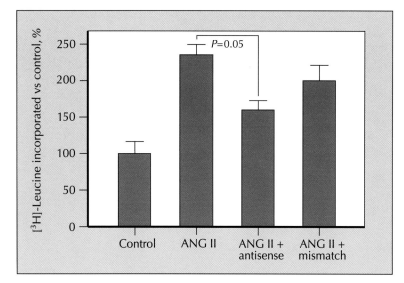

FIGURE 4-35. There is evidence that endothelin-1 (ET-1) may serve as an autocrine or paracrine regulator of the molecular and cellular effects of angiotensin II (ANG II) on cardiac myocyte growth. In cultured neonatal rat cardiac myocytes, ANG II induces the expression of ET-1. By using an antisense oligonucleotide directed against preproendothelin-1 mRNA (ppET-1, the precursor of ET-1), it was shown that cells treated with antisense to ppET-1 to block ET-1 synthesis have a significantly reduced growth response to ANG II, as reflected by leucine incorporation into protein. In other experiments, an antagonist for ET-1 receptors was similarly shown to inhibit the growth effects of ANG II. These observations raise the intriguing possibility that in cardiac myocytes, ET-1 plays a critical autocrine role in the cellular response to ANG II. Data are mean ± SD. (*Adapted from* Ito and coworkers [32]; with permission.)

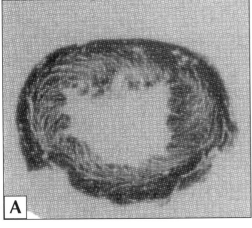

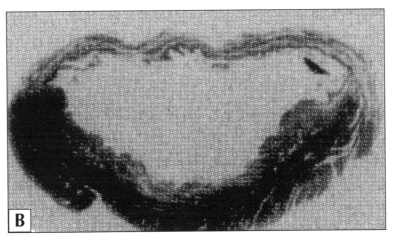

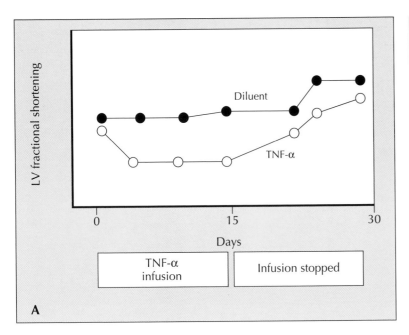

FIGURE 4-36. Role of endothelin in heart failure. Because endothelin can stimulate myocyte growth and regulate extracellular matrix turnover *in vitro* and is increased in the plasma of patients with heart failure, it has been suggested that it might play a pathophysiologic role in myocardial failure. Sakai *et al.* [33] examined this thesis by treating rats with BQ-123, an endothelin receptor antagonist, or placebo after myocardial infarction. Rats treated with BQ-123 had improved left ventricular (LV) function and better survival than placebo-treated animals. Masson trichrome–stained section of LV from Sham-operated rat (**A**), infarcted rat (**B**), and infarcted rat treated with BQ-123 (**C**) showing less LV dilation in the treated animals. These effects are similar to those observed by other investigators with angiotensin-converting enzyme inhibitors. At this time it is unclear whether endothelin and angiotensin exert independent effects on ventricular remodeling or whether they are act in series, as suggested by Figure 4-35. (*From* Sakai and coworkers [33]; with permission.)

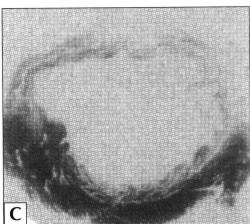

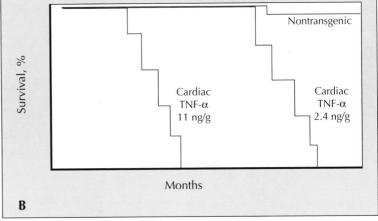

FIGURE 4-37. Tumor necrosis factor (TNF)-α in heart failure. Circulating levels of cytokines including TNF-α are elevated in patients with heart failure. There is now reason to believe that these levels play a role in the pathogenesis of heart failure, although the mechanism by which this occurs remains unclear. Bozkurt *et al.* [34] were able to demonstrate a decrease in left ventricular (LV) fractional shortening as assessed by serial echocardiograms in rats subjected to a continuous infusion with TNF-α (**A**). (*continued*)

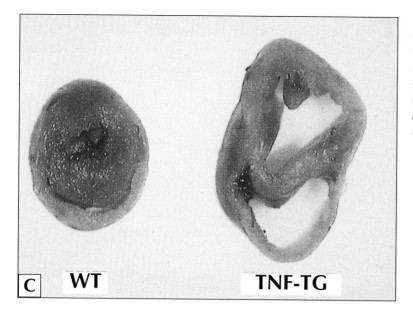

FIGURE 4-37. (*continued*) Interestingly, this decrease in LV function was completely reversed 30 days after the infusion was stopped. When Bryant *et al.* [35] caused overexpression of TNF-α in transgenic mice, there was ventricular dilation and impaired survival of mice that was related to the intensity of TNF-α expression (**B** and **C**). TG—transgenic; WT—wild type. (Part A *adapted from* Bozkurt and coworkers [34]; parts B and C *from* Bryant and coworkers [35]; with permission.*)

Oxidative Stress

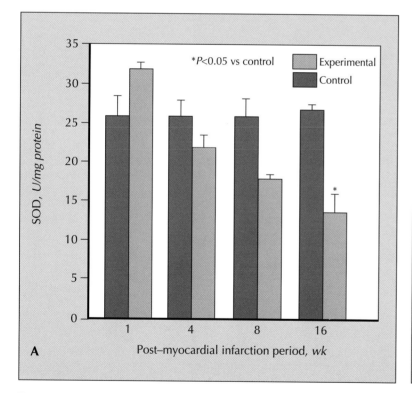

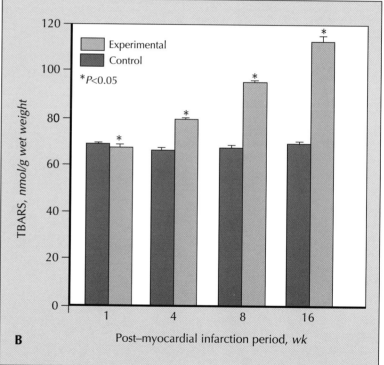

FIGURE 4-38. Role of oxidative stress in progression of myocardial failure. There is evidence that oxidative stress is increased in heart failure and may play a role in progression of the underlying myocardial failure. **A,** In the rat myocardial infarction model, Hill and Singal [36] found that increased oxidative stress in the myocardium was associated with decreased activity of antioxidant enzymes such as superoxide dismutase (SOD). **B,** In the same animals, the myocardial level of thiobarbituric acid reactive substances (TBARS), an index of oxidative stress, was elevated. In guinea pigs with pressure overload–induced myocardial failure, these same investigators were able to prevent the transition from hypertrophy to failure by supplementation of the diet with vitamin E, a lipid-soluble antioxidant. (*Adapted from* Hill and Singal [36]; with permission.)

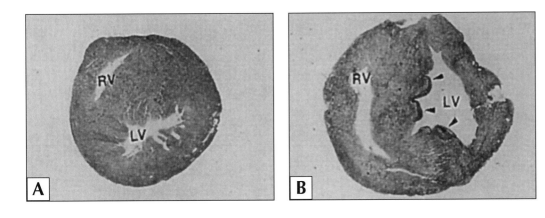

FIGURE 4-39. A and **B,** Transgenic animals offer further evidence for the importance of antioxidant enzymes in the control of cardiac function and remodeling. Removal of a functional copy of the enzyme manganese superoxide dismutase (MnSOD), the main form of superoxide dismutase (SOD) in the mitochondria, results in death of mice at a young age. These mice have anatomic evidence of heart failure, with dilated ventricles and thrombus formation on the ventricular wall (*arrowheads*), consistent with poor systolic function. LV—left ventricle; RV—right ventricle. (*From* Li and coworkers [37]; with permission.)

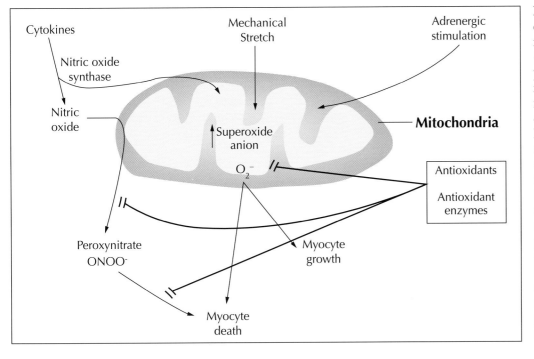

FIGURE 4-40. Oxidative stress as a mediator of the failure phenotype. Oxidative stress resulting from superoxide anion, nitric oxide (NO), and their reaction product, peroxynitrite, may act as important intracellular mediators for remodeling stimuli such as mechanical overload, inflammatory cytokines, and catecholamines. Mitochondria are the major source of superoxide anion in ventricular myocytes, although there are other potentially important oxidase systems in the cytoplasm. Superoxide anions that are unquenched by superoxide dismutase (SOD) or soluble antioxidants result in formation of hydrogen peroxide and hydroxyl radicals. In the presence of nitric oxide, peroxynitrite is also formed. These reactive oxygen species may cause sublethal cell injury that can activate apoptotic pathways, as well as activate growth pathways through oxidative stress–responsive transcription factors.

REFERENCES

1. Swynghedauw B, Moalic JM, Delcayre C: The origins of cardiac hypertrophy. In *Research in Cardiac Hypertrophy and Failure*. Edited by Swynghedauw B. London: INSERM/John Libbey Eurotext; 1990:23–50.

2. Gerdes AM, Kellerman SE, Moore JA, *et al.*: Structural remodeling of cardiac myocytes in patients with ischemic cardiomyopathy. *Circulation* 1992, 86:426–430.

3. Takahashi T, Allen PD, Izumo S: Expression of A-, B-, and C-type natriuretic peptide genes in failing and developing human ventricles. *Circ Res* 1992, 71:9–17.

4. Sadoshima J-I, Jahn L, Takahashi T, *et al.*: Molecular character-izations of the stretch-induced adaptation of cultured cardiac cells: an *in vitro* model of load-induced cardiac hypertrophy. *J Biol Chem* 1992, 267:10551–10560.

5. Simpson P, McGrath A: Norepinephrine-stimulated hypertrophy of cultured rat myocardial cells is an α_1 adrenergic response. *J Clin Invest* 1983, 72:732–738.

6. Sadoshima J-I, Izumo S: Molecular characterization of angiotensin II-induced hypertrophy of cardiac myocytes and hyperplasia of cardiac fibroblasts: critical role of the AT_1 receptor subtype. *Circ Res* 1993, 73:413–423.

7. Shubeita HE, McDonough PM, Harris AN, *et al.*: Endothelin induction of inositol phospholipid hydrolysis, sarcomere assembly, and cardiac gene expression in ventricular myocytes: a paracrine mechanism for myocardial cell hypertrophy. *J Biol Chem* 1990, 265:20555–20562.

8. Thaik CM, Calderone A, Takahashi N, Colucci WS: Interleukin-1β modulates the growth and phenotype of neonatal rat cardiac myocytes. *J Clin Invest* 1995, 96:1093–1099.

9. Calderone A, Thaik CM, Takahashi N, *et al.*: Nitric oxide, atrial natriuretic peptide, and cGMP inhibit the growth-promoting effects of norepinephrine in cardiac myocytes and fibroblasts. *J Clin Invest* 1998, 101:812–818.

10. Beuckelmann DJ, Nabauer M, Erdmann E: Intracellular calcium handling in isolated ventricular myocytes from patients with terminal heart failure. *Circulation* 1992, 85:1046–1055.

11. Takahashi T, Allen PD, Lacro RV, *et al.*: Expression of dihydropy-ridine receptor (Ca^{2+} channel) and calsequestrin genes in the myocardium of patients with end-stage heart failure. *J Clin Invest* 1992, 90:927–935.

12. Hasenfuss G, Meyer M, Schillinger W, *et al.*: Calcium handling proteins in the failing human heart. *Basic Res Cardiol* 1997, 92 (suppl 1):87–93.

13. Hajjar RJ, Schmidt U, Matsui T, *et al.*: Modulation of ventricular function through gene transfer *in vivo*. *Proc Natl Acad Sci USA* 1998, 95:5251–5256.

14. Katz AM: *Physiology of the Heart*, edn 2. New York: Raven Press; 1992.

15. Nakao K, Minobe W, Roden R, *et al.*: Myosin heavy chain gene expression in human heart failure. *J Clin Invest* 1997, 100:2362–2370.

16. Anderson PAW, Malouf NN, Oakeley AE, *et al.*: Troponin T isoform expression in the normal and failing human left ventricle: a correlation with myofibrillar ATPase activity. *Basic Res Cardiol* 1992, 87:175–185.

17. Olivetti G, Abbi R, Quaini F, *et al.*: Apoptosis in the failing human heart. *N Engl J Med* 1997, 336:1131–1141.

18. Unverferth DV, Magorien RD, Unverferth BP, *et al.*: Human myocardial morphologic and functional changes in the first 24 hours after doxorubicin administration. *Cancer Treat Reports* 1981, 65:1093–1097.

19. Cheng W, Li B, Kajistura J, *et al.*: Stretch-induced programmed myocyte cell death. *J Clin Invest* 1995, 96:2247–2259.

20. Communal C, Singh K, Pimentel DR, Colucci WS: Norepinephrine stimulates apoptosis in adult rat ventricular myocytes by activation of the β-adrenergic pathway. *Circ Res* 1998, in press.

21. Weber KT, Brilla CG: Pathological hypertrophy and cardiac interstitium: fibrosis and renin-angiotensin-aldosterone system. *Circulation* 1991, 83:1849–1865.

22. Thomas CV, Coker ML, Zellner JL, *et al.*: Increased matrix metallo-proteinase activity and selective upregulation in LV myocardium from patients with end-stage dilated cardiomyopathy. *Circulation* 1998, 97:1708–1715.

23. Bristow MR: Changes in myocardial and vascular receptors in heart failure. *J Am Coll Cardiol* 1993, 22:61A–71A.

24. Ungerer M, Bohm M, Elce JS, *et al.*: Altered expression of β-adrenergic receptor kinase and β_1-adrenergic receptors in the failing human heart. *Circulation* 1993, 87:454–463.

25. Koch WJ, Rockman HA, Samama P, *et al.*: Cardiac function in mice overexpressing the beta-adrenergic receptor kinase or a βARK inhibitor. *Science* 1995, 268:1350–1353.

26. Hare JM, Givertz MM, Creager MA, Colucci WS: Increased sensitivity to nitric oxide synthase inhibition in patients with heart failure: potentiation of β-adrenergic inotropic responsiveness. *Circulation* 1998, 97:161–166.

27. Schunkert H, Jackson B, Tang SS, *et al.*: Distribution and functional significance of cardiac angiotensin converting enzyme in hyper-trophied rat hearts. *Circulation* 1993, 87:1328–1339.

28. Hirsch AT, Talsness CE, Schunkert H, *et al.*: Tissue-specific activation of cardiac angiotensin converting enzyme in experimental heart failure. *Circ Res* 1991, 69:475–482.

29. Lindpaintner K, Lu W, Niedermajer N, *et al.*: Selective activation of cardiac angiotensinogen gene expression in post-infarction ventricular remodeling in the rat. *J Mol Cell Cardiol* 1993, 25:133–143.

30. Meggs LG, Coupet J, Huang H, *et al.*: Regulation of angiotensin II receptors on ventricular myocytes after myocardial infarction in rats. *Circ Res* 1993, 72:1149–1162.

31. Sadoshima J-I, Xu Y, Slayter HS, Izumo S: Autocrine release of angiotensin II mediates stretch-induced hypertrophy of cardiac myocytes in vitro. *Cell* 1993, 75:977–984.

32. Ito H, Hirata Y, Adachi S, *et al.*: Endothelin-1 is an autocrine/paracrine factor in the mechanism of angiotensin II-induced hypertrophy in cultured rat cardiomyocytes. *J Clin Invest* 1993, 92:398–403.

33. Sakai S, Miyauchi T, Kobayashi M, *et al.*: Inhibition of myocardial endothelin pathway improves long-term survival in heart failure. *Nature* 1996, 384:353–355.

34. Bozkurt B, Kribbs SB, Clubb FJ, *et al.*: Pathophysiologically relevant concentrations of tumor necrosis factor-α promote progressive left ventricular dysfunction and remodeling in rats. *Circulation* 1998, 97:1382–1391.

35. Bryant D, Becker L, Richardson J, *et al.*: Cardiac failure in transgenic mice with myocardial expression of tumor necrosis factor-α. *Circulation* 1998, 97:1375–1381.

36. Hill MF, Singal PK: Antioxidant and oxidative stress changes during heart failure subsequent to myocardial infarction in rats. *Am J Pathol* 1996, 148:291–300.

37. Li Y, Huang T-T, Carlson EJ, *et al.*: Dilated cardiomyopathy and neonatal lethality in mutant mice lacking manganese superoxide dismutase. *Nat Genet* 1995, 11:376–381.

CARDIAC REMODELING AND ITS PREVENTION

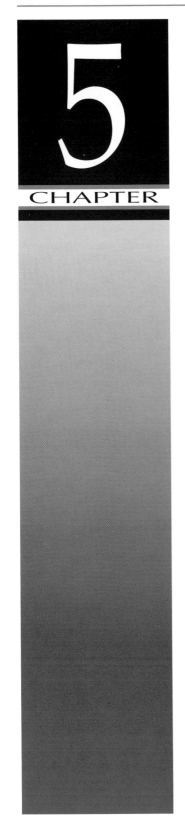

5

CHAPTER

Marc A. Pfeffer

Cardiac chambers have the capacity to alter (remodel) their size and configuration in response to a chronic change in their hemodynamic load. Whether across or within species, the mass and volume of the ventricular chambers maintain a close relationship with the required external work. The changes in chamber volume and mass that accompany normal growth provide the most striking example of the heart's intrinsic capacity to remodel in response to the insidious alterations in demand that take place as a consequence of body growth. Under pathologic conditions of chronic pressure or volume overload, the chamber remodels in direct relation to the imposed hemodynamic burden. The mass increase is attributable to fiber hypertrophy. However, the manner of rearrangement of these additional contractile tissues can lead to either an eccentric (chamber volume > mass) or a concentric (chamber mass > volume) pattern of ventricular growth. Although remodeling in response to a pathologic condition can in one sense be considered adaptive because it permits the restoration of pump function in the face of an imposed hyperfunctional condition, the extent of ventricular remodeling is nevertheless an important marker for a less than optimal prognosis.

A specific type of chamber remodeling can occur as the result of myocardial infarction (MI). In this situation the left ventricle (LV) can undergo an immediate contour change as a result of thinning and elongation of the region affected by myocardial necrosis. This topographic alteration in the infarcted region, termed *infarct expansion*, is a consequence of slippage between muscle fiber bundles, resulting in a reduction across the ventricular wall of the number of myocytes in the noncontractile region. This regional stretching and thinning can continue until connective tissue elements within the infarcted region provide sufficient resistance to oppose further deformation. Both the initial loss of contractile tissues and this subsequent distortion combine to augment the effect of workload and wall stress on the remaining viable myocardium. These events, which occur relatively early during acute MI, provide the substrate for the more insidious global process of subsequent progressive ventricular enlargement.

As with other forms of systolic dysfunction, the greater the degree of ventricular enlargement, the more guarded the prognosis. This is particularly true for survivors of MI in whom a small quantitative augmentation of ventricular volume is associated with a great increase in the relative risk for death. Current methods of noninvasive imaging enable serial assessments of ventricular size and shape to be obtained and have thus delineated the progressive nature of the remodeling that occurs in the impaired LV. Remodeling after MI is a multifactorial process that can be influenced by infarct size and transmurality, the degree of histologic healing in the infarcted region, and ventricular wall stress. Prompt restoration of myocardial flow by thrombolytic therapy or primary coronary angioplasty reduces infarct size and transmurality and diminishes the risk for postinfarction ventricular remodeling. Therapy with anti-inflammatory agents during the early phase of MI can prolong the phase during which the ventricle is vulnerable to infarct expansion. Therefore, avoidance of these agents may reduce the extent of local distortion. Infarct expansion and

the more insidious process of global ventricular enlargement have been successfully attenuated by chronic therapy with angiotensin-converting enzyme (ACE) inhibitors. These factors that influence ventricular remodeling after MI have practical value because they can be modified, and favorable alterations in ventricular size and shape have been shown to result in improved clinical outcome. Indeed, limiting the extent of ventricular remodeling in asymptomatic patients after MI can be considered as preventive therapy for symptomatic congestive heart failure.

CARDIAC GROWTH AND REMODELING

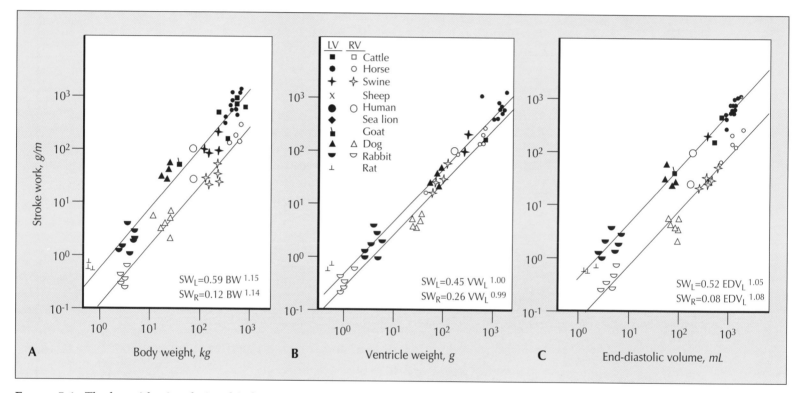

FIGURE 5-1. The logarithmic relationship between ventricular stroke work (SW) and body weight (BW; *panel A*), stroke work and ventricular weight (VW; *panel B*), and stroke work and end-diastolic volume (EDV; *panel C*) [1]. These relationships between external work, ventricular chamber weight, and volume were developed across 10 mammalian species ranging in size from rats to cattle and provide an excellent example of the close association between workload and structure. LV—left ventricle; RV—right ventricle. (*Adapted from* Holt and coworkers [1]; with permission.)

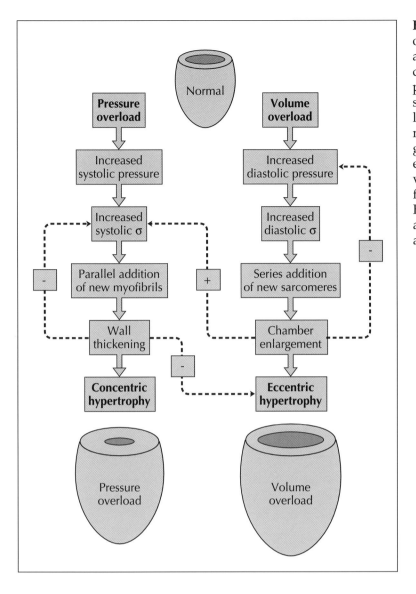

FIGURE 5-2. Patterns of ventricular hypertrophy. Specific patterns of ventricular remodeling occur in response to the imposed augmentation in workload. A pattern of hypertrophic growth characterized as concentric, in which increased mass is out of proportion to chamber volume, is particularly effective in reducing systolic wall stress (σ) under conditions of heightened pressure load. In contrast, in volume overload conditions, in which the major stimulus is diastolic loading, a predominant finding is a great increase in the cavity size or volume. Although there can be extensive increases in mass, the relationship between mass and volume is either preserved or, in severe cases, reduced. The fundamental response is generated by cellular hypertrophy. However, the configuration of the new contractile tissue is specific and offsets the major mechanical stimulus. (*Adapted from* Grossman and coworkers [2]; with permission.)

VENTRICULAR REMODELING: ALTERATION IN CONTOUR OR VOLUME OF VENTRICULAR CAVITY THAT IS NOT ATTRIBUTED TO ACUTE CHANGES IN DISTENDING PRESSURE

Remodeling with preservation of mass/volume ratio
Remodeling with alteration in mass/volume ratio
  Alteration in mass/volume relationship
   ↑ Concentric hypertrophy
  Mass/volume
   ← ↓ Eccentric hypertrophy
   ↓ Failure

FIGURE 5-3. Definition of ventricular remodeling. In a definition of ventricular remodeling, it is important to note that these alterations in size and volume or shape are not related to acute changes in distension [3]. Although alterations in filling pressure change chamber volume, these acute changes do not reflect a true structural modification. Systolic dysfunction impairs ventricular emptying and initially leads to a predominant condition of volume overload. With chamber enlargement, systolic load is also increased. With left ventricular dysfunction and enlargement, the chamber volume may increase out of proportion to mass. This sets up a pathophysiologic condition in which, at any comparable intraventricular pressure, the wall stress is increased compared with that of a ventricle with a preserved mass-to-volume ratio. Although ventricular mass is increased in all three situations, the relationship between the augmented mass and volume differs.

EARLY REMODELING AFTER MYOCARDIAL INFARCTION AND INFARCT EXPANSION

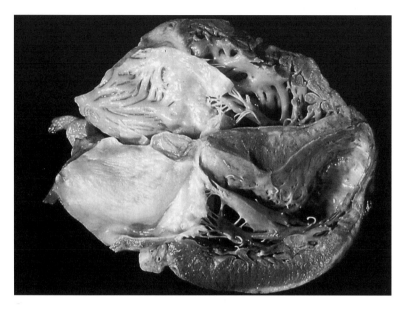

FIGURE 5-4. Pathologic specimen of a human heart that experienced a prior infarction leading to marked apical infarct expansion. Thinning and elongation of the involved apical region have resulted in distortion and enlargement of the ventricular cavity. The scarred apex not only would be unable to contract but would lead to a distortion of the ventricular cavity, resulting in hypertrophy of the remaining viable myocardium. (*Courtesy of* Frederick Schoen, MD, PhD, Boston, MA.)

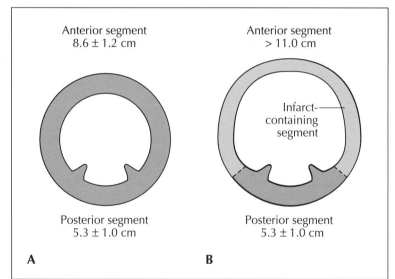

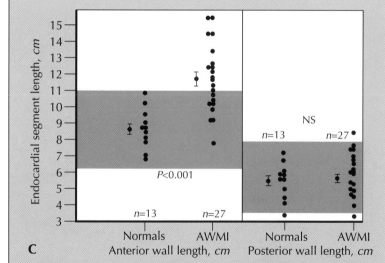

FIGURE 5-5. *In vivo* echocardiographic diagnosis of remodeling. The echocardiographic diagnosis of remodeling was made from the short-axis plane at the level of the papillary muscle. Using the internal landmarks provided by the papillary muscle, the ventricle was divided into two segments, anterior and posterior. **A,** Whereas the normal anterior segment length is 8.6±1.2 cm, the posterior segment is 5.3±1 cm. **B,** In patients with first myocardial infarcts, the segment with the noncontractile region is the obvious infarct-containing segment. Patients who experience infarct expansion develop elongation of this segment within the first week of the infarction. **C,** Actual data points from 27 patients with acute anterior wall myocardial infarction (AWMI) demonstrate that almost 60% of patients with an anterior infarct developed an elongation of the anterior segment that was greater than 2 SD from normal. In these patients, the posterior wall length was not increased 3 days after the infarction. Conversely, in patients with posterior infarcts, one can anticipate that the anterior segment would be normal and that a proportion would have elongation of the posterior segment. *Shaded areas* indicate normal ranges ± SD. (*Adapted from* Erlebacher and coworkers [4]; with permission.)

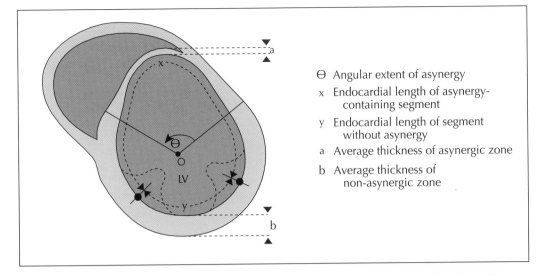

- Θ Angular extent of asynergy
- x Endocardial length of asynergy-containing segment
- y Endocardial length of segment without asynergy
- a Average thickness of asynergic zone
- b Average thickness of non-asynergic zone

FIGURE 5-6. A more extensive method of quantitating infarct expansion developed by Jugdutt and Michorowski [5]. The length of the infarct-containing segment is, of course, determined. However, in this method, which also utilizes two-dimensional short-axis echocardiography, at the mid-papillary muscle level the thickness of the infarcted segment is related to the wall thickness of the noninfarcted region to provide a thinning ratio, the other major component of infarct expansion. Expansion index is calculated by dividing the length of the asynergy-containing segment by the length of the segment without asynergy (x/y). Thinning ratio is determined by dividing average thickness of the asynergic zone by average thickness of the non-asynergic zone (a/b). LV—left ventricle. (*Adapted from* Jugdutt and Michorowski [5]; with permission.)

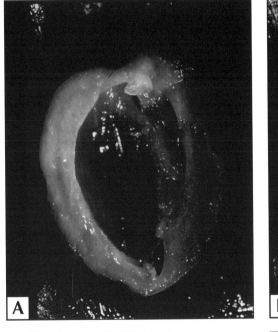

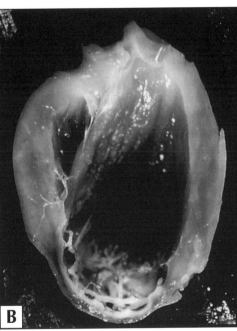

FIGURE 5-7. Predilection of the left ventricular apex for expansion. The left ventricular apex is particularly vulnerable to infarct expansion and initiation of global enlargement. **A,** A normal apex has the greatest radius (r) of curvature and therefore, by the Law of Laplace, has the lowest wall tension (T). **B,** When this region undergoes expansion and thinning, the elongation produces a marked distortion and greatly increases the radius of curvature. Because this area usually has the least wall thickness (h), it is the most vulnerable to any increase in the radius. P—pressure.

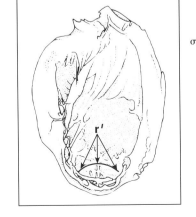

Law of Laplace

$$T = \frac{P \times r}{2}$$

Wall stress (σ)

$$\sigma = \frac{T}{h} = \frac{P \times r}{2h}$$

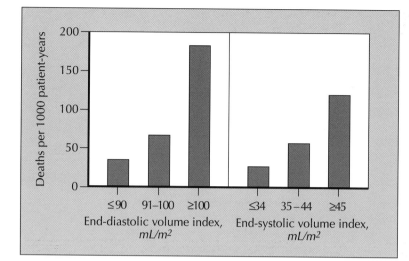

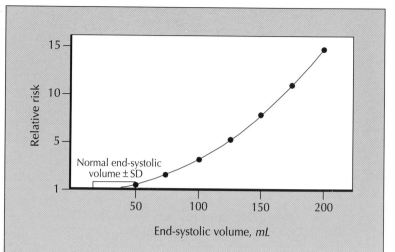

FIGURE 5-8. Mortality rate as related to left ventricular size. In an extensive database that included clinical demographics, catheterization data, and exercise capacity of 733 patients with coronary artery disease, the most powerful predictor of long-term outcome was left ventricular size as measured by volume biplane left ventriculography. The relationship between deaths per thousand patient- years and left ventricular size in either end-diastole or end-systole illustrates the major increase in risk for death that occurs with relatively small changes in left ventricular volume. (*Adapted from* Hammermeister and coworkers [6]; with permission.)

FIGURE 5-9. Relative risk for death in survivors of myocardial infarction. End-systolic volume has been found to be a most important prognostic factor for determinations of long-term survival after myocardial infarction. For each 25-mL increment in end-systolic volume, the risk for death increased exponentially over that of other survivors of myocardial infarction with preserved left ventricular volume. (*Adapted from* White and coworkers [7].)

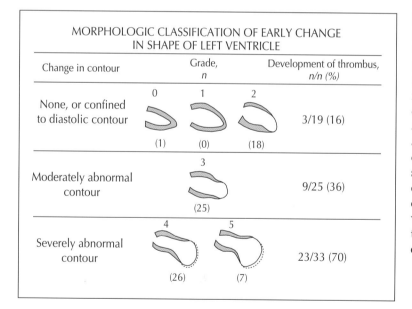

FIGURE 5-10. Morphologic classification of early change in shape of left ventricle (LV). A myocardial infarction (MI) can alter left ventricular LV shape as well as volume. Although much more difficult to quantitate, this scheme has been developed to characterize the distortion that occurs after an MI. LV shape is an important determinant of outcome. Meizlish *et al.* [8] developed a classification for LV shape changes based on radionuclide angiograms and found that greater degrees of distortion were associated with a higher likelihood of death even when adjustment was made for comparable LV ejection fractions. In the above grading system, shape abnormalities of grades 1 and 2 are confined to the diastolic contour. Grades 3 through 5 involve overt alterations in the LV contour that are present in diastole as well as systole. In patients with a first anterior MI, the greater the shape distortion, the higher the likelihood of ventricular thrombus. (*Adapted from* Meizlish and coworkers [8] and Lamas and coworkers [9]; with permission.)

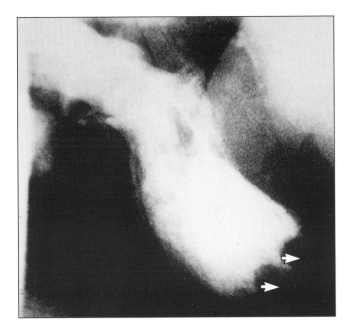

FIGURE 5-11. Contrast left ventriculogram of a patient with a first anterior infarct. This frame in end-systole shows enlargement and distortion of the cavity, with apical expansion. Intraluminal thrombi (*arrows*) are detected as filling defects. (*From* Lamas and coworkers [9]; with permission.)

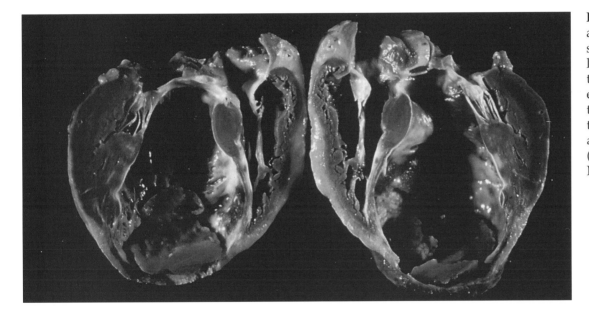

FIGURE 5-12. A heart removed from a cardiac transplant recipient. This specimen, from a survivor of one large anterior septal apical infarction, demonstrates the thinning and elongation of the infarcted region, the cavity enlargement, and hypertrophy of the remaining segment, as well as a large apical thrombus. (*Courtesy of* Lynda Biedrzycki, MD, Boston, MA.)

PROGRESSIVE ENLARGEMENT AFTER MYOCARDIAL INFARCTION

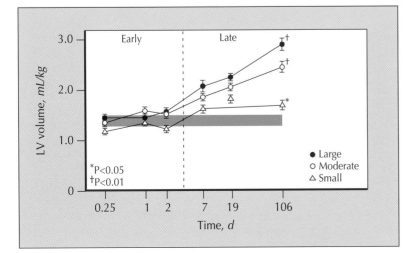

FIGURE 5-13. Progressive ventricular remodeling in a rat model of myocardial infarction. Left ventricular (LV) volumes in rats with various degrees of histologic damage were studied in the acute to chronic period after coronary ligation. The *shaded area* represents mean values ± 2 SEM from normal (not infarcted) animals. Volumes were obtained from the pressure/volume relationship and are compared at the common distending pressure of 20 mm Hg. Therefore, under these conditions, a change in volume is caused by true remodeling rather than altered distention. The extent of this remodeling is a function of both the duration and the degree of histologic damage. Although infarct expansion has been noted as an early process, when filling pressure is taken into account it becomes apparent that the bulk of the global enlargement occurs in the weeks to months after an infarction, when fibrous connective tissue has been established in the infarcted region. (*Adapted from* Pfeffer and coworkers [10]; with permission.)

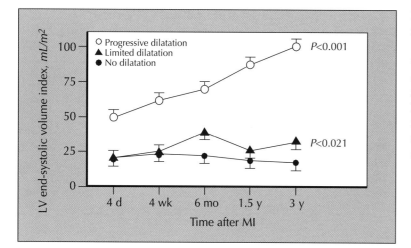

FIGURE 5-14. Progressive ventricular enlargement after myocardial infarction (MI) in humans. In a sequential study of left ventricular (LV) volumes of 99 patients from 4 days to 3 years after acute MI, Gaudron *et al.* [11] demonstrated that progressive enlargement continued in about 25%. Those who experienced progressive and marked changes in ventricular size were more likely to have had large anterior infarctions with limited collateral flow. Recurrent infarction was excluded in this patient population as a potential explanation for this late enlargement. (*Adapted from* Gaudron and coworkers [11]; with permission.)

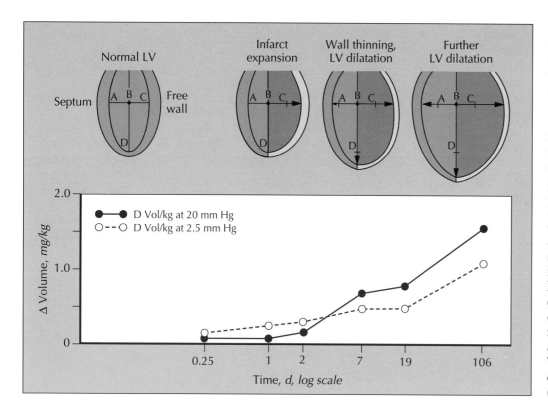

FIGURE 5-15. Time course and components of remodeling after experimental infarction. Changes in volume per kilogram of body weight at common distending pressures indicate a true structural change. *Numerical values* represent actual experimental data. *Upper diagrams*, although not drawn to scale, illustrate the various components of remodeling after infarction. Lengths BA and BC represent the minor radius at the midpoint of the left ventricle (LV), and length BD represents the major radius. In the initial period there is thinning and elongation of the infarcted region, and axis B to C increases. The change in the shape of the perimeter leads to a net increase in ventricular volume. During the early healing period there is further thinning and elongation. However, there is an additional component of chamber enlargement that now involves the viable myocardium, as axes B to A and B to D are also increased. This more global process of enlargement continues long after histologic resolution. (*Adapted from* Pfeffer [12]; with permission.)

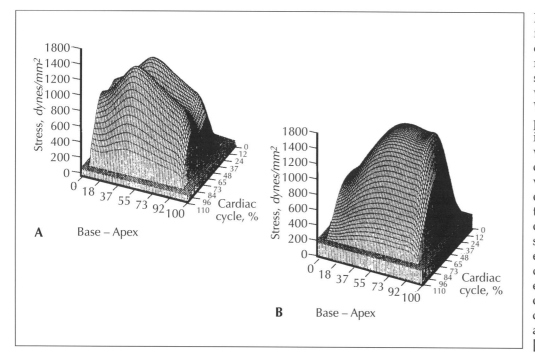

FIGURE 5-16. Regional midwall circumferential wall stress from base to apex calculated during the cardiac cycle in a rat model of myocardial infarction (MI), showing the regionality and complexity of wall stress over the entire cardiac cycle. **A,** Wall stress declines during the early ejection phase in a normal ventricle, despite the increased pressure caused by both systolic wall thickening and a marked decrease in chamber radius. **B,** The infarcted (dilated) ventricle starts from a greater diastolic radius or volume and wall stress. During ejection, there is a much lesser reduction in the radius of the enlarged ventricle (even for the same stroke volume) so that wall stress is actually exacerbated rather than relieved with the development of systolic pressure during early ejection. Also shown is the regionality of abnormal wall stress, consistent with the clinical observation that the base is least affected. (*Adapted from* Capasso and coworkers [13]; with permission.)

MODIFICATION OF REMODELING AFTER MYOCARDIAL INFARCTION

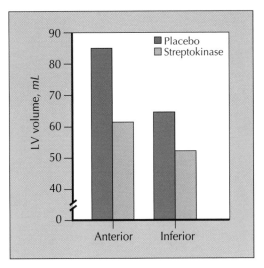

MODIFIABLE FACTORS FOR INTERVENTIONS TO LIMIT ENLARGEMENT AFTER MYOCARDIAL INFARCTION

INTERDEPENDENT FACTORS	INTERVENTIONS
Infarct	Restoration of infarct vessel patency
Size	Thrombolytic therapy + aspirin
Transmurality	Mechanical PTCA
Location	Avoid NSAIDs, steroids
Scar formation	Nitroglycerin
Ventricular wall stress	ACE inhibition

FIGURE 5-17. Modifiable factors for limitation of postinfarction ventricular remodeling. The extent of the infarction, in terms of both the amount of wall motion abnormality and the degree of transmurality, plays a major role in determining the risk for progressive ventricular enlargement. Primary prevention measures should be considered as the major key to reducing the initial risk for myocardial infarction (MI) and subsequent distortion of the left ventricle. During an acute MI, prompt attention to the supply-and-demand balance, with restoration of coronary artery flow, preserves myocardium and reduces infarct size and transmurality. Infarct vessel patency is an independent factor that reduces the risk for late enlargement. Interference with the connective fibers that buttress the infarct region can prolong the vulnerable period for infarct expansion and worsen this condition. Nonsteroidal anti-inflammatory drugs (NSAIDs) and steroids should be avoided. Aspirin does not appear to have this same detrimental effect on infarct expansion. Heightened ventricular wall stress should be viewed as a long-term inciting stimulus for progressive remodeling in both the infarcted and the noninfarcted regions. Although several studies have demonstrated beneficial effects of nitroglycerin on infarct expansion, there is consistent information that angiotensin-converting enzyme (ACE) inhibition therapy favorably alters this process and is associated with improved clinical outcome. PTCA—percutaneous transluminal coronary angioplasty.

FIGURE 5-18. Effects of thrombolytic therapy (streptokinase) on left ventricular (LV) volumes in survivors of acute myocardial infarction (MI). Thrombolytic therapy is associated with less LV enlargement, as assessed in this randomized, double-blind trial that used biplanar left ventriculography 3 weeks after the MI. This study also illustrates that patients with anterior MI are at greater risk for enlargement than patients with inferior infarctions. However, in both instances, the use of thrombolytic therapy led to a reduction in ventricular enlargement. (*Adapted from* White and coworkers [14].)

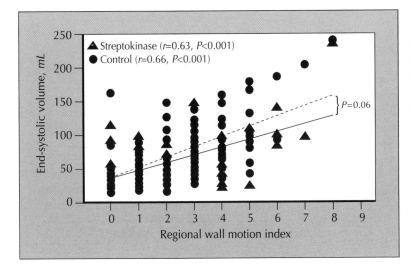

FIGURE 5-19. Echocardiographic substudy from the GISSI (Gruppo Italiano per lo Studio della Streptochinasi nell'Infarto Miocardico) trial. This study demonstrated that left ventricular enlargement 6 months after myocardial infarction is a function of the extent of the wall motion abnormality and that thrombolytic therapy resulted in a strong trend toward smaller ventricular volumes for every degree of abnormality. (*Adapted from* Marino and coworkers [15].)

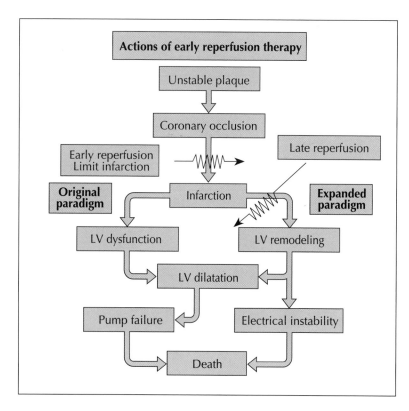

FIGURE 5-20. Expansion of the paradigm of the beneficial actions of early reperfusion therapy. The original paradigm appears on the *left* and the expanded paradigm is on the *right*. Restoration of coronary flow during the early (salvage) phase of acute myocardial infarction (MI) is administered to reduce MI size and transmurality. This preservation of myocardium was anticipated to reduce the wall motion abnormality, improve the ejection fraction, and ultimately lead to a reduction in mortality. Although these observations are accurate, the reduction in death appears to be out of proportion to the improvement in ejection fraction observed in the large placebo-controlled trials [16]. However, recent observations of the influence of infarct vessel patency on left ventricular (LV) remodeling and electrical stability led to an expansion of the original paradigm. The favorable effects of reperfusion therapy in reducing LV dilatation have a prominent role in the more current hypothesis explaining the beneficial actions of reperfusion therapy. (*Adapted from* Kim and Braunwald [17]; with permission.)

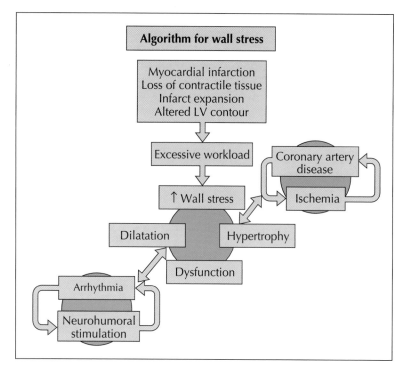

FIGURE 5-21. Algorithm for wall stress. This algorithm for wall stress underscores the central importance of excessive workload and wall stress in the progressive structural alterations in a positive-feedback cycle whereby the structural alterations of left ventricular (LV) dilatation lead to further augmentations in wall stress, reinforcing the progression of the cycle. This scheme is central to understanding the progressive nature of dysfunction, with and without symptoms. This construct provided the rationale for the use of an angiotensin-converting enzyme inhibitor in asymptomatic patients with LV dilatation to prevent further structural changes and reduce the risk for development of congestive heart failure.

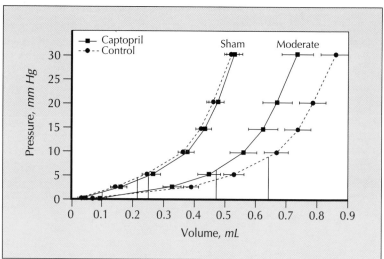

FIGURE 5-22. Pressure-volume relationship in rats with moderate-sized infarctions, demonstrating the effects of captopril therapy. Rats with chronic infarctions have a passive pressure-volume relationship, which is shifted to the right of normal. Such a shift defines a larger ventricle at any common filling pressure (*ie,* postinfarction remodeling). Chronic therapy with captopril, an angiotensin-converting enzyme (ACE) inhibitor, resulted in less enlargement, even when compared for the same amount of histologic damage. The captopril-treated animals also had a lower filling pressure than untreated controls, and therefore the operating volume (*circles*) was reduced with ACE inhibition therapy because of the structural change (*ie,*attenuation of remodeling) and the reduced distending pressure. *Sham* rats were operated and noninfarcted; *moderate* rats had histologic infarct sizes ranging from greater than 20% to less than 40% surface area. (*Adapted from* Pfeffer and coworkers [18]; with permission.)

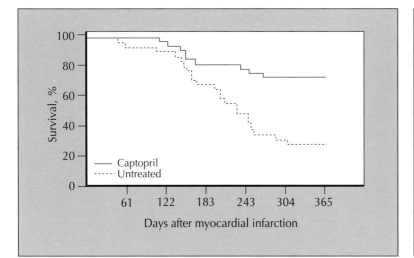

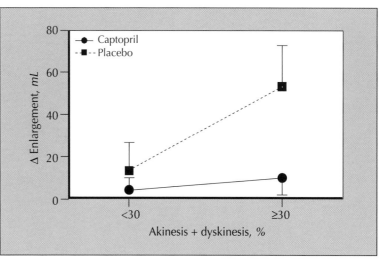

FIGURE 5-23. Influence of angiotensin-converting enzyme (ACE) inhibition therapy (captopril) on survival in the rat myocardial infarction model. Long-term improvement in survival with ACE inhibition was seen in rats with moderate (<40%, >20% surface area) infarctions. In infarcts within this size range, therapy was most effective in prolonging survival. Of interest is that the benefits of ACE inhibition therapy increased with the duration of administration. (*Adapted from* Pfeffer and coworkers [19].)

FIGURE 5-24. Late volume enlargement after first anterior infarction. In asymptomatic patients with left ventricular (LV) dysfunction, late (*ie*, from 3 weeks to 1 year) volume enlargement occurred with administration of conventional therapy. The magnitude of this increase in LV end-diastolic volume was greatest in patients with an occluded infarct-related vessel and a higher degree of wall motion abnormality, as assessed by percent akinesis plus dyskinesis of the baseline left ventriculogram. In a randomized, placebo-controlled study, administration of the angiotensin-converting enzyme (ACE) inhibitor captopril was effective in attenuating the late LV enlargement observed in these selected survivors of myocardial infarction. (*Adapted from* Pfeffer and coworkers [20]; with permission.)

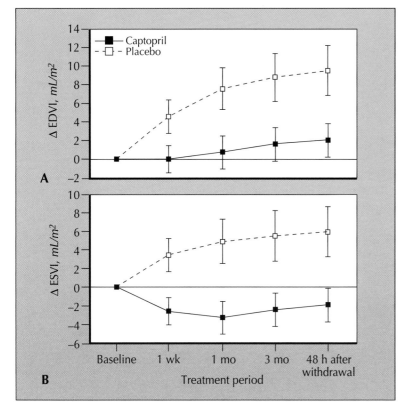

FIGURE 5-25. Change in end-diastolic volume index (EDVI; *panel A*) and end-systolic volume index (ESVI; *panel B*) in patients with Q-wave infarctions as assessed by serial echocardiography. A study by Sharpe [21] has extended prior observations to an earlier time period and has expanded the patient group to include both inferior and anterior Q-wave infarctions. Once again, progressive enlargement is seen with conventional therapy, and this alteration in left ventricular (LV) volume was significantly reduced by the addition of the angiotensin-converting enzyme (ACE) inhibitor captopril. This study also measured LV volume after withdrawal of the ACE inhibitor, demonstrating that the observed differences are not merely a consequence of acute unloading. (*Adapted from* Sharpe [21].)

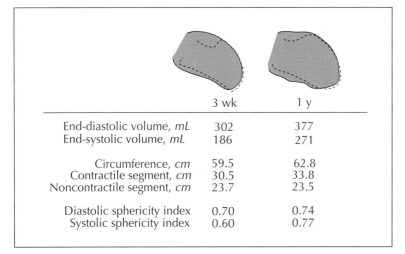

	3 wk	1 y
End-diastolic volume, *mL*	302	377
End-systolic volume, *mL*	186	271
Circumference, *cm*	59.5	62.8
Contractile segment, *cm*	30.5	33.8
Noncontractile segment, *cm*	23.7	23.5
Diastolic sphericity index	0.70	0.74
Systolic sphericity index	0.60	0.77

FIGURE 5-26. Components of late enlargement. Late (*ie*, 3 weeks to 1 year) ventricular enlargement in patients with first anterior myocardial infarction is shown. Although major changes in the noncontractile region characterized the early process of infarct expansion, the increase in volume during the later phase is a consequence of lengthening of the contractile portion and a further shape change, resulting in a more spherical contour. (*Adapted from* Mitchell and coworkers [22].)

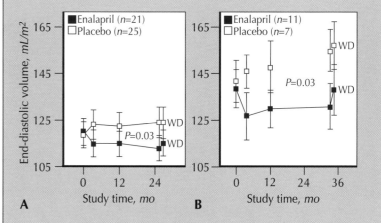

FIGURE 5-27. Serial left ventricular (LV) end-diastolic volume changes in SOLVD (Studies of Left Ventricular Dysfunction) study participants. In an ancillary trial of the SOLVD study, both the prevention (*panel A*) and the treatment (*panel B*) arms demonstrated significant reductions in LV volume in the patients randomized to receive long-term angiotensin-converting enzyme (ACE) inhibitor therapy with enalapril. In general, the asymptomatic patients in the prevention arm experienced less LV enlargement than the symptomatic patients in the treatment arm. In both study groups, enalapril therapy was effective in attenuating progressive LV enlargement. An interesting component of this study was withdrawal data (WD). The ACE inhibitor was withheld for a minimum of 5 days, and the difference in LV end-diastolic volume was sustained, indicating that this therapy was influencing structural enlargement rather than merely an acute unloading effect. (*Adapted from* Konstam and coworkers [23]; with permission.)

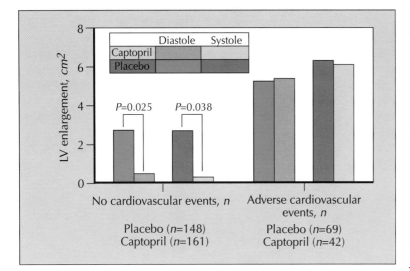

FIGURE 5-28. Changes in left ventricular (LV) area related to adverse cardiovascular events and therapy with captopril. The echocardiographic substudy of the Survival and Ventricular Enlargement trial did indeed confirm that chronic angiotensin-converting enzyme (ACE) inhibition therapy was associated with less ventricular enlargement 1 year after myocardial infarction. Importantly, this study extended previous observations to indicate that patients who had experienced an adverse cardiovascular event were much more likely to demonstrate progressive LV enlargement. Although ACE inhibitor therapy reduced the number of patients who experienced adverse cardiovascular events by approximately 20%, those who experienced either cardiovascular death, heart failure, or MI despite therapy were as likely as patients receiving placebo to demonstrate LV enlargement. These observations point to an important link between LV enlargement and adverse clinical outcome. (*Adapted from* St. John Sutton and coworkers [24]; with permission.)

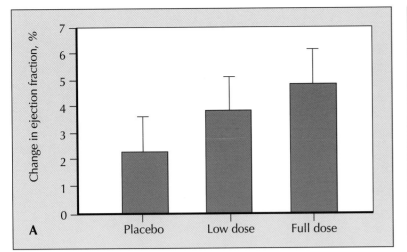

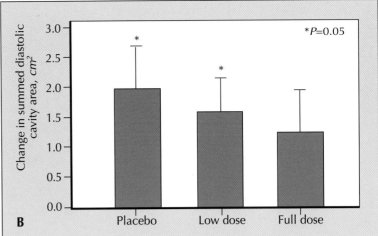

FIGURE 5-29. Change in ejection fraction in the first 14 days after an anterior myocardial infarction. In the cohort of 299 patients with paired studies on day 1 and day 0, there was an overall improvement in ejection fraction. **A,** Those who received an angiotensin-converting enzyme (ACE) inhibitor had a greater benefit, particularly those who were randomized to a full dose of the ACE inhibitor ramipril. **B,** Despite the general improvement in

ejection fraction, there was evidence of left ventricular enlargement, which was most prominent in the patients who were not treated with an ACE inhibitor during the first 14 days of an infarction. These data indicate a relative dissociation between a measure of ventricular performance (*ie,* ejection fraction) and the assessment of remodeling (*ie,* diastolic cavity area). (*Adapted from* Pfeffer and coworkers [25]; with permission.)

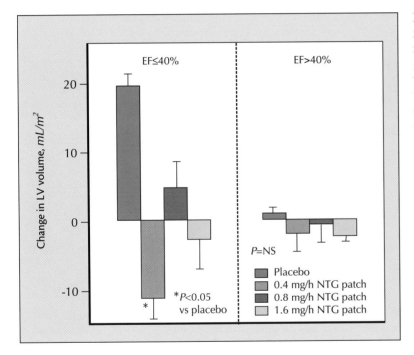

FIGURE 5-30. Changes in left ventricular (LV) end-systolic volume from the early phase (first 3 days to 6 months) after myocardial infarction and the influence of randomization to a transdermal nitro-glycerin (NTG) patch. Chronic therapy with nitroglycerin reduced ventricular enlargement. In this randomized study, it is of interest that, consistent with prior studies, most of the ventricular enlargement occurred in placebo-treated patients who had an LV ejection fraction (LVEF) of 40% or less than in those with an LVEF greater than 40%. The favorable influence of nitroglycerin was demonstrated in the group with LVEF of 40% or less. The authors are careful to indicate that their study was designed to address the LV remodeling influence of nitrates and was not powered to address the issue of clinical outcomes. The observations do support the notion that remodeling is mainly a problem for larger infarcts and that factors that favorably influence filling pressures, such as angiotensin-converting enzyme inhibitors and nitroglycerin, can have long-term benefits on structure. (*Adapted from* Mahmarian and coworkers [26].)

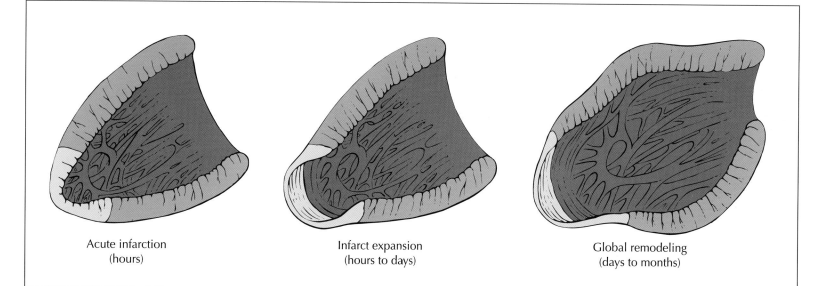

| Acute infarction (hours) | Infarct expansion (hours to days) | Global remodeling (days to months) |

FIGURE 5-31. Left ventricular remodeling after myocardial infarction (MI). During the critical initial hours of MI when acute ischemia progresses to true necrosis, regional systolic dysfunction is already present. However, in this particularly crucial period, measures to restore the balance between O_2 demand and delivery can lead to salvage of contractile tissue. Once cell death has occurred, and particularly if there is a transmural infarction involving the ventri-cular apex, there is a high likelihood that this initially functional distortion of ventricular contour will become structural for infarct expansion. The distorted ventricle undergoes further remodeling as a consequence of heightened wall stress on the remaining viable myocardium, which leads to further cavity enlargement and shape distortion. The latter insidious process is associated with a greater likelihood of cardiovascular morbidity and mortality.

REFERENCES

1. Holt J, Rhode E, Kines H: Ventricular volumes and body weight in mammals. *Am J Physiol* 1968, 215:704–715.

2. Grossman W, Carabello BA, Gunther S, *et al.*: Ventricular wall stress and the development of cardiac hypertrophy and failure. In *Perspectives in Cardiovascular Research. Myocardial Hypertrophy and Failure*, vol 7. Edited by Alpert NR. New York: Raven Press; 1993:1–15.

3. Hutchins GM, Bulkley BH: Infarct expansion versus extension: two different complications of acute myocardial infarction. *Am J Cardiol* 1978, 41:1127–1132.

4. Erlebacher JA, Weiss JL, Weisfeldt ML, *et al.*: Early dilation of the infarcted segment in acute transmural myocardial infarction: role of infarct expansion in acute left ventricular enlargement. *J Am Coll Cardiol* 1984, 4:201–208.

5. Jugdutt BI, Michorowski BL: Role of infarct expansion in rupture of the ventricular septum after acute myocardial infarction: a two-dimensional echocardiographic study. *Clin Cardiol* 1987, 10:641–652.

6. Hammermeister KE, DeRouen TA, Dodge HT: Variables predictive of survival in patients with coronary disease: selection by univariate and multivariate analyses from the clinical, electrocardiographic, exercise, arteriographic, and quantitative angiographic evaluations. *Circulation* 1979, 59:421–430.

7. White HD, Norris RM, Brown MA, *et al.*: Left ventricular end-systolic volume as the major determinant of survival after recovery from myocardial infarction. *Circulation* 1987, 76:44–51.

8. Meizlish JL, Berger HJ, Plankey M, *et al.*: Functional left ventricular aneurysm formation after acute anterior transmural myocardial infarction: incidence, natural history, and prognostic implications. *N Engl J Med* 1984, 311:1001–1006.

9. Lamas GA, Vaughan DE, Pfeffer MA: Left ventricular thrombus formation after first anterior wall acute myocardial infarction. *Am J Cardiol* 1988, 62:31–35.

10. Pfeffer JM, Pfeffer MA, Fletcher PJ, *et al.*: Progressive ventricular remodeling in rat with myocardial infarction. *Am J Physiol* 1991, 29 (suppl H):1406–1414.

11. Gaudron P, Eilles C, Kugler I, *et al.*: Progressive left ventricular dysfunction and remodeling after myocardial infarction: potential mechanisms and early predictors. *Circulation* 1993, 87:755–763.

12. Pfeffer JM: Progressive ventricular dilatation in experimental myocardial infarction and its attenuation by angiotensin converting enzyme inhibition. *Am J Cardiol* 1991, 68:17D–25D.

13. Capasso J, Zhang P, Anversa P: Heterogeneity of ventricular remodeling after acute myocardial infarction in rats. *Am J Physiol* 1992, 262(suppl H):486–495.

14. White HD, Norris RM, Brown MA, *et al.*: Effect of intravenous streptokinase on left ventricular function and early survival after acute myocardial infarction. *N Engl J Med* 1987, 317:850–855.

15. Marino P, Zanolla L, Zardini P: Effect of streptokinase on left ventricular modeling and function after myocardial infarction: the GISSI (Gruppo Italiano per lo Studio della Streptochinasi nell'Infarto Miocardico) Trial. *J Am Coll Cardiol* 1989, 14:1149–1158.

16. Braunwald E: Myocardial reperfusion, limitation of infarct size, reduction of left ventricular dysfunction, and improved survival: should the paradigm by expanded? *Circulation* 1989, 79:441–444.

17. Kim C, Braunwald E: Potential benefits of late reperfusion of infarcted myocardium: the open artery hypothesis. *Circulation* 1993, 88:2426–2436.

18. Pfeffer JM, Pfeffer MA, Braunwald E: Influence of chronic captopril therapy on the infarcted left ventricle of the rat. *Circ Res* 1985, 57:84–95.

19. Pfeffer MA, Pfeffer JM, Steinberg C, Finn P: Survival after an experimental myocardial infarction: beneficial effects of long-term captopril therapy. *Circulation* 1985, 72:406–412.

20. Pfeffer MA, Lamas GA, Vaughan DE, *et al.*: Effect of captopril on progressive ventricular dilatation after anterior myocardial infarction. *N Engl J Med* 1988, 319:80–86.

21. Sharpe N: Early preventive treatment of left ventricular dysfunction following myocardial infarction: optimal timing and patient selection. *Am J Cardiol* 1991, 68(suppl D):64–69.

22. Mitchell GF, Lamas GA, Vaughan DE, *et al.*: Left ventricular remodeling in the year following first anterior myocardial infarction: a quantitative analysis of contractile segment lengths and ventricular shape. *J Am Coll Cardiol* 1992, 19:1136–1144.

23. Konstam M, Kronenberg M, Rousseau M, *et al.*: Effects of the angiotensin converting enzyme inhibitor enalapril on the long-term progression of left ventricular dilatation in patients with asymptomatic systolic dysfunction. *Circulation* 1993, 88:2277–2283.

24. St. John Sutton M, Pfeffer M, Plappert T, *et al.*: Quantitative two dimensional echocardiographic measurements are major predictors of adverse cardiovascular events following acute myocardial infarction: the protective effects of captopril. *Circulation* 1994, 89:68–75.

25. Pfeffer MA, Greaves SC, Arnold JMO, *et al.*: Early versus delayed angiotensin-converting enzyme inhibition therapy in acute myocardial infarction: the Healing and Early Afterload Reducing Therapy Trial. *Circulation* 1997, 95:2643–2651.

26. Mahmarian JJ, Moyé LA, Chinoy DA, *et al.*: Transdermal nitro-glycerin patch therapy improves left ventricular function and prevents remodeling after acute myocardial infarction: results of a multicenter prospective randomized, double-blind, placebo-controlled trial. *Circulation* 1998, 97:2017–2024.

Neurohumoral, Renal, and Vascular Adjustments in Heart Failure

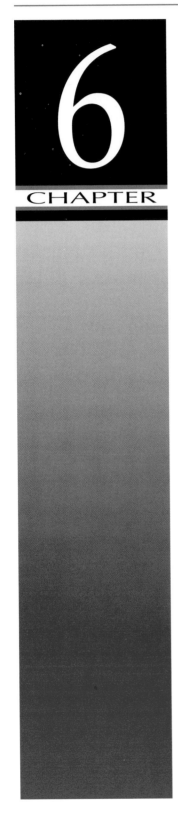

6

CHAPTER

Jorge A. Cusco and Mark A. Creager

Congestive heart failure resulting from left ventricular dysfunction is accompanied by peripheral circulatory changes that influence cardiac function and contribute to the clinical manifestations of heart failure. Neurohumoral systems that modulate both vascular tone and the retention of salt and water are activated. These include the sympathetic nervous system, the renin-angiotensin-aldosterone system, arginine vasopressin, and the natriuretic peptides. In addition, the peripheral circulation undergoes local changes in response to heart failure that are fundamental to the pathophysiology of this disease state. Such changes include an increased release of endothelin and prostaglandins, as well as a possible decrease of activity in the endothelium-derived relaxing factor, nitric oxide. In addition, there may be enhanced local production of angiotensin II.

Taken together, these systemic and local vasoactive systems modulate vascular resistance and determine the regional distribution of the cardiac output. Whereas blood flow to the limb, kidneys, and splanchnic bed may decrease, blood flow to the heart and brain is usually preserved. Diminished exercise capacity in patients with congestive heart failure may be due in part to chronically diminished limb blood flow and failure to increase blood flow normally with metabolic stimulation. Renal hypoperfusion alters intrarenal hemodynamics and may contribute to sodium and water retention.

This chapter reviews the mechanisms in congestive heart failure that underlie systemic activation of the sympathetic nervous system, the renin-angiotensin system, and circulatory neurohormones such as arginine vasopressin and natriuretic peptides. It also focuses on local vasodilator and vasoconstrictor mechanisms that are mediated by the endothelium and the vascular smooth muscle.

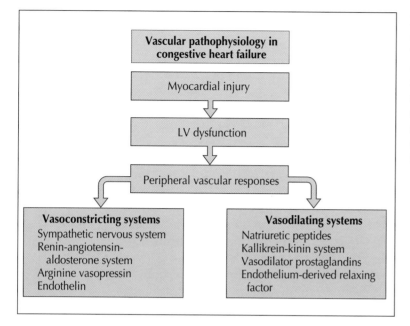

FIGURE 6-1. Myocardial injury causes left ventricular (LV) dysfunction. This activates or alters a variety of peripheral vasomotor mechanisms that are both beneficial (compensatory) and deleterious. Vasoconstrictor systems such as the sympathetic nervous system, the renin-angiotensin-aldosterone system, arginine vasopressin, and endothelin increase afterload and contribute to salt and water retention. Vasodilating systems such as the natriuretic peptides, the kallikrein-kinin system, endothelium-derived relaxing factor, and prostaglandins unload the left ventricle and may facilitate natriuresis.

SYMPATHETIC NERVOUS SYSTEM

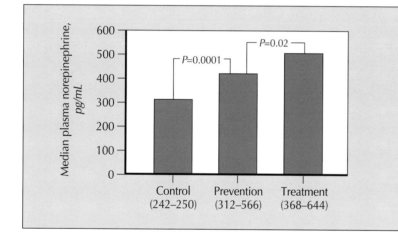

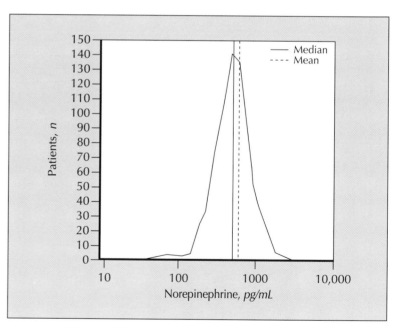

FIGURE 6-2. Sympathetic nervous system activity is increased in patients with congestive heart failure (CHF). In a substudy of the SOLVD (Studies of Left Ventricular Dysfunction) trial, plasma norepinephrine was measured in 54 control subjects, 151 patients with left ventricular dysfunction but no evidence of CHF (prevention group), and 81 patients with left ventricular dysfunction and mild to moderate CHF (treatment group). The median plasma norepinephrine levels for these groups were 317 pg/mL, 422 pg/mL, and 507 pg/mL, respectively (interquartile ranges are shown in parentheses). Mean values for plasma norepinephrine were significantly higher in patients with left ventricular dysfunction compared with those in normal subjects ($P=0.0001$). Levels were significantly higher in patients with overt heart failure compared with those in asymptomatic patients with left ventricular dysfunction ($P=0.02$). This study demonstrates that sympathetic nervous system activation occurs in the early stages of CHF. (*Adapted from* Francis and coworkers [1].)

FIGURE 6-3. Data from the Veterans Administration Heart Failure Trial II (VHeFT II) showed a wide distribution in baseline values of plasma norepinephrine in patients with moderately severe congestive heart failure. The baseline values of plasma norepinephrine are presented on a logarithmic scale for 743 patients with congestive heart failure enrolled in VHeFT II. The median plasma norepinephrine was 490 pg/mL (range, 48 to 3849; mean, 568 pg/mL). Values in most patients were substantially higher than those usually obtained for normal subjects, which averaged 150±100 pg/mL. (*Adapted from* Francis and coworkers [2].)

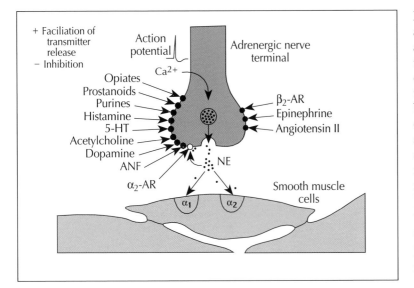

FIGURE 6-4. Sympathetic nerve terminal. Sympathetic nerve activity can be measured directly by measuring the electrical activity in the peripheral nerves and indirectly by measuring the plasma norepinephrine (NE) concentration. Plasma NE is derived from sympathetic nerves, but the amount that reaches the circulation depends on several processes. Plasma NE can be increased by increased nerve release, decreased local uptake, or reduced systemic clearance. Neurotransmitter release at the sympathetic neuroeffector junction is also modulated locally by a variety of hormones and other substances that act on specific receptors located on the presynaptic nerve ending. Several α_2-receptor agonists, including NE itself (via α_2-adrenergic receptors [α_2-AR]), opioids, prostanoids, purines, histamine, 5-hydroxy-tryptamine (5-HT), atrial natriuretic factor (ANF), dopamine, and acetylcholine, *inhibit* NE release. In contrast, epinephrine (via β_2-adrenergic receptors [β_2-AR]) and angiotensin II *increase* NE release from the neuroeffector junction. (*Adapted from* Vanhoutte and Luscher [3]; with permission.)

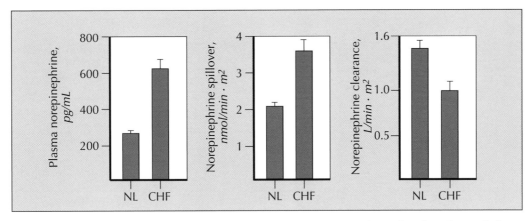

FIGURE 6-5. To determine whether elevated plasma norepinephrine levels in heart failure occur secondary to increased neural release of norepinephrine, decreased clearance, or both, Davis *et al.* [4] used a radiotracer technique to measure plasma norepinephrine levels, spillover, and clearance in 18 normal subjects (NL) and 19 patients with severe New York Heart Association functional class III to IV congestive heart failure (CHF). Patients with CHF had significantly higher baseline plasma norepinephrine levels (249±20 pg/mL vs 628±68 pg/mL; $P<0.001$). A 73% greater spillover of norepinephrine and a 33% reduction in clearance were found in the CHF group. These studies of norepinephrine kinetics demonstrated that both increased spillover and decreased clearance contribute to the higher norepinephrine levels observed in CHF patients. (*Adapted from* Davis and coworkers [4].)

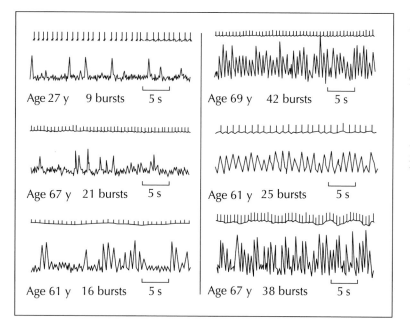

FIGURE 6-6. Microneurography. Sympathetic neural activity can be measured directly in humans by microneurography. Leimbach *et al.* [5] used microneurography for direct recording of intraneural sympathetic nerve activity from the peroneal nerve in normal subjects and patients with congestive heart failure. This figure illustrates microneurographic recordings from three normal subjects (*left*) and three patients with congestive heart failure (*right*). A burst represents a summation of nerve action potentials from multiple fibers. Note the increased sympathetic burst frequency in patients with congestive heart failure. (*Adapted from* Leimbach and coworkers [5]; with permission.)

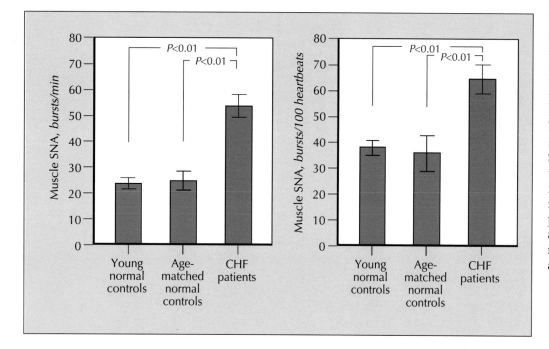

FIGURE 6-7. Muscle sympathetic nerve activity (SNA) was measured in 19 young normal control subjects, nine normal control subjects who were age-matched to patients with congestive heart failure (CHF), and 16 patients with CHF. Muscle SNA is expressed in terms of bursts per minute as well as bursts per 100 heartbeats, thereby correcting for heart rate. In patients with CHF, muscle SNA was significantly higher than in the two control groups. These data provide further evidence that SNA is increased in patients with CHF and that elevated plasma norepinephrine levels occur as a consequence of increased sympathetic neural activity. (*Adapted from* Leimbach and coworkers [5]; with permission.)

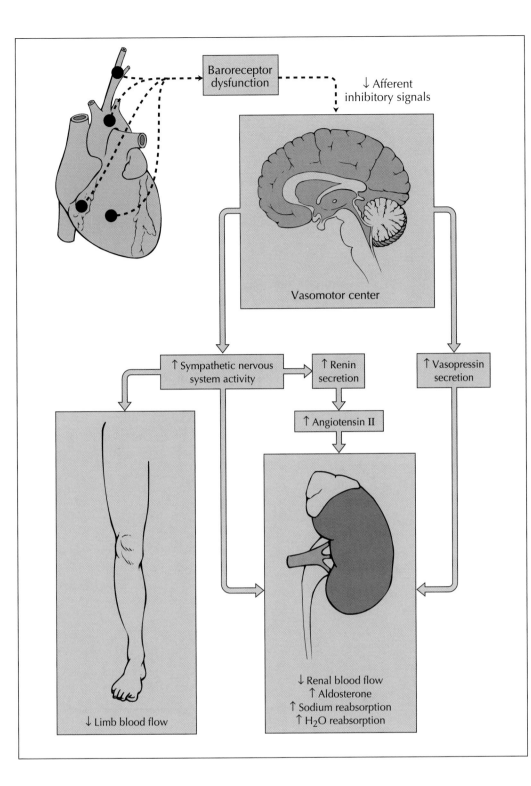

FIGURE 6-8. Baroreceptor dysfunction may account for increased sympathetic and reduced parasympathetic nervous system activity in most patients with congestive heart failure. Normally, autonomic balance is regulated by afferent input from multiple peripheral receptors, including baroreceptors in the heart, lungs, and great vessels, chemoreceptors in the carotid bodies, metaboreceptors in skeletal muscle, sensory receptors in skin, a variety of visceral receptors, and from signals originating in the central nervous system. Of these, the baroreceptors are the principal modulators of sympathetic and parasympathetic activity during changes in intravascular volume or pressure. Mechanoreceptors in the heart and pulmonary vasculature (cardiopulmonary baroreceptors) and in the aortic arch and carotid sinus (arterial baroreceptors) respond to stretch by relaying afferent neural signals to the central system via branches of the vagus and glossopharyngeal nerves. These signals *inhibit* sympathetic and *augment* parasympathetic efferent activity. In plasma volume depletion or hypotension, decreased receptor stretch reduces the afferent stimuli, thus decreasing parasympathetic activity and increasing sympathetic activity. Because baroreceptor function is impaired in heart failure, inhibitory input from arterial and cardiopulmonary baroreceptors is decreased, thereby leading to excessive sympathetic and reduced parasympathetic activity. Abnormal baroreceptor function may also facilitate vasopressin release from the neurohypophysis and stimulate renal release of renin. (*Adapted from* Paganelli and coworkers [6]; with permission.)

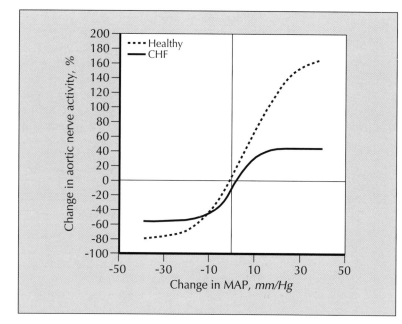

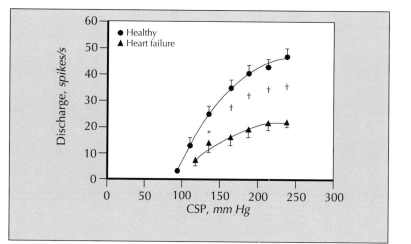

FIGURE 6-9. Abnormalities of arterial baroreceptor function have been demonstrated in animal models of heart failure. Dibner-Dunlap and Thames [7] measured the effect of changes in mean arterial pressure (MAP) on aortic nerve activity (nerve signals from aortic baroreceptors) in healthy dogs and in dogs with congestive heart failure (CHF) secondary to rapid ventricular pacing. Baroreceptor dysfunction is indicated by the observation that, for comparable increases in blood pressure induced by phenylephrine, there was a lesser increase in aortic nerve activity in dogs with CHF compared with that in healthy dogs. (*Adapted from* Dibner-Dunlap and Thames [7].)

FIGURE 6-10. Carotid sinus baroreceptor sensitivity in experimental heart failure. Wang *et al.* [8] measured carotid sinus nerve activity (nerve signals from carotid baroreceptors) during changes in carotid sinus pressure (CSP) in healthy dogs and dogs with heart failure induced by rapid ventricular pacing. With incremental pressure in CSP, there was lessened neural discharge from the carotid sinus nerve in dogs with heart failure compared with healthy dogs. *Asterisk* indicates *P*<0.01; *daggers*, *P*<0.001. (*Adapted from* Wang and coworkers [8].)

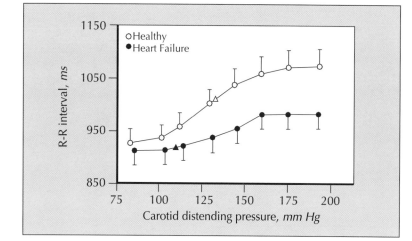

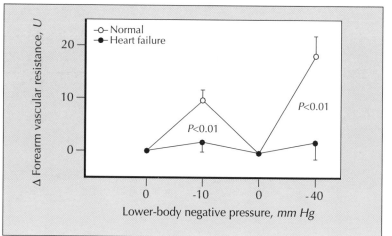

FIGURE 6-11. Abnormalities in arterial baroreceptor reflex function have also been demonstrated in humans. Using a custom-designed neck chamber, Sopher *et al.* [9] applied progressive suction to the carotid sinus of healthy subjects and patients with congestive heart failure (CHF). Neck suction increases transmural pressure across the carotid sinus and simulates an increase in blood pressure, thereby stimulating the carotid sinus baroreceptors. The heart rate (R-R interval) was measured to assess the reflex response to carotid sinus baroreceptor stimulation. The heart rate slowed to a greater extent with increasing carotid distending pressure in healthy subjects compared with patients with CHF. The operational point (*triangle*), also known as the set point, is the starting or resting point of each group on the stimulus response curve. In patients with CHF, the operational point was shifted to the left. The shift in the baroreflex response curve defines an abnormality in the receptor firing function. These findings indicate that in patients with CHF, as shown in animal models, carotid sinus baroreceptor reflex function is impaired. (*Adapted from* Sopher and coworkers [9].)

FIGURE 6-12. Cardiopulmonary baroreceptor reflex function in humans can be assessed by encasing the lower part of the body in a rigid cylinder and subjecting the individual to negative pressure. Normally, increasing levels of lower-body negative pressure reduce cardiac filling pressures, inhibit cardiopulmonary baroreceptors, and increase sympathetic efferent nervous activity, thereby causing vasoconstriction. Whereas low levels of lower-body negative pressure (-10 mm Hg) selectively unload cardiopulmonary baroreceptors, high levels (-40 mm Hg) unload both cardiopulmonary and arterial baroreceptors (by reducing stroke volume and blood pressure). Forearm vasoconstriction occurs during lower-body negative pressure in normal subjects but not in patients with congestive heart failure. These data indicate that cardiopulmonary baroreceptor function is abnormal in patients with congestive heart failure, providing additional evidence for a mechanism that causes sympathetic activation in these individuals. (*Adapted from* Creager [10].)

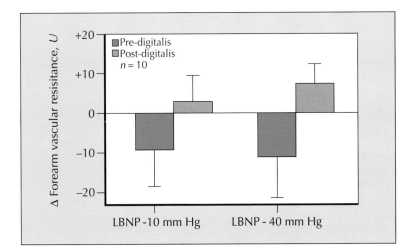

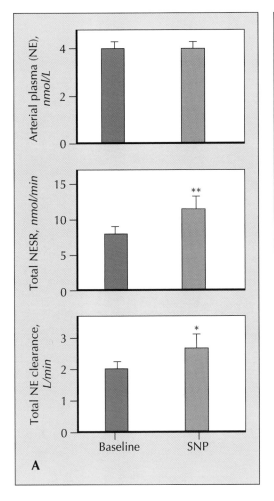

FIGURE 6-13. Some forms of therapy for patients with congestive heart failure favorably affect baroreceptor function. Ferguson *et al.* [11] administered a digitalis glycoside, lanatoside C, to patients with congestive heart failure and subjected them to lower-body negative pressure (LBNP). Before administration of digitalis, LBNP at -10 mm Hg and -40 mm Hg caused paradoxical forearm vasodilatation, indicating impaired baroreceptor function. After administration of digitalis, LBNP at -10 mm Hg and -40 mm Hg caused a more normal forearm vasoconstrictor response. These data suggest that part of the beneficial effect of digitalis in patients with congestive heart failure may be secondary to improvement in baroreceptor function, leading to withdrawal of sympathetic activity. (*Adapted from* Ferguson and coworkers [11].)

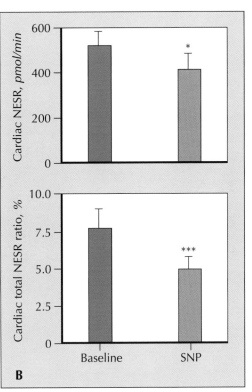

FIGURE 6-14. Baroreceptor unloading may affect sympathetic nervous system function in patients with congestive heart failure (CHF). Kaye *et al.* [12] used sodium nitroprusside (SNP) in doses sufficient to reduce both cardiac filling pressures and arterial pressure in patients with CHF. Nitroprusside infusion increased total body norepinephrine (NE) spillover rate (NESR) as well as total norepinephrine clearance (**A**). In contrast, nitroprusside decreased cardiac NESR (**B**). These findings indicate a differential effect of acute baroreceptor unloading on systemic and cardiac sympathetic activity in patients with heart failure, increasing the former but decreasing the latter. The clinical implication of these observations is that therapeutic interventions that reduce cardiac filling pressures would potentially impart a beneficial effect on survival by reducing cardiac sympathetic efferent activity. (*Adapted from* Kaye and coworkers [12].)

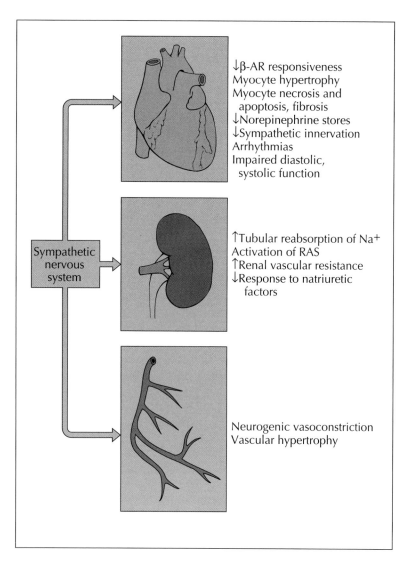

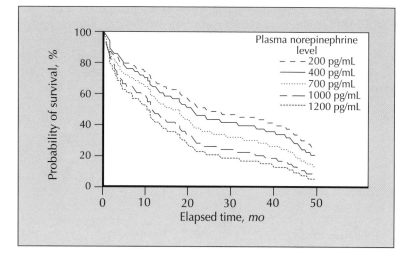

FIGURE 6-15. Increased sympathetic nervous system activity may contribute to the pathophysiology of congestive heart failure by multiple mechanisms involving cardiac, renal, and vascular function [13]. In the heart, increased sympathetic nervous system outflow may lead to desensitization of postsynaptic β-adrenergic receptors (β-AR), nonuniform depletion of norepinephrine stores, nonuniform destruction of sympathetic innervation, arrhythmias, and impairment of diastolic and systolic function, and act directly on myocardial cells, causing myocyte hypertrophy, necrosis, apoptosis, and fibrosis. In the kidneys, increased sympathetic activation induces arterial and venous vasoconstriction, activation of the renin-angiotensin system (RAS), increase in salt and water retention, and an attenuated response to natriuretic factors. In the peripheral vessels, neurogenic vasoconstriction and vascular hypertrophy are induced by increased sympathetic nervous activity. (*Adapted from* Floras [13].)

FIGURE 6-16. Activation of sympathetic nervous system activity, as reflected by elevated plasma norepinephrine levels, has been associated with a poor prognosis in patients with congestive heart failure. Cohn *et al.* [14] measured supine plasma norepinephrine levels in 106 patients with moderate to severe congestive heart failure. A multivariate analysis found that resting plasma norepinephrine levels were a significant independent predictor of mortality among these patients ($P<0.002$). In addition, the norepinephrine level was higher in patients who died from progressive heart failure (1014±699 pg/mL) than in those who died suddenly (619±238 pg/mL). The figure illustrates predicted survival curves for groups of patients with different baseline plasma norepinephrine levels. (*Adapted from* Cohn and coworkers [14].)

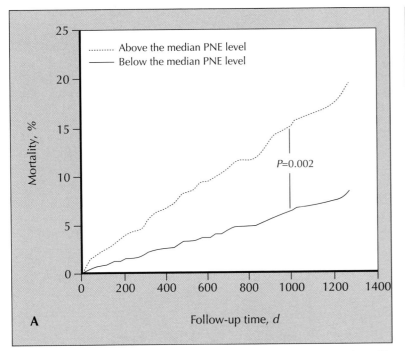

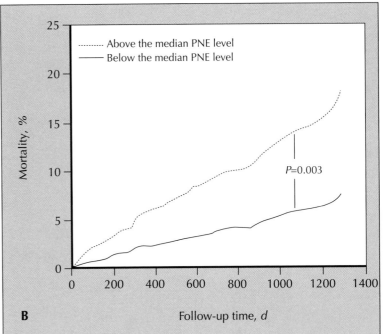

FIGURE 6-17. Plasma norepinephrine (PNE) levels also predict all cause and cardiovascular mortality in patients with asymptomatic left ventricular dysfunction. An analysis [15] from the Studies of Left Ventricular Dysfunction (SOLVD) trial found that PNE was the strongest predictor of clinical events in patients with asymptomatic left ventricular dysfunction. Adjusted all-cause mortality (**A**) and adjusted cardiovascular mortality (**B**) were significantly higher in patients with pre-randomization (*ie*, prior to placebo vs enalapril therapy) norepinephrine concentrations above or below the median value of 393 pg/mL. Plasma norepinephrine levels greater than 393 pg/mL were associated with a relative risk of 2.59 for all-cause mortality, 2.55 for cardiovascular mortality, 2.55 for hospitalization for heart failure, 1.88 for development of heart failure, 1.92 for ischemic events, and 2.59 for myocardial infarction. (*Adapted from* Benedict and coworkers [15].)

THE RENIN-ANGIOTENSIN-ALDOSTERONE SYSTEM

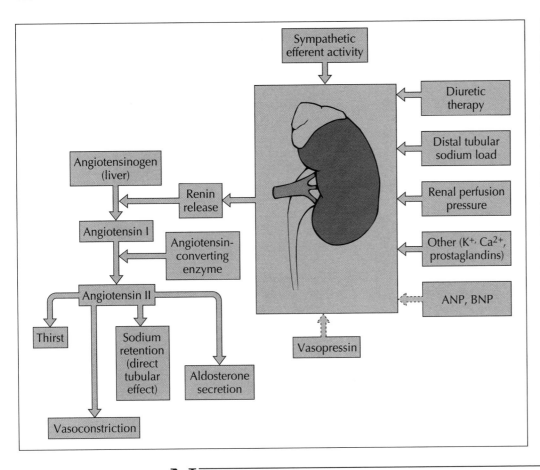

FIGURE 6-18. The renin-angiotensin system is activated in patients with congestive heart failure. The major site of release of circulating renin is the juxtaglomerular apparatus of the kidney, where multiple stimuli may contribute to renal release of renin into the systemic circulation, including increased renal sympathetic efferent activity, decreased distal tubular sodium delivery, reduced renal perfusion pressure, and diuretic therapy. Natriuretic peptides (ANP, BNP),and vasopressin (*dashed arrows*) may inhibit the release of renin. Renin enzymatically cleaves angiotensinogen, a tetrapeptide produced in the liver, to form the inactive decapeptide angiotensin I. Angiotensin I is converted to the octapeptide angiotensin II by the angiotensin-converting enzyme. Angiotensin II is a potent vasoconstrictor; it promotes sodium reabsorption by increasing aldosterone secretion and by a direct effect on the tubules, and it stimulates water intake by acting on the thirst center. Angiotensin II causes vasoconstriction directly and may also facilitate the release of norepinephrine by acting on sympathetic nerve endings. (*Adapted from* Paganelli and coworkers [6]; with permission.)

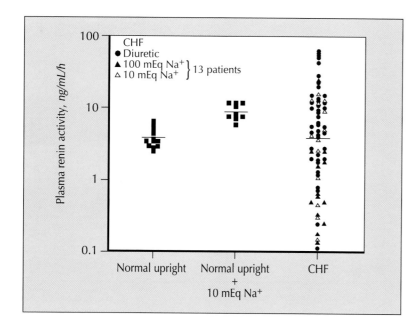

FIGURE 6-19. Cody and Laragh [16] evaluated the role of the renin-angiotensin system in patients with congestive heart failure (CHF). They studied 17 normal subjects in the upright position receiving an unrestricted sodium diet; 12 normal upright subjects receiving a low-sodium diet (10 mEq); and 52 patients with CHF receiving a low-sodium diet (10 mEq), a normal-sodium diet (100 mEq), or diuretics. The mean plasma renin activity in CHF did not differ significantly from that of normal subjects whose plasma renin activity was stimulated by upright position and a low-sodium diet. Nevertheless, many of the patients with CHF had marked elevation of plasma renin activity, as suggested by this logarithmic scale. (*Adapted from* Cody and Laragh [16]; with permission.)

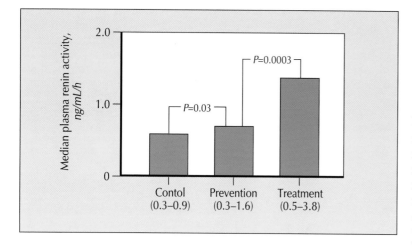

FIGURE 6-20. In the Studies of Left Ventricular Dysfunction (SOLVD), activation of the renin-angiotensin system was evaluated in patients with asymptomatic left ventricular dysfunction or mild congestive heart failure. Plasma renin activity was measured in 56 control subjects, 151 patients with left ventricular dysfunction but no evidence of congestive heart failure (prevention group), and 80 patients with left ventricular dysfunction with mild to moderate congestive heart failure (treatment group). The median plasma renin activity was 0.60 ng/mL/h in the prevention group and 1.4 ng/mL/h in the treatment group (interquartile ranges are shown in parentheses). Mean values for plasma renin activity were marginally increased in the prevention group compared with those in normal subjects. When the data were reanalyzed according to diuretic use, plasma renin activity was normal in patients in both the prevention and the treatment groups not taking diuretics. Therefore, there was no increase in the plasma renin activity in patients with asymptomatic left ventricular dysfunction or mild congestive heart failure who were not receiving diuretics. (*Adapted from* Francis and coworkers [1].)

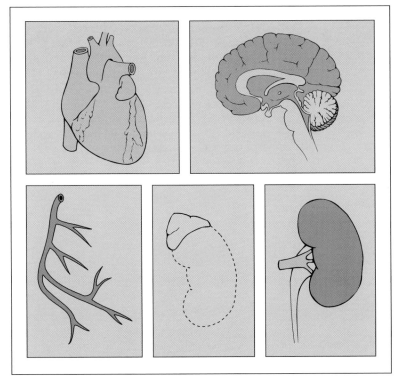

FIGURE 6-21. Tissue renin-angiotensin systems. In addition to the hormonal effects of circulating angiotensin, many or all components of the renin-angiotensin system are present in several organs, including the heart, blood vessels, kidney, brain, and adrenal glands. Angiotensin produced within these tissues may act in a paracrine or autocrine manner to regulate cellular function, independent of the circulating hormone.

POTENTIAL CONTRIBUTIONS OF THE CARDIAC RENIN-ANGIOTENSIN SYSTEM TO THE PATHOPHYSIOLOGY OF HEART FAILURE

POTENTIAL TISSUE EFFECT	PATHOPHYSIOLOGIC CONSEQUENCES
Direct cellular angiotensin II effects	Positive inotropic effect Diastolic dysfunction
Facilitates adrenergic state	Positive inotropic effect Dysrhythmia induction
Coronary vasoconstriction	Subendocardial ischemia
Proto-oncogene expression	Cardiac hypertrophy and remodeling

FIGURE 6-22. Potential effects of the cardiac renin-angiotensin system on the pathophysiology of heart failure. The direct effects of angiotensin II on cardiac tissue include increased inotropy, decreased lusitropy, and coronary artery vasoconstriction. These effects may secondarily promote dysrhythmias and cause subendocardial ischemia. There is also evidence (*see* Chapter 4) that angiotensin contributes to myocardial hypertrophy and remodeling by acting directly on cardiac myocytes and fibroblasts. (*Adapted from* Hirsch and coworkers [17].)

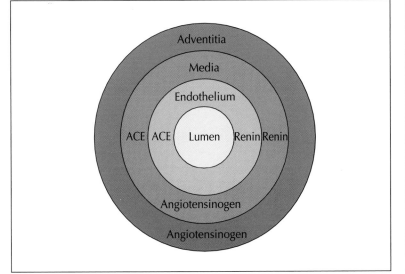

FIGURE 6-23. Distribution of the renin-angiotensin system components within the blood vessel wall. Angiotensinogen can be found in the adventitia and media. Renin, either synthesized locally or taken up from the circulation, has been found in the media and endothelium. Angiotensin-converting enzyme (ACE) has been localized in the media and endothelium. Thus, all of the components necessary for the generation of angiotensin are present in the vessel wall [18].

POTENTIAL CONTRIBUTIONS OF THE VASCULAR RENIN-ANGIOTENSIN SYSTEM TO THE PATHOPHYSIOLOGY OF HEART FAILURE

POTENTIAL TISSUE EFFECT	PATHOPHYSIOLOGIC CONSEQUENCES
Decreased conduit vessel compliance and increased arteriolar resistance	Increased afterload
Venoconstriction	Increased preload
Renal and splanchnic vasoconstriction	Regional blood flow redistribution

FIGURE 6-24. Potential contributions of the vascular renin-angiotensin system to the pathophysiology of heart failure. These contributions include decreased compliance, increased regional and systemic vascular resistance, and venoconstriction. Decreased compliance and increased resistance are due to both vasoconstriction and structural remodeling. (*Adapted from* Hirsch and coworkers [17].)

COMPONENTS OF THE INTRARENAL RENIN-ANGIOTENSIN SYSTEM

LOCALIZATION	COMPONENTS	POSSIBLE FUNCTION
Blood vessels (including vasa recta)	Renin	Intrarenal hemodynamics
	Angiotensinogen	Sodium-water homeostasis
	ACE	
	Angiotensin II receptors	
Glomerulus	Renin	Glomerular hemodynamics
	Angiotensin II receptors	
Proximal tubules	Renin (reabsorbed, interstitium)	Sodium reabsorption
	Angiotensinogen (synthesized)	
	ACE	
	Angiotensin II receptors	

FIGURE 6-25. Components of the intrarenal renin-angiotensin system. These components contribute to the regulation of renal hemodynamic function and sodium reabsorption. Angiotensinogen, renin, angiotensin-converting enzyme (ACE), and angiotensin II receptors are found in many portions of the kidney, including blood vessels, the glomerulus, and the proximal tubules. (*Adapted from* Dzau [19].)

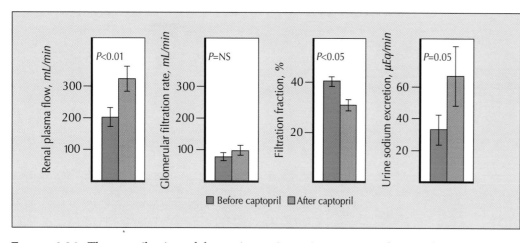

FIGURE 6-26. The contribution of the renin-angiotensin system to abnormal renal hemodynamics and sodium excretion in patients with congestive heart failure. The angiotensin-converting enzyme inhibitor captopril was administered to 12 patients with congestive heart failure. Captopril increased renal plasma flow but had no effect on glomerular filtration rate. Therefore, the filtration fraction, representing the ratio of glomerular filtration rate to renal plasma flow, decreased. In heart failure, renal sodium avidity is associated with a high filtration fraction, which has been postulated to increase peritubular oncotic pressure. After use of captopril, a decrease in filtration fraction, as well as a decrease in the plasma concentration of aldosterone, contributes to the increase in urine sodium excretion. These findings indicate that the renin-angiotensin system contributes importantly to renal vasoconstriction and sodium retention in patients with heart failure. (*Adapted from* Creager and coworkers [20].)

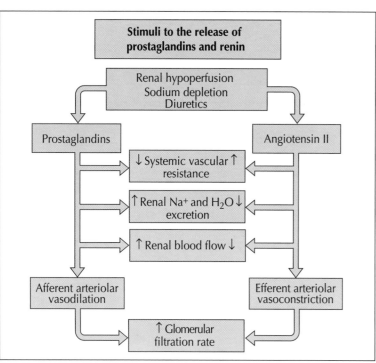

FIGURE 6-27. Stimuli to the release of prostaglandins and renin. Renal hypoperfusion, sodium depletion, and diuretics are potent stimuli for the release of both renin and prostaglandins from the kidney. The release of renal prostaglandins constitutes an adaptive response that counteracts the deleterious effects of the renin-angiotensin system in patients with congestive heart failure. The opposing effects on systemic vascular resistance and sodium and water excretion are also shown. (*Adapted from* Packer [21]; with permission.)

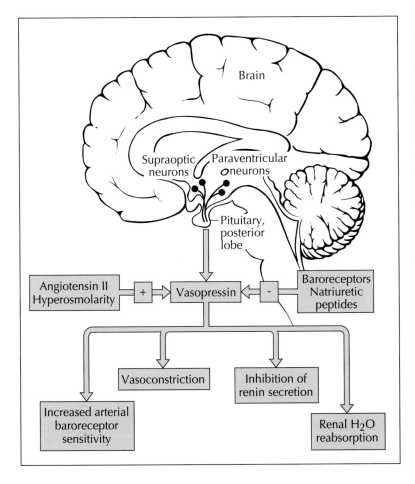

FIGURE 6-28. Arginine vasopressin is a peptide synthesized by the hypothalamic magnocellular neurons of the supraoptic and paraventricular nuclei and is released into the circulation by axon terminals of the posterior pituitary gland. Osmotic and non-osmotic stimuli modulate vasopressin release. Whereas stimulation of hypothalamic osmoreceptors and elevated concentrations of angiotensin II stimulate vasopressin release, baroreceptor activation and natriuretic peptides (ANP, BNP) inhibit vasopressin secretion. Vasopressin acts at the tissue level by binding to specific receptors. It causes vasoconstriction via vasopressin 1 receptors and renal reabsorption of water, renal secretion of renin, and synthesis of renal prostaglandins via vasopressin 2 receptors. In addition, vasopressin may mediate vasodilatation via vasopressin 2 receptors by increasing the release and synthesis of endothelium-derived relaxing factor and vasodilator prostaglandins. Vasopressin also sensitizes baroreceptors, and thus may cause vasodilatation by withdrawing sympathetic activity.

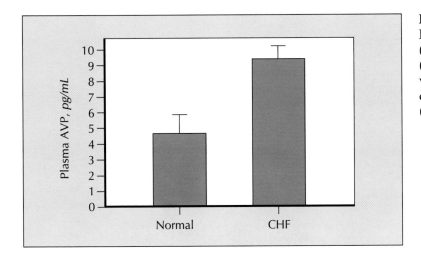

FIGURE 6-29. Plasma vasopressin in patients with heart failure. Francis *et al.* [22] measured basal levels of arginine vasopressin (AVP) in 31 patients with advanced congestive heart failure (CHF) and 11 age-matched normal control subjects. The mean vasopressin level was 9.5±0.89 pg/mL in the CHF group compared with 4.7±0.66 pg/mL in the control group ($P<0.001$). (*Adapted from* Francis and coworkers [22].)

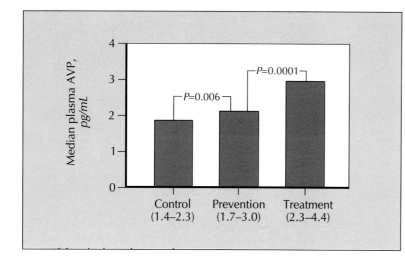

FIGURE 6-30. In a substudy of the Studies of Left Ventricular Dysfunction (SOLVD), arginine-vasopressin (AVP) levels were measured in patients with asymptomatic left ventricular dysfunction (ALVD) or mild congestive heart failure. Plasma AVP levels were measured in 54 control subjects, 147 patients with ALVD (prevention group), and 80 patients with left ventricular dysfunction and mild congestive heart failure (treatment group). The median plasma AVP was 1.9 pg/mL in the control group, 2.2 pg/mL in the prevention group, and 3.0 pg/mL in the treatment group (interquartile ranges are shown in parentheses). Mean values for plasma AVP were significantly higher in patients with left ventricular dysfunction compared with normal control subjects and significantly higher in patients with overt heart failure compared with patients with ALVD. (*Adapted from* Francis and coworkers [1].)

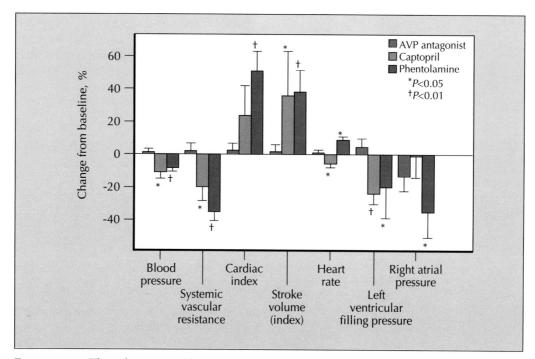

FIGURE 6-31. The relative contributions of the sympathetic nervous system, renin-angiotensin system, and arginine-vasopressin (AVP) system to systemic vascular resistance in patients with congestive heart failure (CHF) was studied by administering an antagonist of each system. Shown are the hemodynamic responses to a V1 AVP antagonist, an angiotensin-converting enzyme inhibitor (captopril), and an α-receptor antagonist (phentolamine) in 10 patients with CHF. The AVP antagonist had relatively little effect on systemic vascular resistance and cardiac function. In contrast, both phentolamine and captopril caused significant decreases in systemic vascular resistance and, consequently, increases in stroke volume and cardiac output. The effect of phentolamine was more profound than that of captopril. These findings suggest that of these three neurohormonal systems, the sympathetic nervous system activity contributes the greatest amount to vasoconstriction in patients with CHF. Whereas the renin-angiotensin system is also important, vasopressin probably contributes little to vasoconstriction in most patients with CHF. Vasopressin may contribute to vasoconstriction in heart failure only when the levels are extremely high. (*Adapted from* Creager and coworkers [23]; with permission.)

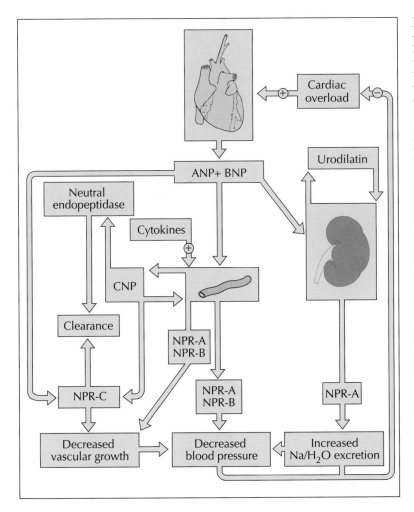

Figure 6-32. The natriuretic peptide family. The natriuretic peptides include atrial natriuretic peptide (ANP), brain natriuretic peptide (BNP), C-type natriuretic peptide (CNP), and urodilatin. ANP is derived from a prohormone composed of 126 amino acids, and it is secreted primarily from cardiac atria. The prohormone is cleaved into an *N*-terminal fragment (ANP1-98) and a C-terminal fragment (ANP99-126). BNP, identified initially in brain, is secreted from both atria and ventricles, particularly the latter. CNP has been identified primarily in brain but is also present in vascular endothelial cells. Urodilatin, or ANP95-126, is found in urine. Stretch receptors in the atria and ventricles detect changes in cardiac chamber volume related to increased cardiac filling pressures, resulting in release of both ANP and BNP but not CNP. The natriuretic peptides are inactivated by neutral endopeptidases. The actions of the natriuretic peptides are mediated by natriuretic peptide receptors (NPRs), designated NPR-A, NPR-B, and NPR-C. Both NPR-A and NPR-B are particulate guanylate cyclases, activation of which increases levels of cGMP. Natriuretic peptide receptors have been localized in vascular smooth muscle, endothelium, platelets, the adrenal glomerulosa, and the kidney. ANP and BNP increase urine volume and sodium excretion, decrease vascular resistance, and inhibit release of renin and secretion of aldosterone and vasopressin. CNP reduces vascular resistance but despite its name, does not have natriuretic properties. (*Adapted from* Wilkins and coworkers [24]; with permission.)

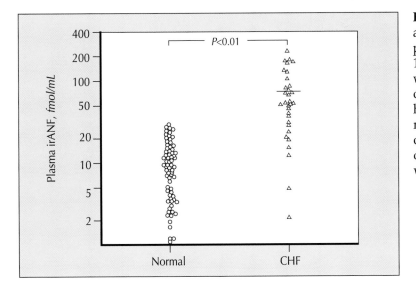

Figure 6-33. Cody *et al.* [25] measured plasma immunoreactive atrial natriuretic factor (irANF) in 70 normal subjects and 31 patients with congestive heart failure (CHF). Plasma irANF was 11±0.9 fmol/mL in normal subjects and 71±9.9 fmol/mL in patients with CHF (*P*<0.01). These results demonstrate a significant elevation of circulating atrial natriuretic factor in patients with CHF. Despite high circulating levels of ANF, patients with CHF demonstrate marked sodium retention, possibly reflecting downregulation of ANF receptors or a persistent imbalance between ANF and opposing mechanisms. (*Adapted from* Cody and coworkers [25]; with permission.)

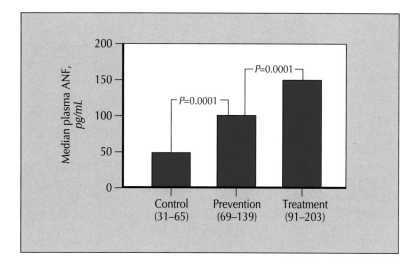

FIGURE 6-34. In the Studies of Left Ventricular Dysfunction (SOLVD), atrial natriuretic factor (ANF) levels were measured in patients with asymptomatic left ventricular (LV) dysfunction and mild congestive heart failure. Plasma ANF was measured in 54 control subjects, 147 patients with LV dysfunction but no evidence of congestive heart failure (prevention group), and 80 patients with mild congestive heart failure (treatment group). The median ANF level was 48 pg/mL in the control group, 103 pg/mL in the prevention group, and 146 pg/mL in the treatment group (interquartile ranges are shown in parentheses). Mean values for plasma ANF were significantly higher in patients with LV dysfunction compared with normal control subjects and were higher in the treatment arm compared with the prevention. Thus, increased release of ANF may be an early response to LV dysfunction. (*Adapted from* Francis and coworkers [1].)

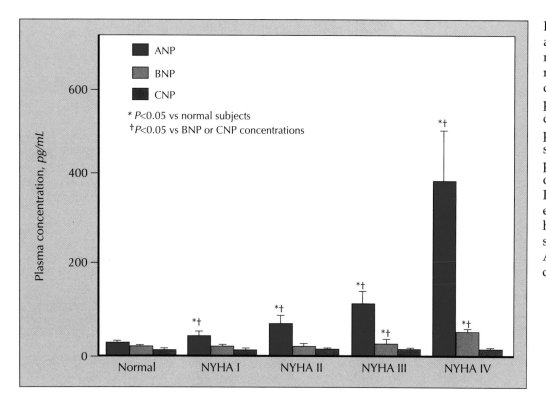

FIGURE 6-35. Plasma concentrations of atrial natriuretic peptide (ANP), brain natriuretic peptide (BNP), and C-type natriuretic peptide (CNP) in patients with congestive heart failure and in normal persons. Whereas plasma ANP concentration was elevated in groups of patients with heart failure whose symptoms ranged from mild to severe, plasma BNP concentration was increased only in patients with severe heart failure. Plasma CNP concentrations were not elevated in any group of patients with heart failure compared with normal subjects. NYHA—New York Heart Association. (*Adapted from* Wei and coworkers [26].)

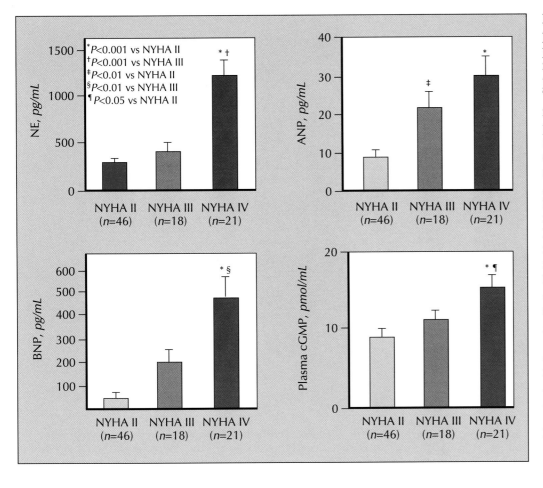

FIGURE 6-36. Measurement of natriuretic peptides in patients with heart failure. The prognostic information derived from measurement of natriuretic peptides in patients with heart failure was assessed by Tsutamoto *et al.* [27]. Plasma levels of atrial natriuretic peptide (ANP), brain natriuretic peptide (BNP), cGMP, and norepinephrine (NE) were measured in 85 patients with chronic congestive heart failure who were followed for 2 years. The concentrations of ANP, BNP, cGMP and norepinephrine increased proportionally with the functional severity of heart failure. In a Kaplan-Meyer analysis of the cumulative rates of survival in patients with heart failure stratified into two groups on the basis of the median plasma concentration of BNP (73 pg/mL), it was shown that survival was significantly worse in the group with the higher plasma BNP levels (*see* Fig. 8-10*B*). A stepwise multivariate analysis, which included ANP, BNP, norepinephrine, New York Heart Association (NYHA) Functional Class, selected hemodynamic indices, and demographic features, found that only a high concentration of plasma BNP (*P*<0.0001) and pulmonary capillary wedge pressure (*P*=0.003) were significant independent predictors of mortality. (*Adapted from* Tsutamoto and coworkers [27]; with permission.)

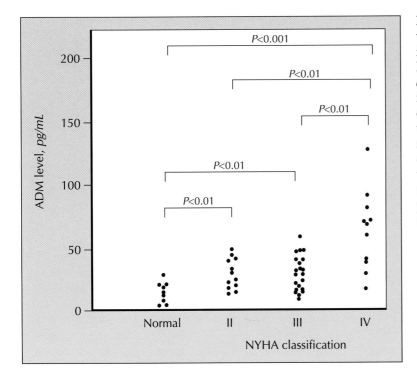

FIGURE 6-37. Adrenomedullin (ADM). ADM is a peptide with vasodilating and natriuretic properties. It was initially isolated from extracts of human pheochromocytoma. It is present in heart, kidney, vascular smooth muscle, and endothelial cells. Jougasaki *et al.* [28] measured circulating AMD levels in normal subjects and in patients with congestive heart failure and found that the plasma concentration of ADM increased as the severity of heart failure worsened. Moreover, the study demonstrated evidence of cardiac secretion of ADM based on measurement of plasma samples obtained in the aorta, coronary sinus, and anterior interventricular vein. This study raises the possibility that ADM may participate in the regulation of vascular function and sodium excretion in patients with heart failure. NYHA—New York Heart Association. (*Adapted from* Jougasaki and coworkers [28].)

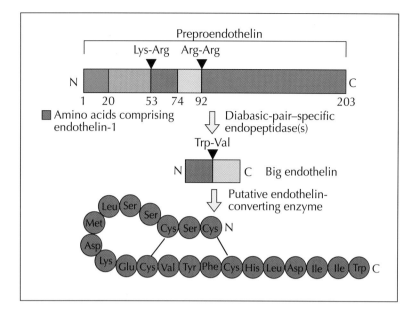

FIGURE 6-38. Endothelin, a 21-amino-acid peptide hormone, is a potent endogenous vasoconstrictor substance produced by endothelial cells. Preproendothelin, a 203-amino-acid peptide, is the endothelin precursor. Initial cleavage by endogenous endopeptidases forms a 39-amino-acid residue called *proendothelin* or *big endothelin*, which is then cleaved to the active endothelin-1 by an endothelin-specific converting enzyme. This enzyme is predominantly bound to the cell membrane but is also present within the cytoplasm. C—carboxyl terminal; N—amino terminal. (*Adapted from* Yanagisawa and coworkers [29]; with permission.)

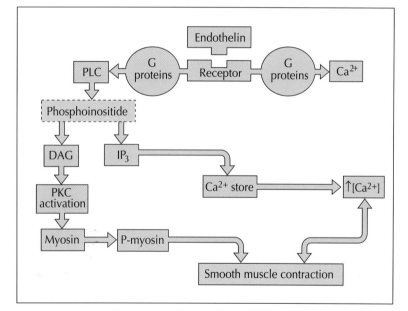

FIGURE 6-39. Endothelin exerts its action via binding with a specific receptor on the cell membrane, which is linked via guanine nucleotide regulatory binding proteins (G proteins) to stimulation of phospholipase C (PLC) and opening of voltage-dependent calcium channels. Activation of PLC degrades phosphoinositide to form inositol trisphosphate (IP$_3$) and diacylglycerol (DAG), second messengers that release calcium from intracellular stores and promote the activation of protein kinase C (PKC), respectively. (*Adapted from* Masaki and coworkers [30]; with permission.)

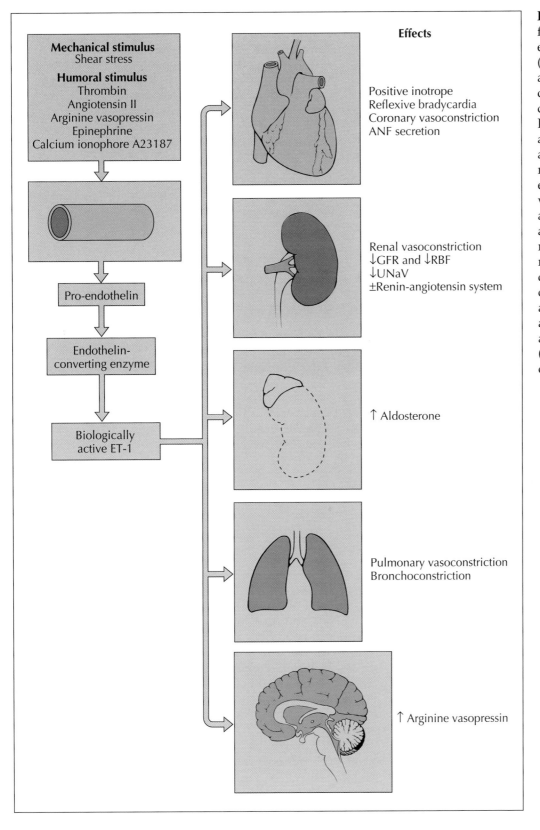

Effects

Positive inotrope
Reflexive bradycardia
Coronary vasoconstriction
ANF secretion

Renal vasoconstriction
↓GFR and ↓RBF
↓UNaV
±Renin-angiotensin system

↑ Aldosterone

Pulmonary vasoconstriction
Bronchoconstriction

↑ Arginine vasopressin

Mechanical stimulus
Shear stress

Humoral stimulus
Thrombin
Angiotensin II
Arginine vasopressin
Epinephrine
Calcium ionophore A23187

Pro-endothelin

Endothelin-
converting enzyme

Biologically
active ET-1

FIGURE 6-40. Summary of the stimuli for endothelin secretion and effects of endothelin in several organs. Mechanical (shear stress) and humoral (thrombin, angiotensin II, vasopressin, epinephrine, calcium ionophore A23187) stimuli may cause the release of endothelin-1 (ET-1). Endothelin increases circulating levels of atrial natriuretic factor (ANF), vasopressin, and aldosterone. It also modulates renin release. Endothelin has a positive inotropic effect and produces coronary and systemic vasoconstriction. These responses produce an increase in blood pressure that is associated with a reflex decrease in heart rate. ET-1 constricts human pulmonary resistance vessels and has a potent bronchoconstrictor effect. Furthermore, ET-1 causes renal vasoconstriction, leading to a reduction in renal blood flow (RBF) and glomerular filtration rate (GFR) and a decrease in urinary sodium excretion (UNaV). (*Adapted from* Underwood and coworkers [31]; with permission.)

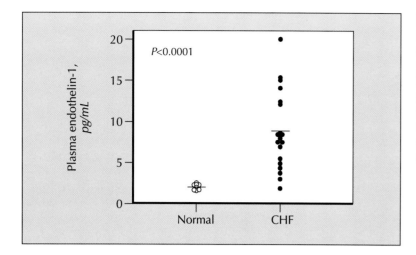

FIGURE 6-41. Cody *et al.* [32] measured immunoreactive circulating endothelin-1 in 12 normal control subjects and in 20 patients with congestive heart failure (CHF). Plasma endothelin-1 was 3.7±0.6 pg/mL in the control group and 9.1±4.1 pg/mL in the CHF group. Increased endothelin synthesis by angiotensin I and vasopressin stimulation and decreased endothelin clearance may contribute to the increased plasma endothelin levels in CHF. Of note, there was a strong positive correlation between endothelin levels and the severity of pulmonary hypertension. (*Adapted from* Cody and coworkers [32]; with permission.)

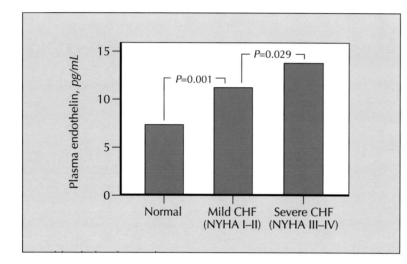

FIGURE 6-42. Rodeheffer *et al.* [33] measured plasma endothelin in 71 normal subjects, 24 patients with mild congestive heart failure (CHF), and 32 patients with severe congestive heart failure (New York Heart Association [NYHA] functional classes are shown in parentheses). The mean plasma concentration of endothelin was 7.1±0.1 pg/mL in the control group, 11.1±0.7 pg/mL in the mild heart failure group, and 13.8±0.9 pg/mL in the severe heart failure group. These data demonstrate that plasma endothelin is significantly increased in patients with CHF and that the level is correlated with the severity of the disease. (*Adapted from* Rodeheffer and coworkers [33].)

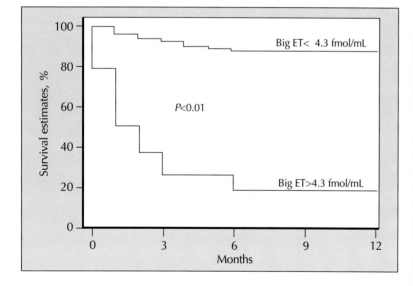

FIGURE 6-43 The prognostic implications of endothelin-1 for patients with congestive heart failure. Pacher *et al.* [34] measured plasma big endothelin-1 (Big ET) concentrations and 16 clinical, hemodynamic, and neurohumoral variables in 113 patients with left ventricular ejection fraction (LVEF) less than 20% and related these to 1-year mortality. Of the 113 patients, there were 58 1-year survivors, 29 nonsurvivors, and 26 heart transplant recipients. Plasma Big ET concentrations were lower in 1-year survivors than in nonsurvivors (2.6±0.1 vs 5.9±0.4 fmol/mL; *P*=0.0001). Cumulative rates of survival over 1 year in 87 patients with severe chronic heart failure (excluding 26 transplant recipients) were stratified into two groups according to Big ET concentration. Survival rates were significantly lower in the patients whose plasma endothelin-1 levels were greater than 4.3 fmol/mL. By multivariate analysis, taking into consideration plasma endothelin 1 concentration, functional class, furosemide dose, LVEF, hemodynamic variables, and plasma atrial natriuretic peptide, renin activity, and aldosterone levels, only plasma Big ET and functional class predicted 1-year mortality (*P*<0.0001). (*Adapted from* Pacher and coworkers [34].)

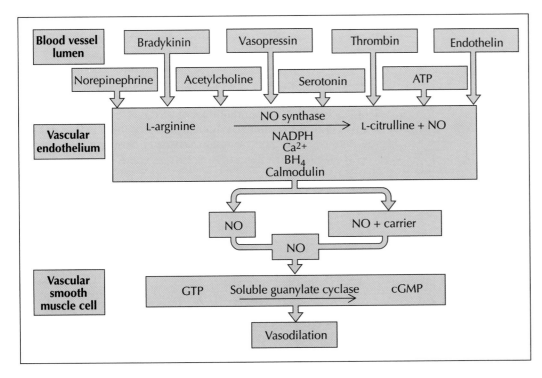

FIGURE 6-44. Vascular endothelial cells synthesize both vasodilators (endothelium-derived relaxing factor [EDRF] and prostacyclin) and vasoconstrictors (*eg*, endothelin and vasoconstrictor prostanoids). EDRF is released in response to a wide variety of stimuli (acetylcholine, norepinephrine, vasopressin, thrombin, endothelin, ATP, serotonin, bradykinin, calcium ionophore A23187). EDRF is nitric oxide (NO), or a related nitroso compound, derived from the metabolism of the amino acid L-arginine, a reaction that is catalyzed by the enzyme NO synthase and requiring the presence of calcium, NADPH (nicotinamide adenine dinucleotide phosphate), tetrahydrobiopterin (BH_4), and calmodulin as cofactors. NO synthase is competitively inhibited by L-arginine analogs. NO is released from the endothelium either as a free radical or combined with a carrier molecule. NO activates the vascular smooth muscle–soluble enzyme guanylate cyclase, increasing cGMP, thereby causing vasodilatation.

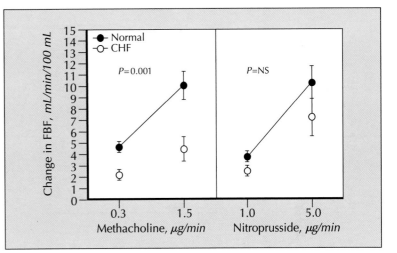

FIGURE 6-46. Abnormal endothelium-dependent relaxation of forearm resistance vessels in patients with congestive heart failure (CHF). Kubo *et al.* [36] measured the forearm blood flow (FBF) response to methacholine, an endothelium-dependent vasodilator, and nitroprusside, an endothelium-independent vasodilator, in eight normal subjects and in 10 patients with CHF. There was a significant decrease in the response to methacholine in heart failure patients compared with normal subjects. There was no significant difference in the response to nitroprusside. These data suggest that endothelium-dependent relaxation is impaired in patients with CHF. (*Adapted from* Kubo and coworkers [36].)

FIGURE 6-45. Endothelium-dependent relaxation of the coronary arteries in congestive heart failure. Treasure *et al.* [35] studied the coronary blood flow responses to serial infusions of acetylcholine and adenosine in seven normal subjects and eight patients with dilated cardiomyopathy (DCM). Infusion of acetylcholine produced a dose-dependent increase in coronary blood flow in normal subjects but not in patients with congestive heart failure. Infusion of adenosine produced a dose-dependent increase in coronary blood flow in both groups. Thus, endothelium-dependent vasodilatation was significantly diminished in heart failure patients, but the maximal vasodilator response to adenosine was similar in both groups. (*Adapted from* Treasure and coworkers [35]; with permission.)

POTENTIAL MECHANISMS FOR IMPAIRED ENDOTHELIUM-MEDIATED VASODILATION IN HEART FAILURE

Impaired endothelial cell receptor function or postreceptor signaling

Deficiency of L-arginine substrate

Abnormal nitric oxide synthase expression or function

Deficient or abnormal nitric oxide synthase cofactors

Impaired release or diffusion of EDRF

Increased degradation of EDRF

Concomitant release of EDCFs

Abnormal cGMP or cGMP-dependent protein phosphorylation

Nonspecifically impaired smooth-muscle vasodilator response

FIGURE 6-47. Potential mechanisms for impaired endothelium-mediated vasodilation in heart failure. The postulated mechanisms for impaired endothelium- mediated vasodilation include impaired endothelial cell receptor function or postreceptor signaling; deficiency of L-arginine substrate; abnormal nitric oxide synthase expression or function; deficient or abnormal nitric oxide synthase cofactor, such as calcium, calmodulin, or NADPH; impaired release or diffusion of endothelium-derived relaxing factor (EDRF); increased degradation of EDRF, concomitant release of endothelium-derived contracting factors (EDCFs), such as thromboxane A_2 and prostaglandin H_2; abnormal cGMP or cGMP-dependent protein phosphorylation; or a nonspecifically impaired smooth-muscle vasodilator response. (*Adapted from* Kubo and Bank [37].)

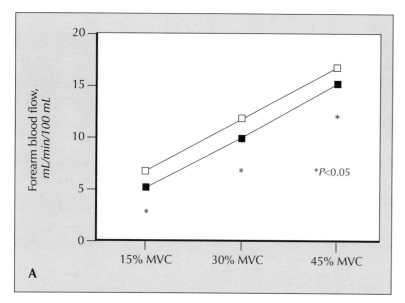

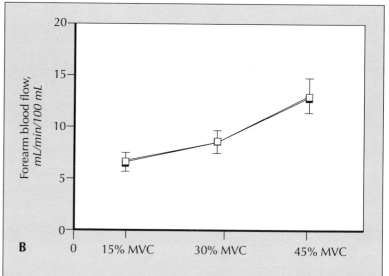

FIGURE 6-48. Endothelium-derived nitric oxide contributes, in part, to exercise-induced vasodilation. Katz *et al.* [38] studied the contribution of nitric oxide–mediated vasodilation during exercise in patients with congestive heart failure. Forearm blood flow was measured at baseline and during rhythmic handgrip exercise before (*open squares*) and after (*closed squares*) regional inhibition of nitric oxide synthesis by N^G-monomethyl-L-arginine (L-NMMA), which was infused into the brachial artery of 17 patients with congestive heart failure and 10 age-matched healthy subjects. Before the administration of L-NMMA, forearm vasodilation during rhythmic handgrip exercise (15%, 30% and 45% maximum voluntary contraction [MVC]) was slightly, albeit not significantly, lower than that in normal subjects. After the administration of L-NMMA, the forearm vasodilator response to exercise decreased in the healthy subjects (**A**) but did not change in the patients with heart failure (**B**). These findings indicate that endothelium-derived nitric oxide contributes to exercise-induced vasodilation in healthy subjects and that exercise-induced vasodilation mediated by nitric oxide is reduced in the forearm circulation of patients with heart failure (*Adapted from* Katz and coworkers [38].)

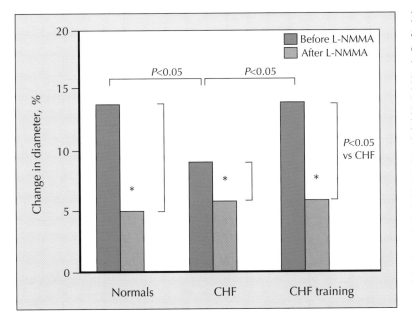

FIGURE 6-49. Increase in shear stress, as occurs when flow is accelerated, stimulates the release of endothelium-derived nitric oxide from blood vessels. Flow-mediated, endothelium-dependent vasodilation, as assessed by vascular ultrasonography, is reduced in limb arteries of patients with congestive heart failure (CHF). Hornig *et al.* [39] studied the effect of physical training on flow-mediated endothelium-dependent vasodilation in patients with heart failure and age-matched healthy subjects. Flow-mediated vasodilation, induced by reactive hyperemia, was assessed in each group of subjects before and after administration of the nitric oxide synthase antagonist, N^G-monomethyl-L-arginine (L-NMMA). Measurements were made at baseline, after 4 weeks of handgrip training, and 6 weeks after the training program was discontinued. Prior to training, flow-mediated vasodilation was reduced in patients with heart failure compared with healthy subjects (8.6%±0.9% versus 13.5% ±0.7%; $P<0.05$). After 4 weeks of handgrip training, flow-mediated vasodilation in the patients with heart failure increased to 13.6%±0.9%. After training, the portion of flow-mediated vasodilation inhibited by L-NMMA was significantly increased compared with baseline and was similar to that observed in healthy subjects. These findings indicate that physical training improves flow-mediated vasodilation in patients with CHF, most likely by enhancing endothelial release of nitric oxide. *Asterisks* indicate $P<0.05$ versus corresponding value before L-NMMA. (*Adapted from* Hornig and coworkers [39].)

REGIONAL BLOOD FLOW

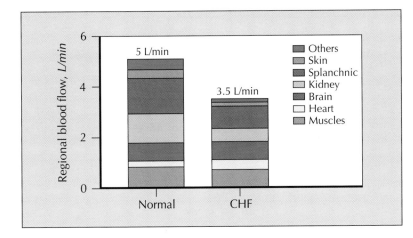

FIGURE 6-50. Distribution of regional blood flow at rest in normal subjects and in patients with congestive heart failure (CHF). The net effect of the various vasoconstricting and vasodilating systems that are activated in CHF is to redistribute the cardiac output. (*Adapted from* Zelis and coworkers [40]; with permission.)

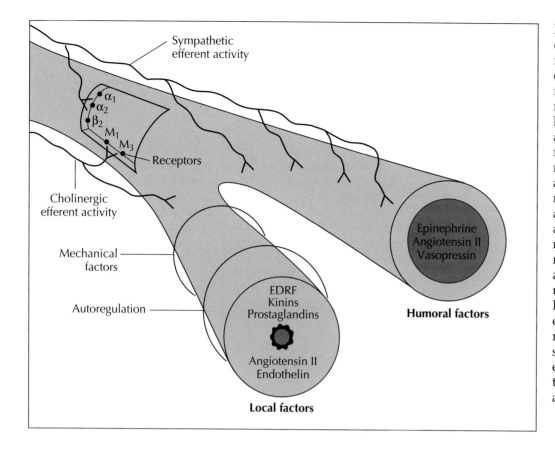

FIGURE 6-51. Peripheral blood flow is determined by the interaction of multiple factors. These factors include sympathetic efferent activity (modulated by baroreceptors, chemoreceptors, and somatic receptors), cholinergic efferent activity, humoral factors (such as epinephrine, angiotensin II, and vasopressin), local factors (such as endothelium-derived relaxing factor [EDRF], endothelin, angiotensin II, prostaglandins, and kinins), mechanical factors (such as muscle activity and cutaneous thermoregulation), and autoregulatory mechanisms (including myogenic reflexes and metabolism-induced responses). Increased sympathetic efferent activity modulated by blunted baroreceptors, systemic increases in angiotensin II and vasopressin, local increases in endothelin and prostaglandins, local reduction of EDRF, and mechanical factors, such as increased arterial wall sodium and extravascular tissue edema, all contribute to the decreased peripheral blood flow associated with congestive heart failure [41].

REFERENCES

1. Francis GS, Benedict C, Johnstone DE, *et al.*: Comparison of neuroendocrine activation in patients with left ventricular dysfunction with and without congestive heart failure. *Circulation* 1990, 82:1724–1729.

2. Francis GS, Cohn JN, Johnson G, *et al.*: Plasma norepinephrine, plasma renin activity and congestive heart failure: relations to survival and the effects of therapy in V-HeFT II. *Circulation* 1993, 87 (suppl V):140–148.

3. Vanhoutte PM, Luscher TF: Peripheral mechanisms in cardiovascular regulation: transmitters, receptors and the endothelium. In *Handbook of Hypertension*, vol 8. Edited by Tarazi RC, Zanchetti A. Amsterdam: Elsevier Science Publishers; 1986:96–123.

4. Davis D, Baily R, Zelis R: Abnormalities in systemic norepinephrine kinetics in human congestive heart failure. *Am J Physiol* 1988, 254(suppl E) :760–766.

5. Leimbach WN Jr, Wallin BG, Victor RG, *et al.*: Direct evidence from intraneural recordings for increased central sympathetic outflow in patients with heart failure. *Circulation* 1986, 73:913–919.

6. Paganelli WC, Creager MA, Dzau VJ: Cardiac regulation of renal function. In *The International Textbook of Cardiology*. Edited by Cheng TO. New York: Pergammon Press; 1986:1010–1020.

7. Dibner-Dunlap ME, Thames MD: Baroreflex control of renal sympathetic nerve activity is preserved in heart failure despite reduced arterial baroreceptor sensitivity. *Circ Res* 1989, 65:1526–1535.

8. Wang W, Chen J-S, Zucker IH: Carotid sinus baroreceptor sensitivity in experimental heart failure. *Circulation* 1990, 81:1959–1966.

9. Sopher SM, Smith ML, Eckberg DL, *et al.*: Autonomic pathophysiology in heart failure: carotid baroreceptor-cardiac reflexes. *Am J Physiol* 1990, 259:H689–H696.

10. Creager MA: Baroreceptor reflex function in congestive heart failure. *Am J Cardiol* 1992, 69:10G–16G.

11. Ferguson DW, Abboud FM, Mark AL: Selective impairment of baroreflex mediated vasoconstrictor responses in patients with ventricular dysfunction. *Circulation* 1984, 69:451–460.

12. Kaye DM, Jennings GL, Dart AM, Esler MD: Differential effect of acute baroreceptor unloading on cardiac and systemic sympathetic tone in congestive heart failure. *J Am Coll Cardiol* 1998, 31:583–587.

13. Floras JS: Clinical aspects of sympathetic activation and parasympathetic withdrawal in heart failure. *J Am Coll Cardiol* 1993, 22:72A–84A.

14. Cohn JN, Levine B, Olivari MT, *et al.*: Plasma norepinephrine as a guide to prognosis in patients with chronic congestive heart failure. *N Engl J Med* 1984, 311:819–823.

15. Benedict CR, Shelton B, Johnstone DE, *et al.* for the SOLVD Investigators: Prognostic significance of plasma norepinephrine in patients with asymptomatic left ventricular dysfunction. *Circulation* 1996, 94:690–697.

16. Cody RJ, Laragh JH: The role of the renin-angiotensin-aldosterone system in the pathophysiology of chronic heart failure. In *Drug Treatment of Chronic Heart Failure*. Edited by Cohn J. New York: Advanced Therapeutics Communications; Yorke Medical Publications; 1983:35–51.

17. Hirsch AT, Pinto YM, Schunkert D, *et al.*: Potential role of the tissue renin-angiotensin system in the pathophysiology of congestive heart failure. *Am J Cardiol* 1990, 66:22D–32D.

18. Hirsch AT, Creager MA: The peripheral circulation in heart failure. In *Congestive Heart Failure*. Edited by Hosenpud JD, Greenberg BH. Heidelberg: Springer-Verlag; 1994:145–160.

19. Dzau VJ: Short- and long-term determinants of cardiovascular function and therapy: contributions of circulating and tissue renin-angiotensin systems. *J Cardiovasc Pharmacol* 1989, 14(suppl 4):T1–T5.

20. Creager MA, Halperin AL, Bernard DB, *et al.*: Acute regional circulatory and renal hemodynamic effects of converting enzyme inhibition in patients with congestive heart failure. *Circulation* 1981, 64:483–489.

21. Packer M: Interaction of prostaglandins and angiotensin II in the modulation of renal function in congestive heart failure. *Circulation* 1988, 77:I64–I73.

22. Francis GS, Goldsmith SR, Levine BT, *et al.*: The neurohumoral axis in congestive heart failure. *Ann Intern Med* 1984, 101:370–377.

23. Creager MA, Faxon DP, Cutler SS, *et al.*: Contribution of vasopressin to vasoconstriction in patients with congestive heart failure: comparison with the renin angiotensin system and the sympathetic nervous system. *J Am Coll Cardiol* 1986, 7:758–765.

24. Wilkins MR, Redondo J, Brown LA: The natriuretic-peptide family. *Lancet* 1997, 349:1307–1310.

25. Cody RJ, Atlas SA, Laragh JH, *et al.*: Atrial natriuretic factor in normal subjects and heart failure patients. *J Clin Invest* 1986, 78:1362–1374.

26. Wei C-M, Lerman A, Rodeheffer RJ, *et al.*: Endothelin in human congestive heart failure. *Circulation* 1994, 89:1580–1586.

27. Tsutamoto T, Wada A, Maeda K, *et al.*: Attenuation of compensation of endogenous cardiac natriuretic peptide system in chronic heart failure. *Circulation* 1997, 96:509–516.

28. Jougasaki M, Rodeheffer RJ, Redfield MM, *et al.*: Cardiac secretion of adrenomedullin in human heart failure. *J Clin Invest* 1996, 97:2370– 2376.

29. Yanagisawa M, Kurihara S, Kimura S, *et al.*: A novel potent vaso-constrictor peptide produced by vascular endothelial cells. *Nature* 1988, 332:411–415.

30. Masaki T, Yanagisawa M, Goto K, *et al.*: Cardiovascular significance of endothelin. In *Cardiovascular Significance of Endothelium-Derived Vasoactive Factors*. Edited by Rubanyi GM. Mt. Kisco, NY: Futura Publishing; 1991:65–81.

31. Underwood RD, Chan DP, Burnett JC: Endothelin: an endothelium derived vasoconstrictor peptide and its role in congestive heart failure. *Heart Failure* 1991, 7:50–58.

32. Cody RJ, Haas GJ, Binkley PF, *et al.*: Plasma endothelin correlates with the extent of the pulmonary hypertension in patients with chronic congestive heart failure. *Circulation* 1992, 85:504–509.

33. Rodeheffer RJ, Lerman A, Heublein DM, *et al.*: Increased plasma concentrations of endothelin in congestive heart failure in humans. *Mayo Clin Proc* 1992, 67:719–724.

34. Pacher R, Stanek B, Hülsmann M, *et al.*: Prognostic impact of big endothelin-1 plasma concentrations compared with invasive hemodynamic evaluation in severe heart failure. *J Am Coll Cardiol* 1996, 27:633–641.

35. Treasure CB, Vita JA, Cox DA, *et al.*: Endothelium dependent dilation of the coronary microvasculature is impaired in dilated cardiomyopathy. *Circulation* 1990, 81:772–779.

36. Kubo SH, Rector TS, Bank AJ, *et al.*: Endothelium dependent vasodilation is attenuated in patients with heart failure. *Circulation* 1991, 84:1589–1596.

37. Kubo SH, Bank AJ: Endothelium dependent vasodilation in heart failure. *Heart Failure* 1992, 8:142–153.

38. Katz SD, Krum H, Khan T, Knecht M: Exercise-induced vasodilation in forearm circulation of normal subjects and patients with congestive heart failure: role of endothelium-derived nitric oxide. *J Am Coll Cardiol* 1996, 28:585–590.

39. Hornig B, Maier V, Drexler H: Physical training improves endothelial function in patients with chronic heart failure. *Circulation* 1996, 93:210–214.

40. Zelis R, Nellis S, Longhurst J, *et al.*: Abnormalities in the regional circulations accompanying congestive heart failure. *Prog Cardiovasc Dis* 1975, 18:181–199.

41. Hirsch AT, Dzau VJ, Creager MA: Baroreceptor function in congestive heart failure: effect on neurohumoral activation and regional vascular resistance. *Circulation* 1987, 75(suppl IV):36–48.

Management of Heart Failure

ASSESSMENT OF HEART FAILURE

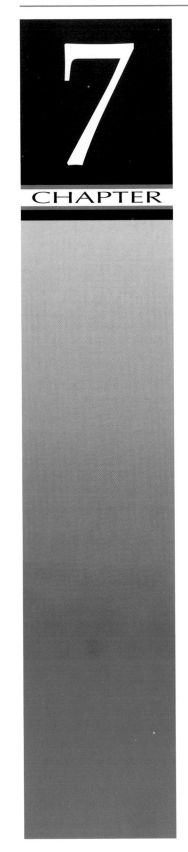

CHAPTER 7

James B. Young

The clinical syndrome of heart failure may result from cardiac disease of many different etiologies. It reflects both the primary hemodynamic abnormalities caused by cardiac dysfunction and the consequences of multiple secondary compensatory systems (*eg*, vasoconstriction, neurohormonal activation, metabolic imbalance). Not surprisingly, the clinical manifestations of heart failure show a striking heterogeneity and, as a consequence, the clinical assessment of patients with heart failure is among the most challenging in medicine [1–3].

Traditionally, physicians have looked for symptoms and signs that reflect abnormal fluid retention or organ congestion [4,5]. Although many patients present with these "congestive" findings, it has become apparent that many more patients with heart failure can be diagnosed earlier in the course of the illness, with symptoms secondary to reduced exercise capacity, fatigue, or arrhythmia [6–10]. Particularly challenging is the treatment of elderly patients [3] and those with occult or minimally symptomatic left ventricular systolic dysfunction [7,10].

The signs and symptoms of heart failure may present acutely, as with the fulminant onset of myocarditis, or they may develop gradually, such as several years after an uncomplicated myocardial infarction. Pulmonary or systemic congestion may appear suddenly in a patient with previously undetected or compensated heart failure (*eg*, due to a change in salt intake or the initiation of a nonsteroidal anti-inflammatory drug). The presentation of signs and symptoms of heart failure may also reflect the nature of the underlying cardiac dysfunction (*eg*, right versus left heart failure), and there is increasing awareness that many patients with heart failure have predominantly diastolic (versus systolic) ventricular dysfunction [11]. Such patients may present with marked clinical symptoms and signs, despite a normal or nearly normal left ventricular ejection fraction. The prevalence of symptomatic heart failure is increasing because of the growing population of elderly individuals predisposed to this condition by the long-term effects of coronary heart disease, valvular disease, or systemic conditions such as hypertension and diabetes mellitus [12–14]. In these patients, heart failure is often due predominantly to diastolic dysfunction and is frequently undetected because the symptoms are attributed to the normal consequences of aging or other coexistent illnesses.

The assessment of patients with heart failure should include efforts to characterize the etiology, determine the severity, and identify factors that may have precipitated clinical decompensation. Several questions should be posed during the evaluation of a patient for heart failure: Are the symptoms and signs caused by heart failure or by any of several noncardiac conditions that can cause similar findings? What is the etiology of cardiac dysfunction? What is the severity of the cardiac dysfunction? What is the level of functional impairment? What is the prognosis? What is the optimal therapeutic approach? Arriving at the correct answers to these questions begins with taking a complete history and conducting a full physical examination, supplemented by appropriate hematologic and blood chemistry determinations, an electrocardiogram, and chest radiograph. In the large majority of patients in whom there is a suspicion of heart failure, an echocardiogram is important to clarify cardiac anatomy and function. An assessment of exercise capacity is also frequently helpful to quantify the level of functional impairment, detect inducible myocardial ischemia, exclude noncardiac (*eg*, pulmonary) causes of dyspnea, and determine prognosis. Additional tests, including radionuclide studies, cardiac catheterization, and myocardial biopsy, may be needed to complete the evaluation in selected patients.

It is now recognized that asymptomatic cardiac dysfunction can be present for long periods prior to the development of clinically evident signs and symptoms of decompensation [7–15]. Because there is evidence (*see* Chapter 5) that treatment of asymptomatic individuals can delay or even prevent the progression to symptomatic disease and improve prognosis, early diagnosis of asymptomatic or minimally symptomatic ventricular dysfunction is of para-mount importance. Because of the growing importance of appropriate diagnosis and treatment of heart failure, the Agency for Health Care Policy and Research (AHCPR) has issued guidelines regarding evaluation and care of patients with symptomatic left ventricular systolic dysfunction [16]. At the heart of these guidelines is proper assessment of patients suspected to have heart failure.

OVERVIEW OF THE ASSESSMENT

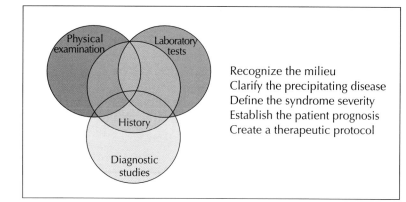

Recognize the milieu
Clarify the precipitating disease
Define the syndrome severity
Establish the patient prognosis
Create a therapeutic protocol

FIGURE 7-1. Specific goals of patient evaluation when heart failure is suspected. First, one must appropriately recognize the heart failure syndrome and differentiate heart and circulatory failure from problems that cause similar complaints and findings. Second, by staging the severity of heart failure, the clinician can establish prognosis with reasonable accuracy. This is important in the design of therapeutic protocols to treat certain aspects of the syndrome. Finally, identifying the primary etiology of myocardial dysfunction and determining the precipitating causes of decompensation are extremely important. The interplay of patient history, physical examination, laboratory tests, and specific diagnostic studies helps the clinician achieve these goals. (*Adapted from* Konstam and coworkers [16].)

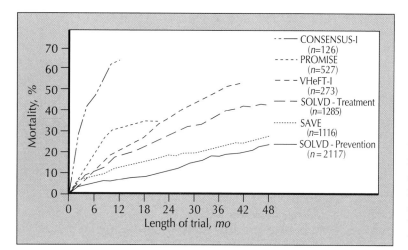

FIGURE 7-2. Clinical heart failure trials: placebo mortality curves. The data from several large, placebo-controlled clinical trials completed in the last few years emphasize that patients with heart failure or asymptomatic ventricular dysfunction represent a wide spectrum of morbidity and mortality risks. The CONSENSUS-I (Cooperative North Scandinavian Enalapril Survival Study) trial evaluated patients with New York Heart Association (NYHA) class

IV congestive heart failure treated with diuretics and digitalis [17]. The placebo cohort demonstrated a mortality at 12 months in excess of 60%. Patients in this trial had ejection fractions of 35% or less.

These patients should be compared with the placebo cohorts of the SOLVD (Studies of Left Ventricular Dysfunction)-Prevention trial [18] and SAVE (Survival and Ventricular Enlargement) Trial [19]. These studies were also performed in patients with ventricular dysfunction (ejection fraction of ≤35% in SOLVD and <40% in SAVE). Patients were asymptomatic after myocardial infarction in SAVE, and either asymptomatic or minimally symptomatic (NYHA class I and II) in SOLVD-Prevention. Twelve-month placebo mortality rates in these groups, in contrast to the CONSENSUS-I cohort, were around 10%. At the 48-month follow-up point, mortality was substantial (about 20%), but was still dramatically less than that typically noted in patients with symptomatic congestive heart failure.

The first Veterans Administration Heart Failure Trial (VHeFT-I) [20], SOLVD Treatment Trial [21], and PROMISE (Prospective Randomized Milrinone Survival Evaluation) Trials [22] included patients with mild to moderate congestive heart failure (usually NYHA class II or III). In these trials, a gradation in placebo group mortality can be noted, with the curves falling between the less ill SAVE or SOLVD-Prevention trial cohorts and the more ill CONSENSUS-I patients.

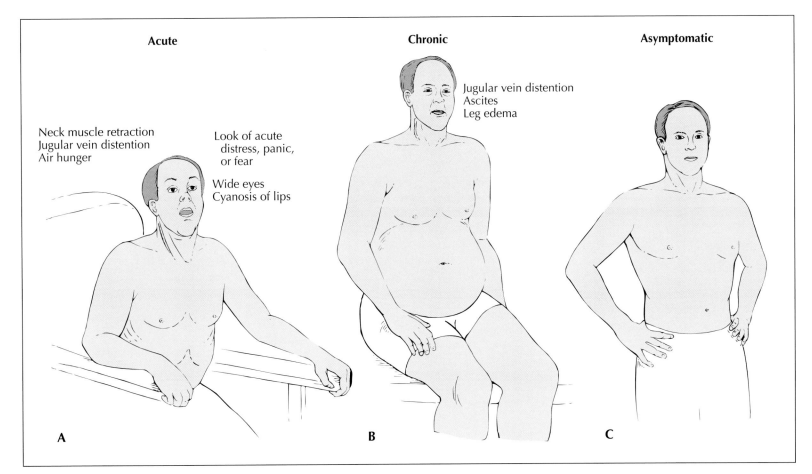

Acute   Chronic   Asymptomatic

Neck muscle retraction
Jugular vein distention
Air hunger

Look of acute
distress, panic,
or fear

Wide eyes
Cyanosis of lips

Jugular vein distention
Ascites
Leg edema

A   B   C

FIGURE 7-3. The varied faces of heart failure. When heart failure is discussed, patients with pulmonary edema, such as the patient with acute, distressing air hunger (**A**), or those with chronic congestive heart failure, such as the patient with edema (**B**), often come to mind. This is not unreasonable, because heart failure traditionally was diagnosed when congestion developed [14].

We now know that the patient who appears fit and has few complaints (**C**) may also have heart failure. In fact, the majority of patients with left ventricular dysfunction do not manifest congestive symptomatology or findings. The detection of heart failure in such patients is challenging.

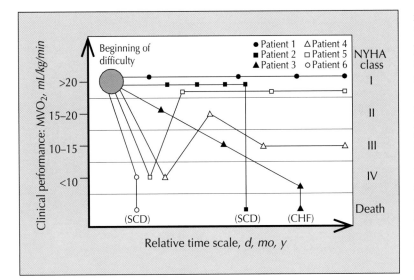

FIGURE 7-4. Variability of natural history of congestive heart failure (CHF). Patients can present at a variety of points during their illness [17–21]. Initial patient contact may be triggered by an episode of acute pulmonary edema caused by severe diastolic dysfunction (perhaps precipitated by hypertension or ventricular ischemia), or symptoms may have been developing insidiously over several

months as the heart dilates slowly in response to chronic alcohol toxicity. A variety of theoretic courses are plotted in this figure; a patient might present at any of the marked points. Patient 1, for example, is one in whom myocardial infarction has caused asymptomatic left ventricular (LV) dysfunction. In this patient, clinical compensation is present, ongoing ischemia is absent, and exercise performance is adequate. The patient is discovered to have systolic LV dysfunction during echocardiography performed before hospital discharge, and remains asymptomatic throughout long-term follow-up. Patient 2 has ischemic heart disease, myocardial infarction, mild to moderate LV dysfunction, and adequate exercise performance. This patient, without preceding congestive decompensation, suffers sudden cardiac death (SCD). Patient 3 is one in whom myocardial injury is steadily progressive over time, causing gradual clinical deterioration until death from CHF ensues. Patients 4 and 5 develop substantive and debilitating CHF but improve with treatment. However, whereas patient 4, despite aggressive therapy, continues to experience moderately severe CHF (New York Heart Association [NYHA] class III), patient 5 does not exhibit recurrence of congestive symptomatology and achieves adequate exercise performance during long-term follow-up. Patient 6 deteriorates dramatically, with SCD occurring soon after the diagnosis of CHF has been made. MVO$_2$—myocardial oxygen consumption.

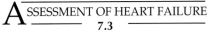

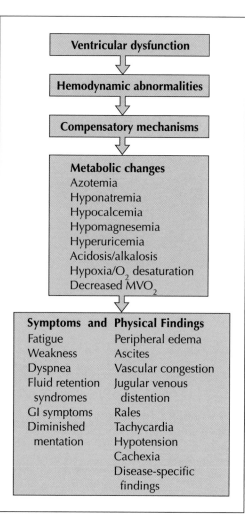

FIGURE 7-5. Clinical presentation of heart failure. The primary myocardial injury (multiple different diseases) produces ventricular dysfunction, resulting in subsequent hemodynamic abnormalities that eventually cause clinical manifestations of heart failure. A period of clinical compensation is often observed, during which patients are asymptomatic. A variety of symptoms, physical findings, and metabolic abnormalities may occur in heart failure. Symptoms can be exacerbated or attenuated, depending on fluctuations in hemodynamic abnormalities, adequacy of physiologic compensatory mechanisms, and the success of therapeutic intervention. Death in patients with heart failure can result from systemic organ failure (caused by hypoperfusion or congestion) or from sudden cardiac death (caused by the lethal arrhythmias that commonly accompany heart failure). Pulmonary embolism, stroke, or concurrent diseases that precipitate heart failure can also cause death. GI—gastrointestinal. MVO_2—myocardial oxygen consumption.

CIRCULATORY FAILURE WITHOUT OVERT MYOCYTE DYSFUNCTION

Sudden pressure or volume overload

Acute systemic afterload increase
(sudden onset of malignant hypertension)

Acute pulmonary hypertension (pulmonary embolism)

Acute volume overload (valvular regurgitation)

Chronic pressure or volume overload

Chronic high cardiac output states
(arteriovenous fistulae, Paget's disease, anemia)

Valvular heart disease (rheumatic aortic stenosis)

Congenital heart disease (ventricular septal defect)

Impaired cardiac filling

Pericardial restrictions (effusion, constriction)

Restrictive myocardial disease
(amyloidosis, hemochromatosis)

Hypertrophic cardiomyopathy (many cases)

Mechanical obstructions (valve stenosis, myxoma)

Arrhythmia (tachycardia, bradycardia, heart block)

FIGURE 7-6. Circulatory failure without overt myocyte dysfunction. Differentiating circulatory failure without overt myocyte dysfunction from primary abnormalities of the myocardium is important because of the therapeutic implications. Sudden pressure or volume overload, as may occur with malignant hypertension, pulmonary embolism, or acute valvular regurgitation, may present with acute heart failure even though myocardial contractility is normal. Likewise, certain types of chronic pressure or volume overload, such as aortic stenosis, arteriovenous fistulae, or septal defects, can cause heart failure with normal myocyte function. Impaired cardiac filling may also cause circulatory failure despite normal myocyte contractile function.

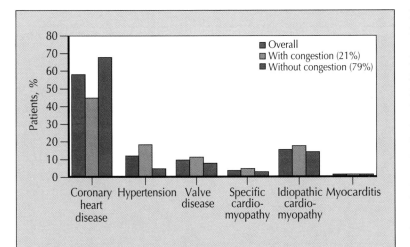

FIGURE 7-7. A contemporary analysis of the etiology of heart failure. The Registry of Studies of Left Ventricular Dysfunction (SOLVD) consisted of 6270 participants who were identified as having either left ventricular systolic dysfunction with an ejection fraction of less than 45% or clinical evidence of congestive heart failure with radiographic confirmation [23,24]. Thirty percent of the patients in the registry had ejection fractions of 35% or greater, and 14% of patients were identified on the basis of clinical congestive heart failure rather than depressed ventricular function. Patients were entered into this registry between January 1, 1988, and February 28, 1989. In the past, patients with congestive heart failure were most likely to have hypertensive or valvular heart disease. Today, however, coronary heart disease is the most common etiology [25]. The relative contributions of various etiologies were similar in patients with and without congestive symptoms. When assessing patients with suspected heart failure, particular attention should be paid to coronary heart disease and hypertension.

ASSESSING THE PATIENT

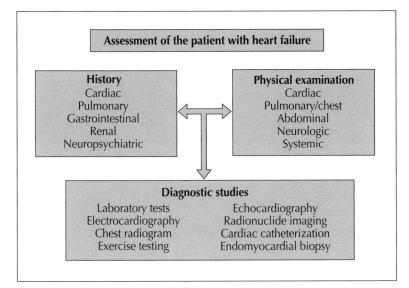

FIGURE 7-8. Approach to the problem of assessing heart failure. To adequately assess patients with heart failure, historical information, data from the physical examination, and diagnostic study information should be obtained and integrated. It should be emphasized that although information from all three categories may be used in the evaluation, not every test needs to be, or should be, performed. In most patients, an electrocardiogram, a chest radiograph, and an echocardiogram are performed. Additional diagnostic studies should be tailored to the patient. Echocardiography could include M-mode, two-dimensional, and Doppler studies. Radionuclide examination might consist of perfusion, performance, or positron emission tomographic studies. Cardiac catheterization could include angiography, hemodynamics, or endomyocardial biopsy in certain circumstances. Computed tomography and magnetic resonance imaging are sometimes useful, as is determination of maximal exercise oxygen consumption. Information obtained from the history and physical examination should dictate the need for and type of ancillary testing.

THE CLINICAL HISTORY IN ASSESSING HEART FAILURE

CARDIOVASCULAR	SYSTEMIC	PULMONARY	RENAL	GASTROENTEROLOGIC	NEUROLOGIC AND NEUROPSYCHIATRIC
Angina pectoris	Edema	Dyspnea on exertion	Nocturia	Abdominal pain	Anxiety or panic attacks
Nonspecific chest pain	Petechiae or ecchymosis	Orthopnea	Oliguria	Abdominal bloating	Depression
Fatigue	Diet	Paroxysmal nocturnal dyspnea	Anuria	Constipation	Syncope
Weakness	Medication use	Pleurisy		Anorexia	Confusion
Orthostatic faintness		Cough		Nausea	Decreased mental activity
Palpitations		Hemoptysis		Vomiting	
		Wheezing		Diarrhea	

FIGURE 7-9. Use of clinical history in assessing heart failure. Gathering historical information that documents and clarifies the clinical presentation is the first important task when heart failure is suspected. Although dyspnea is a hallmark of heart failure, it can also be characteristic of other conditions [26]. During history taking, a cardinal issue is the attempt to quantify the exertion level required to produce symptoms [27]. By eliciting the factors that cause symptoms, insight into the syndrome's severity can be gained. The assessment of heart failure focuses on objectively measured parameters that quantify cardiac dysfunction and subsequent physical limitations. Weakness, fatigue, dyspnea, and edema are considered the most common symptoms of heart failure. Obtaining an ancillary history that elucidates concomitant cardiovascular and noncardiovascular illnesses is also critical, as is assessment of medication use [28]. Many drugs can exacerbate heart failure (*eg*, antiarrhythmic drugs, β-adrenergic blockers, calcium channel blockers, and nonsteroidal anti-inflammatory agents), depending on the clinical situation, and thus their use should be characterized.

PHYSICAL FINDINGS TO PURSUE WHEN EXAMINING PATIENTS WITH HEART FAILURE

VITAL SIGNS	PULMONARY SIGNS
Positional blood pressure	Rales
Pulse rate, rhythm, and quality	Rhonchi
Respiratory rate and pattern	Friction rub
Temperature	Wheezes
Blood pressure response to Valsalva's maneuver	Dullness to percussion
Determination of proportional pulse pressure	Diaphragmatic impairment

CARDIOVASCULAR SIGNS	ABDOMINAL SIGNS
Neck-vein distention	Ascites
Abdominal-jugular neck-vein reflex	Hepatosplenomegaly
Cardiomegaly on palpation or percussion	Decreased bowel sounds
Chest wall pulsatile activity	Ileus
Gallop rhythm on auscultation	
Heart murmurs	NEUROLOGIC SIGNS
Diminished S_1 or S_2	Mental status abnormalities
Prominent P_2	SYSTEMIC SIGNS
Friction rub	Edema
	Cachexia
	Petechiae or ecchymosis
	Rash
	Arthritis

FIGURE 7-10. Physical findings to pursue when examining patients with heart failure. The physical examination of heart failure patients provides critical information that supplements data from the patient's history. Vital signs should be carefully measured. Positional blood pressure is important in patients receiving vasodilator drugs, as are pulse rate and rhythm. The presence of atrial fibrillation or frequent premature ventricular contractions has significant prognostic and therapeutic implications and can be suspected from analysis of the cardiac rhythm. The respiratory rate and pattern are important because tachypnea may reflect the severity of pulmonary congestion or compromise, and certain periodic respiratory patterns can be seen in the later stages of severe circulatory failure (*eg*, Cheyne-Stokes respirations).

Assessment of the blood pressure response to Valsalva's maneuver [29–31], calculation of proportional pulse pressure (pulse pressure divided by systolic pressure) [26], determination of augmented jugular vein distention after abdominal compression (hepatojugular reflux) [2–5,32,33], and thoracic percussion to identify cardiomegaly [34] are simple procedures that should be performed in every patient suspected of having heart failure or ventricular dysfunction. Distension of normally filled jugular veins or further distention of already filled jugular veins after gentle abdominal pressure suggests central venous congestion with volume overload. A proportional pulse pressure less than 0.25 has an 88% accuracy in predicting cardiac index less than 2.21/min/m². Cardiomegaly is suggested by a laterally displaced heart border detected by percussion [34]. The usual abnormalities searched for during cardiac examination, such as murmurs, rubs, and gallop sounds, must be sought.

Many findings that are routinely sought are well known and described, such as pulmonary rales, wheezes ("cardiac asthma"), ascites, and peripheral edema. Other findings, however, may be equally important and can provide insight into both the chronicity and the severity of disease. Cachexia, for example, points to long-standing heart failure that is often end-stage. Petechiae or ecchymoses suggest coagulopathy secondary to hepatic congestion. Examination of the integument can point toward the presence of systemic disease (*eg*, scleroderma, myxedema).

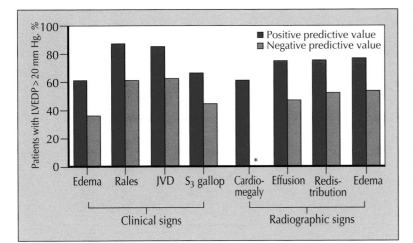

FIGURE 7-11. Predictive values of clinical findings in congestive heart failure (CHF) patients. Many studies have reviewed the clinical and radiographic findings often used to diagnose CHF [2–5,26,35–40].

These reports have consistently emphasized that, although in certain circumstances clinical findings might be quite accurate in the diagnosis of CHF, their reliability in predicting hemodynamics is limited. Absence of radiographic or physical signs of congestion does not necessarily ensure a normal pulmonary capillary wedge pressure, for example, and may lead to either an inaccurate diagnosis of heart failure or inadequate therapy [35].

This figure demonstrates that in one study of 52 consecutive patients with chronic CHF [35], detection of peripheral edema, pulmonary rales, jugular venous distension (JVD), and an S_3 gallop had positive predictive values ranging from 61% to 87%. Chest radiographic findings, such as cardiomegaly, pleural effusion, vascular redistribution suggesting congestion, and frank pulmonary edema, had similar positive and negative predictive values. The negative predictive value of cardiomegaly on chest radiography was not calculated (*asterisk*) because all but three patients had this finding. Thus, no single finding alone can be used to make the diagnosis [36–40]. LVEDP—left ventricular end-diastolic pressure.

FRAMINGHAM CRITERIA FOR DIAGNOSIS OF CONGESTIVE HEART FAILURE

MAJOR CRITERIA	MINOR CRITERIA	MAJOR OR MINOR
Paroxysmal nocturnal dyspnea	Extremity edema	Weight loss ≥4.5 kg over 5 days' treatment
Neck vein distension	Night cough	
Rales	Dyspnea on exertion	
Cardiomegaly	Hepatomegaly	
Acute pulmonary edema	Pleural effusion	
S_3 gallop	Vital capacity reduced by one third from normal	
Increased venous pressure (>16 cm H_2O)	Tachycardia (≥120 bpm)	
Positive hepatojugular reflux		

FIGURE 7-12. A constellation of symptoms and abnormal physical findings should be used in making the diagnosis of congestive heart failure. The Framingham Study results, for example, suggested that several specific clinical criteria be combined and weighted. To establish a clinical diagnosis of congestive heart failure by this method, at least one major and two minor criteria are required [13,14,41].

LABORATORY TESTS TO CONSIDER DURING ASSESSMENT OF PATIENTS WITH HEART FAILURE

Complete blood count (including white blood cell differential and platelet count)
Serum electrolyte level
Blood urea nitrogen
Serum creatinine (and clearance) level
Liver function tests
Prothrombin time
Erythrocyte sedimentation rate
Arterial blood gases (possibly with exercise) levels
Urinalysis
Biochemistry screen (ie, magnesium, uric acid, calcium, and phosphorus levels)
Thyroid function studies
Serum drug levels (ie, digoxin and anti-arrhythmic drugs)

FIGURE 7-13. Laboratory tests for assessment of patients with heart failure. A variety of laboratory studies should be considered during assessment of the patient with heart failure. In general, these studies help in estimating the severity of heart failure and provide information regarding problems that can be anticipated with therapeutic interventions. Some of these studies should be obtained (eg, thyroid function studies) in an attempt to diagnose causes of left ventricular dysfunction. Others are ordered to give insight into therapeutic or toxic effects of drugs commonly administered to patients with heart failure. Not all tests listed are necessary in every patient with heart failure. Ordinarily, sophisticated measures of plasma neurohumors, such as epinephrine, norepinephrine, vasopressin, renin, and so on, are not necessary or helpful in the diagnosis and management of individual patients with heart failure (although their importance with respect to the pathophysiology of the syndrome is unquestioned). Recently, Cowie *et al.* [10] demonstrated that in patients with symptoms suspected by a primary care physician to be due to heart failure, brain natriuretic peptide seemed a useful predictor of which patients are likely to have heart failure and require further clinical evaluation.

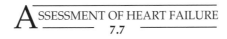

DIAGNOSTIC PROCEDURES TO CONSIDER DURING ASSESSMENT OF PATIENTS WITH HEART FAILURE

Aerobic exercise capacity testing
  Oxygen utilization at maximal exertion
  Time to anaerobic threshold
Cardiac catheterization
  Aortography
  Coronary angiography
  Hemodynamic assessment
  Ventriculography

Chest radiography
  Cardiac fluoroscopy
  Computerized tomographic
    scanning
  Echocardiogram
    M-mode
    Pulsed Doppler
    Two-dimensional

Electrocardiogram
  Ambulatory electrocardiogram
Electrophysiologic study
Magnetic resonance imaging
Positron-emission tomography
Pulmonary function testing
Radionuclide angiogram
Scintigraphic perfusion studies

FIGURE 7-14. Diagnostic procedures for assessment of patients with heart failure. There are many ancillary diagnostic tests to be considered during evaluation of the heart failure patient. These range from rather simple procedures, such as chest radiography and electrocardiography, to sophisticated studies, such as magnetic resonance imaging and positron-emission tomography. Whereas some are noninvasive, others, such as cardiac catheterization, require central vascular access. In planning assessment of the patient with heart failure, the risks, costs, and the type of information they can provide should dictate the selection of diagnostic tests.

DIAGNOSTIC TESTS AND THE INFORMATION THEY PROVIDE DURING ASSESSMENT OF HEART FAILURE

CHEST RADIOGRAPHY AND CARDIAC FLUOROSCOPY

Cardiothoracic ratio
Selective chamber size and shape
Cardiac or great vessel calcification
Pulmonary vascularity and congestion
Pleural effusions
Mass lesions or infiltrates
Mediastinal configuration
Great vessel abnormality

ELECTROCARDIOGRAPHY

Rhythm
  Atrial fibrillation
  Ventricular arrhythmias
  Atrioventricular conduction
Heart rate
Evidence of hypertrophy
Q waves
"P" mitrale or pulmonale
Conduction disturbances
Metabolic and drug effects (ST, T changes)

ECHOCARDIOGRAPHY (TWO-DIMENSIONAL AND M-MODE)

Chamber size and shape
Valve integrity and motion
Fractional shortening of ventricles
Mean circumferential fiber shortening
Mitral E-point to septal separation
Systolic wall thickening
Wall motion analysis
Estimation of wall stress
Endomyocardial biopsy guidance
Exercise and pharmacologic stress (wall motion)
Tissue characterization
Pericardial effusion
Pericardial restriction

DOPPLER ECHOCARDIOGRAPHY (PULSED AND CONTINUOUS WAVE)

Quantification of valve stenosis and regurgitation
  Estimation of pulmonary artery pressure
  Estimation of stroke volume and cardiac output
Determination of diastolic filling characteristics
Detection of shunts

FIGURE 7-15. Common ancillary diagnostic tests. The most commonly requested diagnostic tests in patients with heart failure are chest radiography, electrocardiography, and echocardiography (including M-mode, two-dimensional, and Doppler studies).

The chest radiogram can provide insight into cardiac size, pleural effusions, pulmonary congestion, and mediastinal configuration. Electrocardiography may suggest ischemic heart disease.

Echocardiography (M-mode, two-dimensional, or Doppler) provides an evaluation of the valves, chambers, pericardium, myocardium, and global function. More information is probably gained by echocardiographic examination of heart failure patients than by any other tests available.

A. NONINVASIVE IMAGING TECHNIQUES FOR ASSESSMENT OF PATIENTS WITH HEART FAILURE

OBSERVATION	FIRST-PASS RNVG	EQUILIBRIUM RNVG	MRI	CT
Anatomic relationships	0/+	+	++++	+++
Tissue characterization	0	0	+++	+++
Wall motion	++	++++	+++	+++
Hypertrophy	0	0/+	++++	+++
Wall thickening	0	0	++++	++
Valvular regurgitation and stenosis	0	0	++	+
Hemodynamics	0	0	0	0
Diastolic function	++	++	+	0
Stress exercise	++++	++++	0	0
Pharmacologic stress	++++	++++	+	+
Lower cost and easy availability	+++	+++	+	+

B. NONINVASIVE IMAGING TECHNIQUES FOR ASSESSMENT OF PATIENTS WITH HEART FAILURE

OBSERVATION	M-MODE ECHOCARDIOGRAPHY	TWO-DIMENSIONAL ECHOCARDIOGRAPHY	DOPPLER
Anatomic relationships	+	+++	0/+
Tissue characterization	++	++	0
Wall motion	+	++++	0
Hypertrophy	+++	++++	0
Wall thickening	+++	+++	0
Valvular regurgitation and stenosis	++	++	++++
Hemodynamics	+	+	++++
Diastolic function	++	+++	++++
Stress exercise	++++	++++	++++
Pharmacologic stress	+	++++	++
Lower cost and easy availability	++++	++++	+++

FIGURE 7-16. Noninvasive imaging techniques for assessment of patients with heart failure. A variety of noninvasive techniques can be used to provide greater insight into ventricular performance and to aid in the assessment of heart failure.

A, In addition to radionuclide techniques and echocardiography, magnetic resonance imaging (MRI) and computed tomographic (CT) studies can be valuable. MRI defines cardiac anatomy, clarifies anatomic relationships, characterizes tissue patterns, and may be the best method to quantify cardiac mass and chamber dimensions. It is, however, expensive. The major limitation of CT scans of the heart are the long exposure times required for the motion artifacts to be great. The major advantage of this form of cardiac imaging is that cross-sectional views with spatial and density orientation can

be produced and appear to be better than echocardiographic or radionuclide studies. CT scans also provide precise images of great-vessel orientation. Performance of stress testing, either physiologic or pharmacologic, can be difficult in the MRI or CT facility.

B, In general, echocardiography is readily available and costs less than radionuclide, MRI, or CT procedures. Echocardiography may be valuable and cost-effective when simple questions such as normal versus abnormal ventricular function or presence of pericardial effusion are asked. *Zero* represents no value; *plus signs* represent the relative value, *one plus sign* meaning minimal value and *four plus signs* meaning very valuable. RNGV—radionuclide ventriculography. (*Adapted from* Young and Farmer [1].)

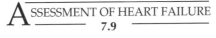

A. EXERCISE TESTING IN PATIENTS WITH HEART FAILURE

NYHA CLASS (SYMPTOM SEVERITY): IV — Severe; III — Moderate to severe; II — Mild to moderate; I — Minimal or asymptomatic

METS (mL O$_2$/kg/min)	WEBER-JANICKI STAGE (min)	SPEED, mph	ELEVATION, %	BRUCE STAGE (min)	SPEED, mph	ELEVATION, %	NAUGHTON STAGE (min)	SPEED, mph	ELEVATION, %
1.0(3.5)									
1.5(5.3)									
2.0(7.0)									
2.5(8.8)	1(2)	1.0	0				1(3)	1.0	0
3.0(10.5)							2(3)	1.5	0
3.5(12.3)	2(2)	1.5	0				3(3)	2.0	0
4.0(14.0)							4(3)	2.0	3.5
4.5(15.8)	3(2)	2.0	3.5				5(3)	2.0	7.0
5.0(17.5)									
5.5(19.3)	4(2)	2.0	7.0	1(3)	1.7	10.0	6(3)	3.0	5.0
6.0(21.0)									
6.5(22.8)	5(2)	2.0	10.5				7(3)	3.0	7.5
7.0(24.5)									
7.5(26.3)	6(2)	3.0	7.5				8(3)	3.0	10.0
8.0(28.0)									
8.5(29.8)	7(2)	3.0	10.0	2(3)	2.5	12.0	9(3)	3.0	12.5
9.0(31.5)									
9.5(33.3)	8(2)	3.0	12.5	3(3)	3.4	14.0	10(3)	3.0	15.0
10.0(35.0)									
10.5(36.8)	9(2)	3.0	15.0						
11.0(38.5)	10(2)	3.4	14.0						
11.5(40.3)									
12.0(42.0)									
12.5(43.8)									
13.0(45.5)				4(3)	4.2	16.0			

FIGURE 7-17. Exercise testing in patients with heart failure. Maximal myocardial oxygen consumption (MVO$_2$) is defined as the greatest amount of oxygen a patient can utilize while performing dynamic aerobic exercise that utilizes large muscle masses. It reflects oxygen transport and cellular metabolism. MVO$_2$ is usually expressed as milliliters of oxygen consumed per kilogram of body weight per minute. Exercise performance can be described in "metabolic equivalents" (METS). One MET is defined as 3.5 mL O$_2$/kg/min and reflects the quantity of oxygen utilized when an individual is sitting or resting quietly. World-class endurance athletes can achieve 18 METS during maximal exercise (reflecting 60 mL O$_2$/kg/min MVO$_2$). Patients with coronary heart disease capable of achieving 10 METS (or 35 mL O$_2$/kg/min MVO$_2$) have excellent prognoses. On the other hand, patients able to obtain peak exercise of 5 METS or less have poor prognoses [42–44]. Exercise testing in heart failure is performed to quantify functional capacity. Shown are six commonly used exercise protocols. In general, the best estimate of MVO$_2$ in a heart failure patient can be accomplished with protocols that increase physical stress loads gradually, such as the Weber-Janicki and Naughton protocols (A), and the Balke and Branching protocols (B). (continued)

NYHA CLASS (SYMPTOM SEVERITY):
IV — Severe
III — Moderate to severe
II — Mild to moderate
I — Minimal or asymptomatic

METS (mL O₂/kg/min)	ELLESTAD STAGE (min)	SPEED, mph	ELEVATION, %	BALKE STAGE (min)	SPEED, mph	ELEVATION, %	BRANCHING STAGE (min)	SPEED, mph	ELEVATION, %
1.0(3.5)									
1.5(5.3)									
2.0(7.0)							BRANCH I		
2.5(8.8)				1(2)	3.0	0	1(2)	1.9	0
3.0(10.5)									
3.5(12.3)							2(2)	2.6	0
4.0(14.0)				2(2)	3.0	2.5	3(2)	2.6	3.0
4.5(15.8)							4(2)	2.6	6.0
5.0(17.5)	1(3)	1.7	10.0	3(2)	3.0	5.0	5(2)	2.6	9.0
5.5(19.3)							6(2)	2.6	12.0
6.0(21.0)				4(2)	3.0	7.5	7(2)	2.6	15.0
6.5(22.8)							8(2)	2.6	17.5
7.0(24.5)	2(2)	3.0	10.0	5(2)	3.0	10.0	9(2)	2.6	20.0
7.5(26.3)							10(2)	2.6	22.0
8.0(28.0)				6(2)	3.0	12.0			
8.5(29.8)	3(2)	4.0	10.0				BRANCH II		
9.0(31.5)				7(2)	3.0	15.0	3.4–4.4 METs		
9.5(33.3)							BRANCH III		
10.0(35.0)				8(2)	3.0	17.5	3.9–4.9 METs		
10.5(36.8)							BRANCH IV		
11.0(38.5)				9(2)	3.0	20.0	4.5–5.3 METs		
11.5(40.3)									
12.0(42.0)				10(2)	3.0	22.5			
12.5(43.8)									
13.0(45.5)	4(3)	5.0	10.0						

FIGURE 7-17. (*continued*) Protocols that rapidly increase stress levels, such as the Bruce (**A**) and Ellstead (**B**) protocols, are more suitable for the screening of patients for the presence of ischemic heart disease than for quantifying functional limitations resulting from ventricular dysfunction. Although values for peak oxygen uptake can be estimated from exercise workload, online measured values of oxygen consumption may more accurately reflect cardiac impairment and allow differentiation between cardiac and pulmonary pathophysiology. Several additional parameters are important to take into consideration during exercise. These include ability to augment systolic blood pressure, the onset of the anaerobic threshold (when gas exchange is measured online), and electrocardiographic changes such as ST-segment abnormalities (possibly reflecting ischemia) or development of cardiac arrhythmias. NYHA—New York Heart Association (*Adapted from* Young and Farmer [1].)

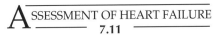

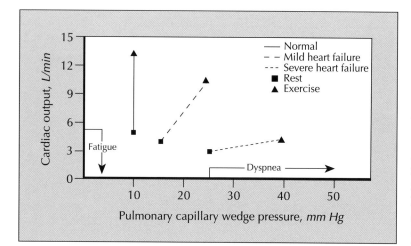

FIGURE 7-18. Pathophysiology of heart failure related to symptoms. Exercise testing is important in patients with heart failure because it may unmask significant symptomatology. In patients with significant systolic ventricular dysfunction, the cardiac output fails to increase normally under the physiologic stress of exertion, and the pulmonary pressures become disproportionately elevated. Diminution in exercise capacity is a cardinal complaint in patients with heart failure [45–47]. The determinants of exercise intolerance have proven complex. For example, the extent of left ventricular functional impairment may have little bearing on the maximal amount of exercise patients can accomplish [48]. Many factors influence the maximal oxygen consumption in patients with heart failure. Myocardial or circulatory abnormalities (*eg*, severity of systolic ventricular dysfunction and its subsequent impact on muscle perfusion) impair exercise capacity by limiting the hemodynamic response to exercise. Peripheral factors have more recently come under scrutiny. These include skeletal muscle metabolism, nutritional state, and physical conditioning. Ventilatory factors control oxygen exchange and therefore affect the maximal oxygen consumption.

SYSTOLIC VERSUS DIASTOLIC DYSFUNCTION IN HEART FAILURE

PARAMETERS	SYSTOLIC	DIASTOLIC
History		
Coronary heart disease	++++	+
Hypertension	++	++++
Diabetes	+++	+
Valvular heart disease	++++	-
Paroxysmal dyspnea	++	+++
Physical examination		
Cardiomegaly	+++	+
Soft heart sounds	++++	+
S₃ gallop	+++	+
S₄ gallop	+	+++
Hypertension	++	++++
Mitral regurgitation	+++	+
Rales	++	++
Edema	+++	+
Jugular venous distention	+++	+
Chest radiograms	+++	+
Cardiomegaly	+++	+++
Pulmonary congestion		
Electrocardiograms	+++	-
Low voltage	++	++++
Left ventricular hypertrophy	+++	+
Q waves	++++	-
Echocardiograms	+++	-
Low ejection fraction	++	++++
Left ventricular dilation		
Left ventricular hypertrophy		

FIGURE 7-19. Systolic versus diastolic dysfunction in heart failure. Although it is common, congestive heart failure in which diastolic dysfunction is preponderant (vs systolic dysfunction) may be difficult to diagnose [49]. It is important to remember that the clinical features of heart failure may be similar whether left ventricular systolic function is normal or is substantively depressed [50]. The pathophysiology of heart failure with normal systolic ventricular function is different, however, from that noted in patients with depressed left ventricular ejection fraction [51,52]. Furthermore, certain aspects of the history and physical examination, along with clinical measurements, help to distinguish diastolic problems from those more often associated with systolic failure. For example, patients with hypertensive heart disease, particularly those with severe left ventricular hypertrophy, often experience heart failure because of diastolic dysfunction. *Plus signs* indicate "suggestive" (the number reflects relative weight); *minus signs* indicate "not very suggestive."

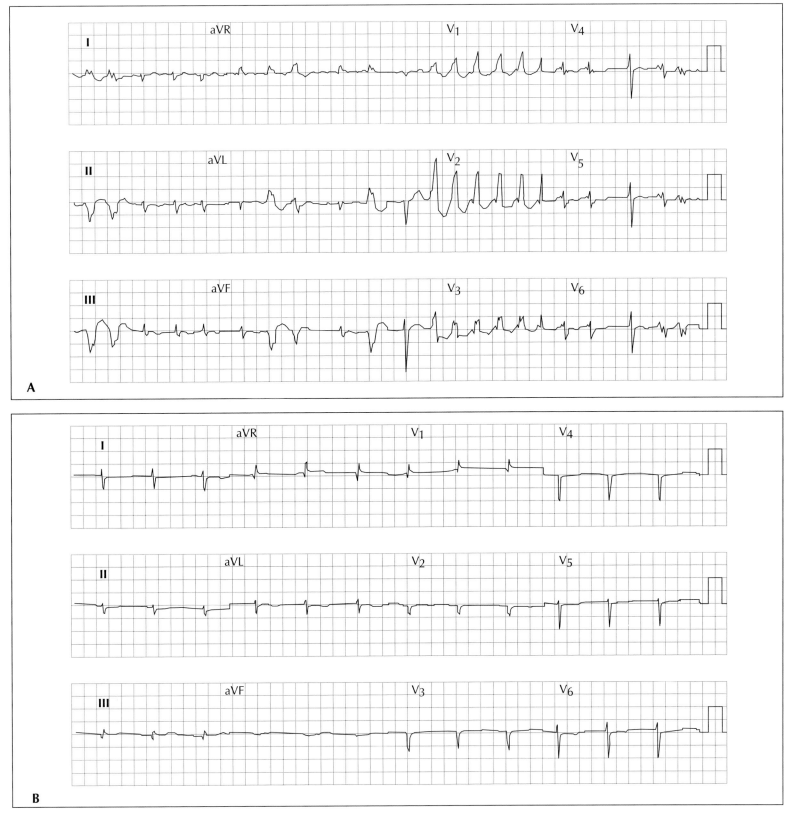

FIGURE 7-20. Electrocardiography in heart failure patients. An electrocardiogram (ECG) can provide valuable information in the assessment of patients with heart failure. These examples represent commonly observed findings in severe heart failure. **A,** Low voltage and arrhythmia. This ECG demonstrates a right bundle branch block pattern and low voltage throughout the limb leads and precordium. Premature ventricular contractions, couplets, and nonsustained ventricular tachycardia are also seen. This patient has severe coronary heart disease with multiple myocardial infarctions and an ejection fraction of 15%. **B,** Cardiomyopathy. Patients with dilated cardiomyopathy may have Q waves (*see* precordial leads), which can lead to the mistaken diagnosis of myocardial infarction. This patient did not have coronary heart disease. The tracing also shows low voltage throughout, an interventricular conduction defect pattern, and nonspecific ST-T wave changes.

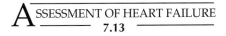

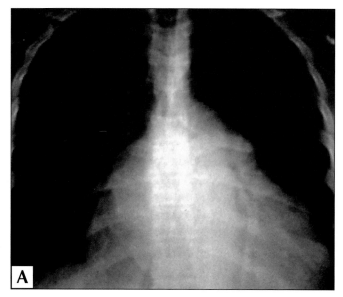

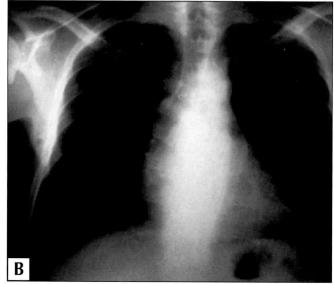

FIGURE 7-21. Chest radiographs of patients with heart failure. **A,** Congestive heart failure with cardiomegaly. This radiograph demonstrates cardiomegaly (cardiothoracic ratio, 0.77), pulmonary congestion, and bilateral pleural effusions (note blunted costophrenic angles). The cardiac silhouette may indicate the existence of a pericardial effusion. Also note the thin chest wall and osteopenia suggesting cachexia.

B, Congestive heart failure with left ventricular hypertrophy. This radiograph demonstrates mild pulmonary congestion with a high-normal cardiothoracic ratio of 0.53. These radiographic findings are typical of patients with hypertensive heart disease or hypertrophic cardiomyopathy resulting in diastolic dysfunction in the presence of a normal ejection fraction.

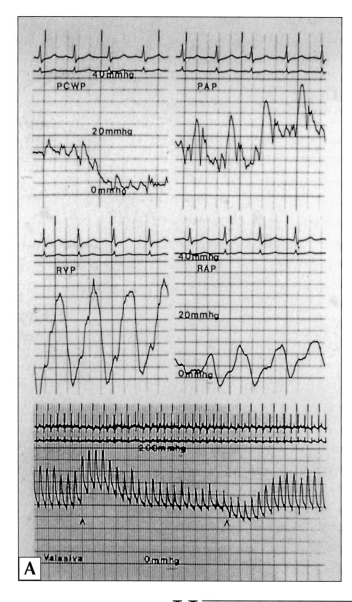

FIGURE 7-22. Hemodynamics in heart failure patients. **A,** Hemodynamic findings obtained during routine surveillance by right heart catheterization and endomyocardial biopsy in a patient 5 years after heart transplantation. The patient complained of mild dyspnea on exertion, but was well compensated and could perform ordinary daily activities. During maximal exercise, he achieved a myocardial oxygen consumption (MVO_2) of 18 mL O_2/kg/min. Although the patient was moderately hypertensive (blood pressure, 170/100 mm Hg), intracardiac and pulmonary pressures were at the upper limits of normal. Right atrial pressure (RAP) was slightly elevated with a paradoxic increase during inspiration, a characteristic finding with orthotopic allografts. The patient's cardiac output was 4.7 L/min. Valsalva's maneuver in this patient is not entirely normal, since it does not exhibit the "overshoot" phenomenon seen in patients with normal ventricular function. This patient's ejection fraction was 47%. *(continued)*

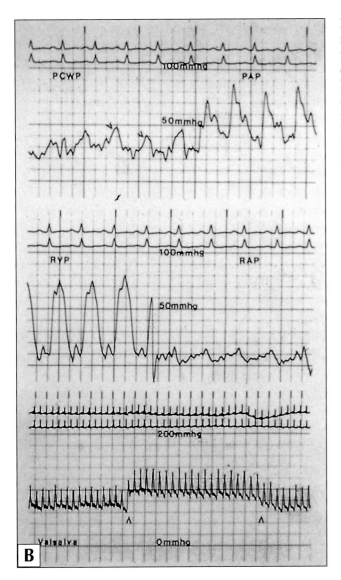

FIGURE 7-22. *(continued)* **B,** Hemodynamic findings from a patient with cardiomyopathy and severe systolic and diastolic dysfunction: a 45-year-old man with end-stage cardiomyopathy believed to be caused by excessive alcohol consumption. The patient's ejection fraction is 15%. Cardiac output is 2.9 L/min, and the systemic blood pressure is 103/82 mm Hg. The patient has severe pulmonary hypertension (pulmonary artery pressure [PAP] of 87/35 mm Hg with pulmonary capillary wedge pressure [PCWP] of 35 mm Hg). Valsalva's maneuver in this patient is markedly abnormal, demonstrating the "square wave" pattern characteristic of severe left ventricular dysfunction. RVP—right ventricular pressure.

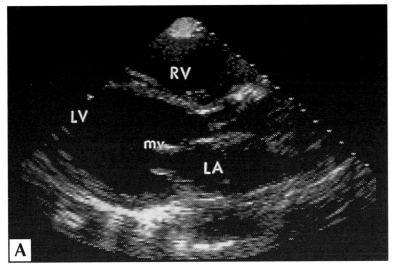

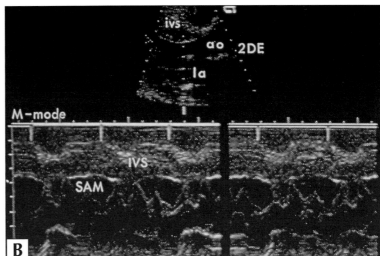

FIGURE 7-23. Echocardiographic patterns in heart failure. Information obtained with an echocardiogram can help clarify a patient's complaints and certain physical findings. **A,** Dilated cardiomyopathy. This long-axis parasternal view from a two-dimensional echocardiogram demonstrates the multichamber enlargement characteristic of dilated cardiomyopathy. No evidence of pericardial effusion is present, even though the patient had a paradoxical drop in systolic blood pressure of 10 mm Hg with inspiration (systolic pressure starting at 90 mm Hg). The left ventricular (LV) wall is symmetrically thin, and in real time, no

focal wall motion abnormalities are seen. Rather, the entire LV is hypokinetic, and the ejection fraction is calculated to be only 15%.

B, Hypertrophic cardiomyopathy. M-mode and two-dimensional (2DE) echocardiographic findings of severe LV hypertrophy with evidence of outflow tract obstruction (systolic anterior motion [SAM] of the mitral valve). In systole, the LV cavity becomes virtually obliterated, and the ejection fraction is calculated to be greater than 75%. The interventricular septum (IVS) is dramatically thickened. The patient complained of chest pain and severe dyspnea on exertion, and he also had syncope. *(continued)*

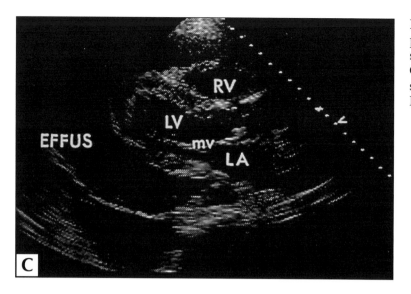

FIGURE 7-23. *(continued)* **C,** Pericardial effusion (EFFUS). This patient has normal right and left ventricular chamber size and systolic function, but a large pericardial effusion is present. Clinically, the patient was hypotensive and complained of shortness of breath. ao—aorta; LA—left atrium; mv—mitral valve; RV—right ventricle.

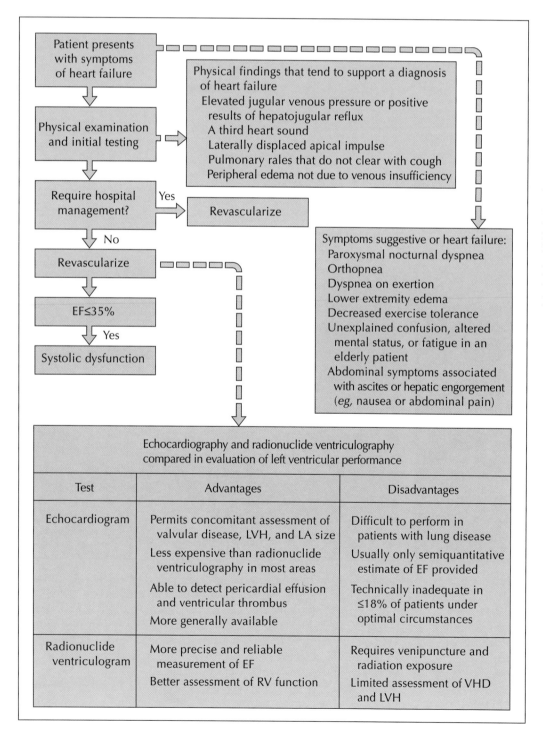

FIGURE 7-24. The Agency for Health Care Policy and Research (AHCPR) recommendations for initial evaluation of patients with heart failure. These guidelines focus on symptomatic individuals presenting with symptoms of heart failure and physical findings that support a clinical diagnosis of congestive heart failure. These guidelines stress the importance of objectively measuring systolic left ventricular function. The link between symptoms, physical findings, and objective assessment of ventricular performance is the key to patient management [16]. EF—ejection fraction; LA—left atrium; LVH—left ventricular hypertrophy; RV—right ventricle; VHD—valvular heart disease. (*Adapted from* Konstam and coworkers [16].)

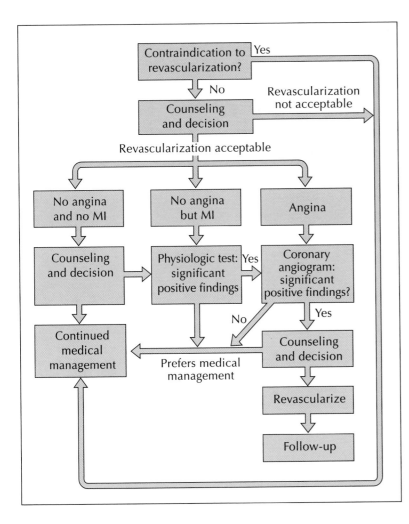

FIGURE 7-25. The Agency for Health Care Policy and Research (AHCPR) patient guidelines for the evaluation and treatment of coronary artery disease (CAD) in patients with heart failure. These guidelines focus heavily on the importance of identifying CAD as an underlying pathology in individuals with symptomatic heart failure [16]. The reason for this is the well-documented response to revascularization that patients have with respect to ventricular function and heart failure. When assessing patients with heart failure, decisions must be made regarding performance of coronary angiography. It is suggested that patients presenting with angina syndromes undergo angiographic study with subsequent revascularization, if possible and appropriate. In patients without angina who do have prior myocardial infarction (MI), physiologic testing to determine whether or not ischemia is present should be performed, and subsequent decisions regarding coronary angiography should be made. (*Adapted from* Konstam and coworkers [16].)

DESIGNING A THERAPEUTIC PLAN

QUESTIONS AFTER ASSESSMENT TO DETERMINE THERAPEUTIC STRATEGY

Is heart failure apparent?

Is the problem primarily systolic or diastolic dysfunction?

What caused the problem?

What precipitated deterioration?

How severe is the heart failure?

What is the prognosis?

What is the best acute therapeutic strategy?

What is the best chronic therapeutic strategy?

Can the initiating/precipitating problem be cured or eliminated, and can the state of heart failure be ameliorated or attenuated?

FIGURE 7-26. Integration of diagnostic evaluation in the assessment of patients with heart failure. Data obtained during the assessment of patients with heart failure can be used to answer several key questions. It is critical to determine if heart failure is present, what caused the difficulty or precipitated deterioration, and how severe the syndrome is. When these questions are answered, insight into the patient's long-term prognosis can be gained and therapeutic strategies can be designed to address both acute and chronic problems as well as the initiating or precipitating causes.

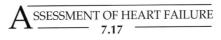

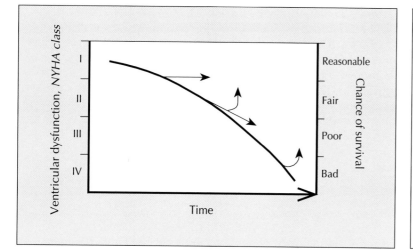

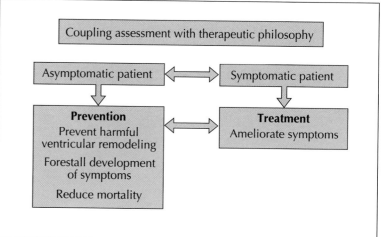

FIGURE 7-27. Assessment of heart failure and timing of therapy. If enhancement of survival is to be achieved in patients with heart failure, it is important that therapy be initiated as early as possible to minimize further deterioration of ventricular function. In the future, it is hoped that diagnostic assessments will allow routine detection of left ventricular dysfunction before symptoms develop [6,7]. *Arrows* demonstrate that it may be easier to prevent a downward disease course when treatment is begun in asymptomatic individuals rather than waiting for class IV failure to develop. At this point, improving the prognosis is very difficult. NYHA— New York Heart Association.

FIGURE 7-28. Coupling heart failure assessment with therapeutic philosophy. Therapy of heart failure should be designed to prevent ventricular remodeling, forestall development of clinical symptoms, ameliorate symptoms, and reduce mortality. Treatment strategies are based on data obtained during clinical assessment, particularly during risk stratification of both symptomatic and asymptomatic patients. Patients sometimes alternate between compensation and decompensation or asymptomatic and symptomatic states, and treatment protocols should reflect an ongoing assessment of a patient's clinical status.

REFERENCES

1. Young JB, Farmer JA: The diagnostic evaluation of patients with heart failure. In *Congestive Heart Failure: Pathophysiology, Diagnosis, and Comprehensive Approach to Management.* Edited by Hosenpud JD, Greenberg BH. New York: Springer-Verlag; 1994:597–621.

2. Badgett RG, Lucey CR, Mujrow CD: Can the clinical examination diagnose left sided heart failure in adults? *JAMA* 1997, 277:1712–1719.

3. Tresch DD: The clinical diagnosis of heart failure in older patients. *J Am Geriatr Soc* 1997, 45:1128–1133.

4. Cohn JN: Jugular venous pressure monitoring: a lost art? *J Cardiac Failure* 1997, 3:71–73.

5. McGee SR: Physical examination of venous pressure: a critical review. *Am Heart J* 1998, 136:10–18.

6. Armstrong PW, Moe GW: Medical advances in the treatment of congestive heart failure. *Circulation* 1994, 88:2941–2952.

7. Cohn JN: The prevention of heart failure: a new agenda [editorial]. *N Engl J Med* 1992, 327:725–726.

8. Feldman AM: Can we alter survival in patients with congestive heart failure? *JAMA* 1992, 267:1956–1961.

9. Parrish DL, Grayburn PA: Use of echocardiography in patients with congestive heart failure. *Cardiol Rev* 1998, 6:203–212.

10. Cowie MR, Struthers AD, Wood DA, *et al.*: Volume of natriuretic peptides in assessment of patients with possible new heart failure in primary care. *Lancet* 1997, 350:1349–1353.

11. Gaasch WH: Diagnosis and treatment of heart failure based on left ventricular systolic or diastolic dysfunction. *JAMA* 1994, 271:1276–1280.

12. Ghali JK, Cooper R, Ford E: Trends in hospitalization rates for heart failure in the United States, 1973–1986. *Arch Intern Med* 1992, 152:649–655.

13. Kannel WB, Belanger AJ: Epidemiology of heart failure. *Am Heart J* 1991, 121:951–957.

14. McKee PA, Castelli WP, McNamara PM, *et al.*: The natural history of congestive heart failure: the Framingham Study. *N Engl J Med* 1971, 285:1441–1446.

15. Braunwald E: ACE inhibitors: a cornerstone of the treatment of heart failure. *N Engl J Med* 1991, 325:351–353.

16. Konstam M, Dracup K, Baker D, *et al.*: Heart failure: evaluation and care of patients with left ventricular systolic dysfunction [Clinical practice guideline No. 11; AHCPR publication 94-0612]. Rockville, MD: Agency for Health Care Policy and Research; June 1994.

17. The CONSENSUS Trial Study Group: Effects of enalapril on mortality in severe congestive heart failure. *N Engl J Med* 1987, 316:1429–1435.

18. The SOLVD Investigators: Effect of enalapril on mortality and the development of heart failure in asymptomatic patients with reduced left ventricular ejection fractions. *N Engl J Med* 1992, 327:685–691.

19. Pfeffer MA, Braunwald E, Moyé LA, *et al.*: Effect of captopril on mortality and morbidity in patients with left ventricular dysfunction after myocardial infarction: results of the Survival and Ventricular Enlargement Trial. *N Engl J Med* 1992, 327:668–677.

20. Cohn JN, Archibald DG, Ziesche S, *et al.*: Effect of vasodilator therapy on mortality in chronic congestive heart failure: results of a Veterans Administration Cooperative Study. *N Engl J Med* 1986, 314:1547–1552.

21. The SOLVD Investigators: Effect of enalapril on survival in patients with reduced left ventricular ejection fractions and congestive heart failure. *N Engl J Med* 1991, 325:293–302.

22. Packer M, Carver JR, Rodeheffer RJ, *et al.*: Effect of oral milrinone on mortality in severe chronic heart failure. *N Engl J Med* 1991, 325:1468–1475.

23. The SOLVD Investigators: Studies of Left Ventricular Dysfunction (SOLVD): rationale, design and methods: two trials that evaluate the effect of enalapril in patients with reduced ejection fraction. *Am J Cardiol* 1990, 66:315–322.

24. Bangdiwala SI, Weiner DH, Bourassa MG, *et al.*: Studies of Left Ventricular Dysfunction (SOLVD) Registry: rationale, design, methods and description of baseline characteristics. *Am J Cardiol* 1992, 70:347–353.

25. Gheorghiade M, Bonow RO: Chronic heart failure in the United States: a manifestation of coronary artery disease. *Circulation* 1998, 97:282–289.

26. Stevenson LW, Perloff JK: The limited reliability of physical signs for estimating hemodynamics in chronic heart failure. *JAMA* 1989, 261:884–888.

27. Szlachcic J, Massie BM, Kramer BL, *et al.*: Correlates and prognostic implication of exercise capacity in chronic congestive heart failure. *Am J Cardiol* 1985, 55:1037–1042.

28. Young JB, Weiner DH, Pratt CM, *et al.*: Relationship of ejection fraction and symptomatic status to medication use in patients with heart failure: a report from Studies of Left Ventricular Dysfunction (SOLVD) Registry. *South Med J* 1994, 88:414–423.

29. Zema MJ, Caccovano M, Kligfield P: Detection of left ventricular dysfunction in ambulatory subjects with the bedside Valsalva maneuver. *Am J Med* 1983, 75:241–248.

30. Zema MJ, Restivo Bernard, Sos T, *et al.*: Left ventricular dysfunction: bedside Valsalva manoeuvre. *Br Heart J* 1980, 44:560–590.

31. Zema MJ, Masters AP, Margouleff D: Dyspnea: the heart or the lungs? Differentiation at bedside by use of the simple Valsalva maneuver. *Chest* 1984, 85:59–64.

32. Ewy GA: The abdominojugular test: technique and hemodynamic correlates. *Ann Intern Med* 1988, 109:456–460.

33. Butman SM, Ewy GA, Standen JR, *et al.*: Bedside cardiovascular examination in patients with severe chronic heart failure: importance of rest or inducible jugular venous distension. *J Am Coll Cardiol* 1993, 22:968–974.

34. Heckerling PS, Wiener SL, Wolfkiel CJ, *et al.*: Accuracy and reproducibility of precordial percussion and palpation for detecting increased left ventricular end-diastolic volume and mass: a comparison of physical findings and ultrafast computed tomography of the heart. *JAMA* 1993, 270:1943–1948.

35. Chakko S, Woska D, Martinez H, *et al.*: Clinical, radiographic, and hemodynamic correlations in chronic congestive heart failure: conflicting results may lead to inappropriate care. *Am J Med* 1991, 90:353–359.

36. Gahli JK, Kadakia S, Cooper RS, Liao Y: Bedside diagnosis of preserved versus impaired left ventricular systolic function in heart failure. *Am J Cardiol* 1991, 67:1002–1006.

37. Goldman L, Hashimoto B, Cook EF, Loscalzo A: Comparative reproducibility and validity of systems for assessing cardiovascular functional class: advantages of a new specific activity scale. *Circulation* 1981, 64:1227–1234.

38. Remes J, Miettinen H, Reunanen A, *et al.*: Validity of clinical diagnosis of heart failure in primary health care. *Eur Heart J* 1991, 12:315–321.

39. Packer M: Clinical trials in congestive heart failure: why do studies report conflicting results [editorial]? *Ann Intern Med* 1988, 109:3–5.

40. Marantz PR, Alderman MH, Tobin JN: Diagnostic heterogeneity in clinical trials for congestive heart failure. *Ann Intern Med* 1988, 109:55–61.

41. Ho KKL, Anderson KM, Kannell WB, *et al.*: Survival after the onset of congestive heart failure in Framingham Heart Study subjects. *Circulation* 1993, 88:107–115.

42. Morris CK, Ueshima K, Kawaguchi T, *et al.*: The prognostic value of exercise capacity: a review of the literature. *Am Heart J* 1991, 122:1423–1431.

43. Mancini DM, Eisen H, Kussmaul W, *et al.*: Value of peak exercise oxygen consumption for optimal timing of cardiac transplantation in ambulatory patients with heart failure. *Circulation* 1991, 83:778–786.

44. Mills RM Jr, Haught WH: Evaluation of heart failure patients: objective parameters to assess functional capacity. *Clin Cardiol* 1996, 19:455–460.

45. Engel PJ: Effort intolerance in chronic heart failure: what are we treating [editorial]? *J Am Coll Cardiol* 1990, 15:995–998.

46. Fowler MB: Exercise intolerance in heart failure [editorial]. *J Am Coll Cardiol* 1991, 17:1073–1074.

47. Francis GS, Rector TS: Maximal exercise tolerance as a therapeutic end point in heart failure: are we relying on the right measure [editorial]? *Am J Cardiol* 1994, 73:304–306.

48. Myers J, Froelicher VF: Hemodynamic determinants of exercise capacity in chronic heart failure. *Ann Intern Med* 1991, 115:377–386.

49. Kessler KM: Heart failure with normal systolic function: update of prevalence, differential diagnosis, prognosis, and therapy [editorial]. *Arch Intern Med* 1988, 148:2109–2111.

50. Goldsmith SR, Dick C: Differentiating systolic from diastolic heart failure: pathophysiologic and therapeutic considerations. *Am J Med* 1993, 95:645–655.

51. Kitzman DW, Higginbotham MB, Cobb FR, *et al.*: Exercise intolerance in patients with heart failure and preserved left ventricular systolic function: failure of the Frank-Starling mechanism. *J Am Coll Cardiol* 1991, 17:1065–1072.

52. Litwin SE, Grossman W: Diastolic dysfunction as a cause of heart failure. *J Am Coll Cardiol* 1993, 22(suppl A):49–55.

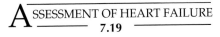

PROGNOSIS, USE OF PROGNOSTIC VARIABLES, AND ASSESSMENT OF THERAPEUTIC RESPONSES

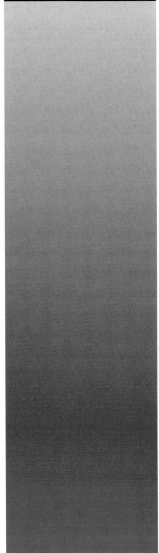

CHAPTER 8

Michael O. Osayamen, Thomas S. Rector, and Jay N. Cohn

The onset of clinically recognized heart failure among patients with various predisposing diseases such as coronary artery disease, valvular heart disease, diabetes, and hypertension marks a significant change in the prognosis for those patients. Despite recent therapeutic advances that improve survival and exercise tolerance, patients with chronic heart failure still have a poor prognosis, with annual mortality rates as high as 50%. Heart failure deaths increase exponentially with age, and death occurs suddenly and unexpectedly without any evidence of recent hemodynamic or functional deterioration in about 30% to 50% of patients with chronic heart disease. The proportion of deaths that are sudden tends to be higher during earlier stages of the disease, *ie*, in patients with mild to moderate symptoms of chronic heart failure. Unfortunately, the identification of chronic heart failure patients who are at increased risk of sudden cardiac death is still an unresolved problem. These grim statistics emphasize the importance of preventing the development of heart failure.

Attempts have been made recently to stratify predictors of pump failure death from predictors of sudden cardiac deaths. Numerous variables have been identified as prognostic markers that can be used to place patients in different risk strata. Hemodynamic, structural, biochemical, and functional variables all offer some prognostic information. Predictions regarding life expectancy are best made by considering several prognostic variables, but useful statistical models are not available. Therefore, in evaluating the cost-effective use of medications and surgical interventions, the clinician must make qualitative assessments of the patient's risk and likelihood of benefiting from therapy.

Assessment of therapeutic response entails the examination of multiple endpoints. Two of the most important potential benefits of medical therapy—the prevention of premature mortality and hospital admissions for heart failure—are impossible for the physician to assess in patient management. Surrogate endpoints for these important benefits would be helpful, but the relationships between changes in surrogate endpoints and favorable clinical outcomes have not been adequately validated. Nevertheless, patients should be treated with interventions that have been shown to reduce the likelihood of death and hospitalization when the potential for benefit outweighs the adverse effects and costs. The effects of heart failure and its treatment on a patient's quality of life can and should be evaluated by systematic inquiry. A self-administered questionnaire has been developed and validated as a measure of therapeutic response. Use of a peak exercise test to evaluate the response to therapy may provide data supporting an effect, but may not necessarily reflect a symptomatic or clinically important benefit of therapy.

MORTALITY IN PATIENTS WITH HEART FAILURE

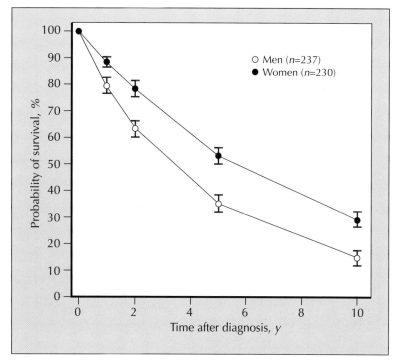

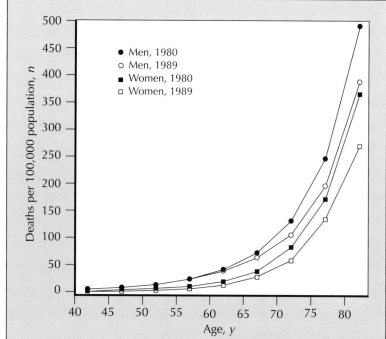

FIGURE 8-1. Survival after the clinical diagnosis of congestive heart failure from 1948 to 1988 in the Framingham Heart Study [1]. Even though individuals who died within 90 days of the diagnosis were excluded, median survival after recognition of heart failure in men was only 3.2 years. Women also had a poor, but better, survival rate, with a median survival time of 5.4 years. Although the difference in survival compared with a control group without heart failure (similar in age and concurrent diseases) was not established, development of clinical heart failure clearly is associated with a poor prognosis. There were no differences in survival between the cohorts who developed heart failure from 1948 to 1974 and those who developed heart failure from 1975 to 1988. Standard error bars are shown.

FIGURE 8-2. Deaths in patients with a primary diagnosis of congestive heart failure (CHF) in 1980 and 1989 based on Canadian statistics [2]. Whereas deaths coded as CHF, left ventricular failure, cardiomyopathy, cardiac enlargement, and hypertensive heart disease were included, deaths coded as ischemic heart disease were not, thereby underestimating the true death rates from heart failure. The exponential increase in the death rate from heart failure in both genders parallels the known age-related increases in the incidence and prevalence of heart failure. Many of the age-specific death rates decreased during the 1980s, suggesting that advances in the prevention and treatment of heart failure may have reduced mortality from heart failure in the population.

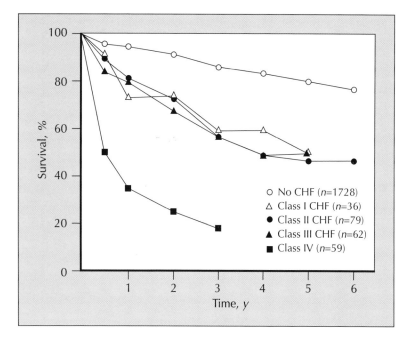

FIGURE 8-3. Survival among patients with different degrees of heart failure symptoms compared with similar patients without congestive heart failure (CHF) [3]. Classification of heart failure was based on the worst clinical condition 6 weeks prior to cardiac catheterization at Duke University Medical Center (1969 to 1981). All patients had coronary artery disease that was managed medically. These data demonstrate the effect, per se, of heart failure on mortality. The difference in survival between groups with a recent history of CHF and patients without overt heart failure was 27% after 3 years of follow-up. Patients who were symptomatic with any physical activity (class IV) had a very poor prognosis. (*Adapted from* Califf and coworkers [3]; with permission.)

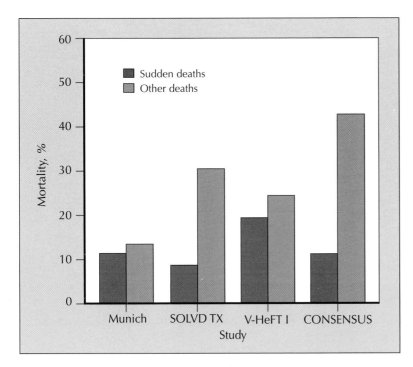

FIGURE 8-4. Proportion of deaths that occurred suddenly in the placebo arms of several large clinical trials that enrolled patients with heart failure [4–7]. *Sudden deaths* were defined generally as those that occurred a short time after the onset of symptoms in the absence of signs or symptoms of worsening heart failure. However, it is likely that there are inconsistencies in the classification of deaths by different investigators. Sudden deaths were common, comprising 20% to 45% of the total deaths. A prognostic variable that is specific for sudden deaths has not been established because the incidences of deaths from both pump failure and sudden deaths, which are presumably caused by abnormal rhythms, tend to increase with the severity of cardiac dysfunction. CONSENSUS—Cooperative North Scandinavian Enalapril Survival Study; SOLVD TX—Studies of Left Ventricular Dysfunction Treatment; V-HeFT I—Vasodilator Heart Failure Trial I.

USE OF PROGNOSTIC VARIABLES

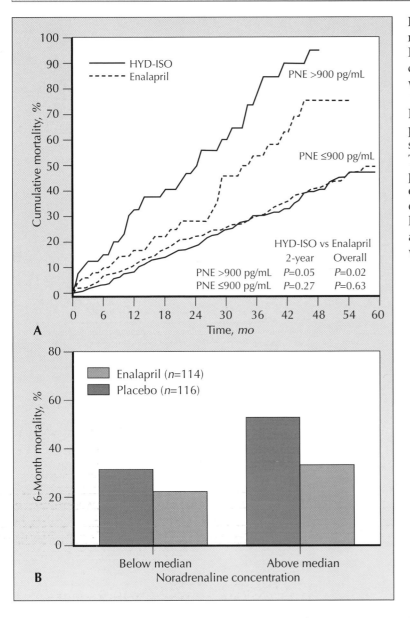

FIGURE 8-5. Effect of enalapril on survival within strata of plasma norepinephrine concentration (PNE). **A,** The Vasodilator Heart Failure Trial (V-HeFT II), in which improved survival with enalapril compared with hydralazine plus isosorbide dinitrate (HYD-ISO) was found in patients with PNE greater than 900 pg/mL [8].

B, In the CONSENSUS (Cooperative North Scandinavian Enalapril Survival Study) Trial, which compared enalapril with placebo [9], the median PNE was 772 pg/mL. Once again, the survival benefit was larger in the group with the highest PNEs. These data suggest that the PNE may be useful in identifying patients who are most likely to gain a survival benefit from enalapril. Further studies are needed to determine whether this observation is related to a specific pharmacologic effect that is most likely seen in patients with a high PNE. (Part A *adapted from* Francis and coworkers [8]; part B *adapted from* Swedberg and coworkers [9]; with permission.)

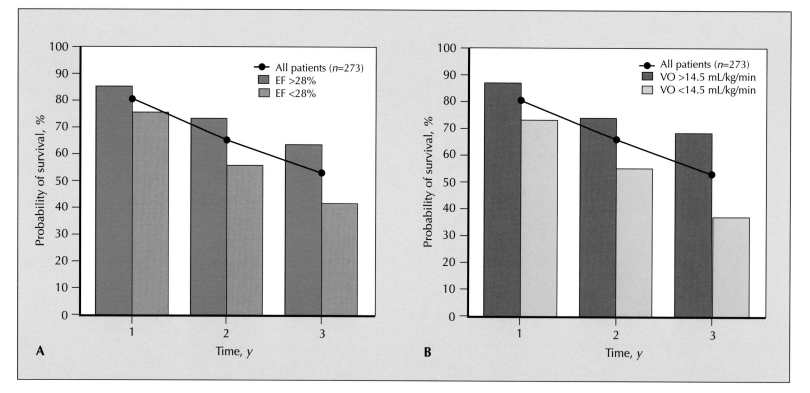

FIGURE 8-6. Examples of the prognostic information available from measurement of the left ventricular ejection fraction (EF; **A**) and peak oxygen consumption (VO$_2$; **B**) in the Vasodilator Heart Failure Trial (V-HeFT I). These data from the placebo group (patients treated with digoxin and diuretic) [10] indicate that the probability of survival over 3 years in different risk strata can differ by 20% to 30%. Strata were defined arbitrarily by the median values in this sample and may not represent the most discriminating cutpoints for these prognostic variables.

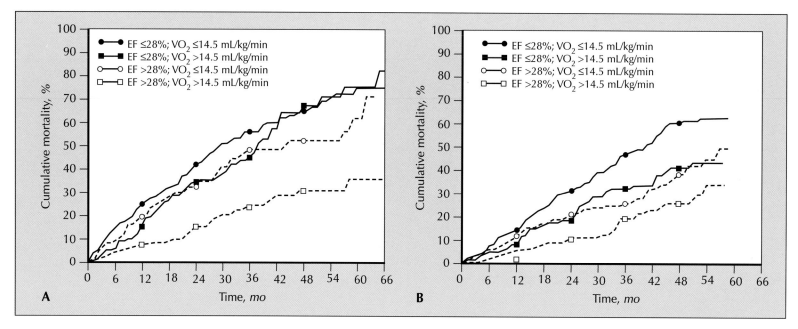

FIGURE 8-7. Prognostic stratification using ejection fraction (EF) and peak oxygen consumption (VO$_2$), which were found to be significant prognostic variables during multivariate analysis. Data are from all patients in the Vasodilator Heart Failure Trials (V-HeFT I; **A** and V-HeFT II; **B**) [10]. Patients who had relatively good EF and VO$_2$ clearly had a better prognosis than those who fell into the higher risk strata of both variables. For example, the difference in the probability of survival between these two strata after 3 years of follow-up was approximately 30%. Patients in the higher risk strata of only one of these prognostic variables had an intermediate survival. These trends were evident in both studies even though the overall prognosis tended to be better in V-HeFT II. This was in part because all patients in V-HeFT II received medications that prolong survival (hydralazine plus isosorbide dinitrate or enalapril), whereas the majority of patients in V-HeFT I received placebo or prazosin, which did not improve survival. (*Adapted from* Cohn and coworkers [10]; with permission.)

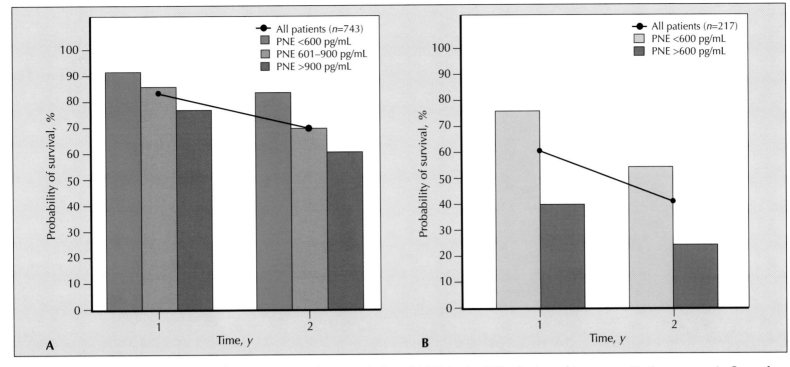

FIGURE 8-8. **A** and **B**, Probability of survival in two studies stratified by measurement of supine resting plasma norepinephrine concentration (PNE) [8,11]. These are among several studies associating PNE with the likelihood of survival in patients with heart failure. The overall prognosis of the group in **B** [11] was worse than that in **A** [8], as was the prognosis within similar strata of PNE. These data highlight the difficulty in making a quantitative prognosis. Several prognostic variables need to be taken into consideration because of the complex pathophysiology and multiple modes of death in patients with heart failure. Multivariate predictive models have not been developed and validated.

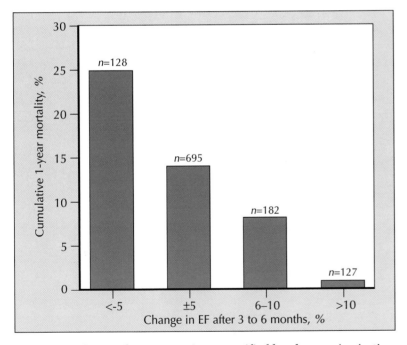

FIGURE 8-9. Survival among patients stratified by changes in ejection fraction (EF) 3 to 6 months after baseline in the Vasodilator Heart Failure Trials (V-HeFT I and II) [12]. EF did not differ by more than 5% in the majority of patients (61%), and mortality 1 year after the second assessment in this subgroup was 14%. The small subgroup whose EF improved by more than 10% had a very low mortality of 1% after 1 year. In contrast, a fall in the EF of more than 5% was associated with a 25% mortality after 1 year. The changes in EF were not strongly associated with several other prognostic variables, including baseline EF and treatment. Furthermore, the second measurement tended to be more informative than the baseline assessment and change from baseline. Data that establish change in any prognostic variable as a surrogate for a beneficial effect of a treatment on survival have not been reported.

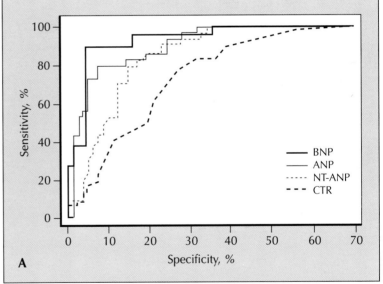

FIGURE 8-10. Survival in patients with congestive heart failure (CHF) stratified by changes in endogenous cardiac natriuretic peptide. **A,** On release, a prohormone, stored in the atria, is cleaved into the active C-terminal atrial natriuretic peptide (ANP) and the inactive, less rapidly cleared N-terminal atrial natriuretic peptide (NT-ATP). Both are mainly secreted from the atria in response to atrial stretch, and BNP (B-type or brain natriuretic peptide) is secreted mainly from the ventricular myocytes in proportion to the degree of the left ventricular dysfunction. Cowie *et al.* [13] suggest that circulating levels of these hormones could be sensitive and specific to survival and ongoing left ventricular dysfunction in patients with CHF. (*continued*)

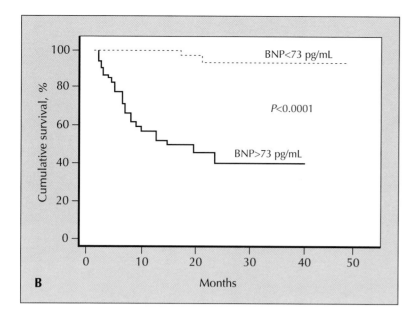

B

FIGURE 8-10. (*continued*) **B,** Patients who have relatively high BNP levels clearly have worse prognosis. These findings suggest that downregulation of natriuretic peptide receptor coupled with the attenuation of the compensatory activity of cardiac natriuretic peptide system may increase the mortality of CHF patients with high levels of plasma cardiac natriuretic peptides, particularly high B-type natriuretic peptide derived from the ventricle [14]. CTR— cardiothoracic ratio. (Part A *adapted from* Cowie and coworkers [13]; part B *adapted from* Tsutamoto and coworkers [14].)

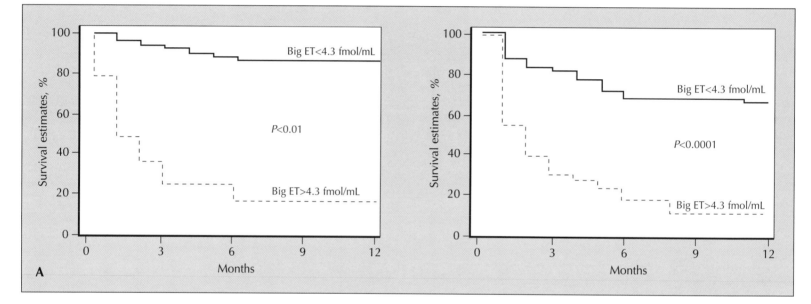

A

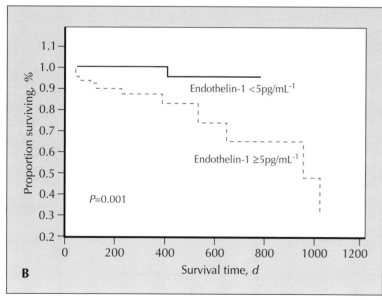

B

FIGURE 8-11. Survival estimates in two studies stratified by assessment of plasma endothelin system [15,16]. These are among several studies associating high plasma levels of both endothelin-1 and the propeptide big endothelin-1 (Big ET) with strong predictors of mortality in severe heart failure. **A,** The overall prognosis of 113 patients was worse in those with higher plasma Big ET (*dashed line*) whether 26 transplants were excluded (*left panel*) or included (*right panel*). **B,** Pousset *et al.* [16] have also shown the association of plasma endothelin-1 as a predictor of cardiac death in 120 congestive heart failure patients with ischemic or non-ischemic cardiomyopathy by using assay with very low cross-reactivity to big endothelin. A large study is currently being conducted to determine the dose-effect characteristics of a nonspecific endothelin receptor antagonist, bosentan, in congestive heart failure patients. (Part A *adapted from* Pacher and coworkers [15]; part B *adapted from* Pousset and coworkers [16].)

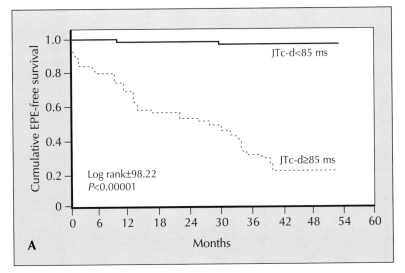

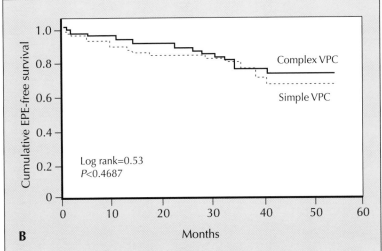

FIGURE 8-12. Sudden death in patients with chronic heart failure. The proportion of sudden deaths in chronic heart failure patients tends to be higher during earlier stages of the disease. **A,** Multivariate predictive models have not been developed and validated in chronic heart failure patients who die suddenly from electrical abnormalities, but several studies have shown that patients who died suddenly had significantly longer QT and repolarization dispersion, *ie*, high interlead variability of JT (J point to end of T wave) and QT intervals in the surface electrocardiogram (ECG) than survivors or those who died from progressive pump failure. Fu *et al.* [17] showed in a retrospective analysis of 163 patients [ischemic (*n*=126) and idiopathic dilated (*n*=37) cardiomyopathy with a left ventricular ejection fraction ≤40%]

that JTc-d (JTc-d dispersion, Jtc=JT/RR) was an important independent predictor of sudden cardiac death and ventricular tachyarrhythmia in patients with chronic heart failure. **B,** The mode of death was unrelated to the incidence of complex ventricular premature contraction (complex VPC) [17]. Smaller studies have suggested that QT/QTc dispersion [18], late potential, heart rate variability, abnormalities of action potential duration, and after-depolarizations on a surface 12-lead ECG can be used as markers for electrical instability, which may bring about sudden death in chronic heart failure patients. Further clinical experience is needed to establish whether they add substantiality to the more conventional prognostic tests. EPE—endpoint event. (*Adapted from* Fu and coworkers [17].)

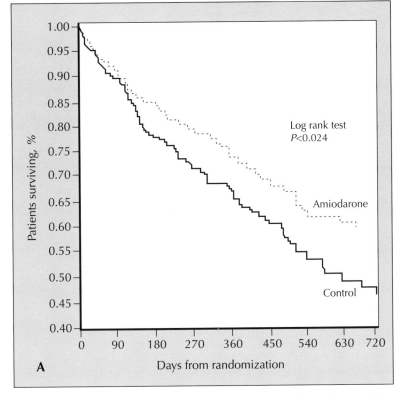

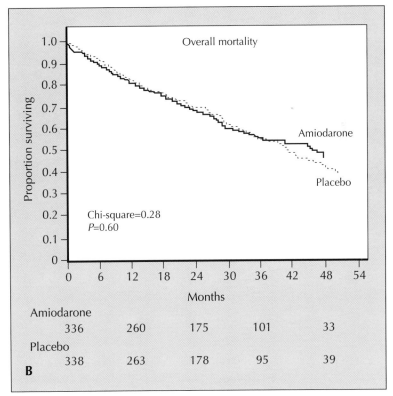

FIGURE 8-13. Two large-scale trials with amiodarone in patients with heart failure have given conflicting results. **A,** The GESICA study demonstrated an amiodarone-related reduction in mortality in a patient popoulation with severe heart failure, 70% of whom had not sustained a prior acute myocardial infarction [19]. Patients were not required to exhibit baseline arrhythmias, and the randomized therapy was not blinded. **B,** In the CHF-STAT study, no overall benefit of amiodarone on mortality was demonstrated [20]. These patients were required to exhibit less than 10 premature ventricular depolarizations

(PVCs) per hour at the time of entry, and 70% were identified as having an ischemic etiology of their heart failure. Subgroup analysis of CHF-STAT suggested a trend for benefit of amiodarone in the nonischemic group. Furthermore, a recent meta-analysis of individual data from 6500 patients in 13 randomized controlled trials of patients with recent myocardial infarction or congestive heart failure showed prophylactic amiodarone to reduce the rate of arrhythmic sudden death and total mortality [21]. (Part A *adapted from* Doval and coworkers [19]; part B *adapted from* Singh and coworkers [20].)

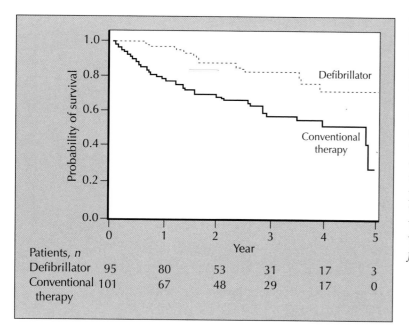

Figure 8-14. Effects of implantable defibrillator (ICD) on survival in patients with ischemic cardiomyopathy. In the MADIT (Multicenter Automatic Defibrillator Implantation Trial) trial, patients with prior myocardial infarction, left ventricular ejection fraction ≤35%, nonsustained ventricular tachycardia, and inducible ventricular tachycardia were stratified into antiarrhythmic drug therapy (n=101) or implanted defibrillator (n=95) groups. During an average follow-up of 27 months, this trial established that ICD therapy is a reasonable alternative for postinfarct patients with compensated heart failure who have nonsustained ventricular tachycardia and inducible ventricular tachycardia at electro-physiologic testing (P=0.009) [22]. Although antiarrhythmic drug therapy was not standardized, 74% of the drug therapy group were receiving amiodarone at 1 month follow-up. Some patients were also stratified to receive class I antiarrhythmic drug. (*Adapted from* Moss and coworkers [22].)

ASSESSMENT OF THERAPEUTIC RESPONSES

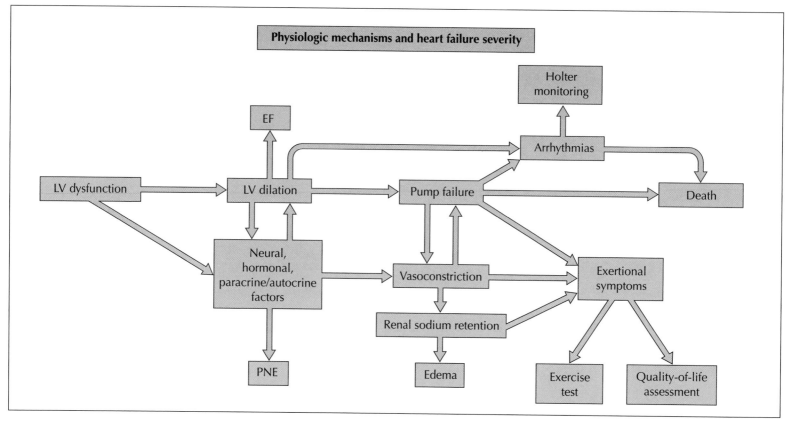

FIGURE 8-15. Physiologic mechanisms leading to markers for the severity of heart failure. Left ventricular (LV) dysfunction progresses through ventricular remodeling to chamber enlargement that can be detected by echocardiographic, radionuclide, or angiographic measurement of reduced LV ejection fraction (EF) or an increased chamber volume. LV dysfunction and chamber dilation result in activation of neural, hormonal, and local tissue paracrine and auto-crine processes, which contribute to vasoconstriction, renal sodium retention, and aggravation of LV dysfunction. The neurohormonal abnormality can be detected by elevated circulating levels of norepi-nephrine, renin activity, atrial natriuretic peptide, or other hormonal markers of the process. The sodium retention is manifested by edema or pulmonary congestion. The LV pump failure combined with the neurohormonal and vasoconstrictor mechanisms contribute to symp-toms that can be quantitated by a formal exercise test, often supple-mented by measurement of gas exchange.

Quality of life instruments provide a more global assessment of the functional impairment produced by the disease and its treatment. Pump failure may progress to death, but ventricular arrhythmias that are frequent accompaniments of LV dilation and pump failure may contribute independently to sudden death and may be detected and quantitated by Holter monitoring. In the treatment of heart failure, an improvement in any of these clinical markers may be used as a guide to a therapeutic response, but the relationship of any of these markers to clinical benefit, including life prolongation, has not yet been validated empirically. PNE—plasma norepinephrine concentration.

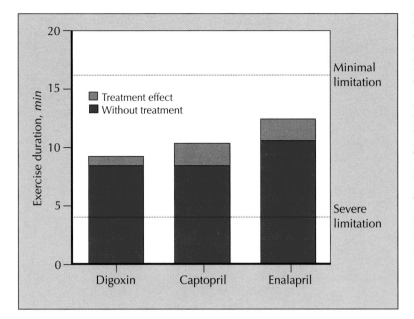

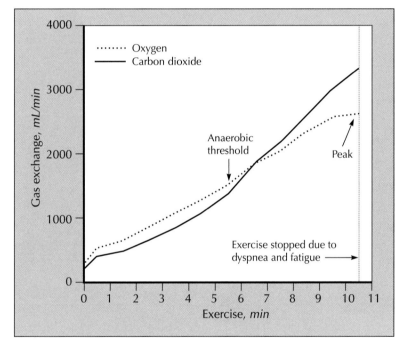

FIGURE 8-16. The magnitude of changes in exercise duration observed after 12 weeks in controlled clinical trials of commonly used medications [23–25]. All of these studies used a modified Naughton treadmill protocol in which the workload was increased every 2 minutes, beginning with a very easy workload of 1 mph (slow walk) on a level grade. Severely limited (able to complete less than two stages) or minimally impaired (able to complete more than eight stages) patients are often excluded from trials in an effort to select those thought to be most amenable to treatment. These particular medications have increased exercise duration by 2 minutes (one stage) or less on average compared with control groups in several studies. However, individual responses have been highly variable. In addition, patients often have substantial intolerance to exercise despite these improvements, and changes in exercise duration have not been established as reliable markers of changes in quality or quantity of life.

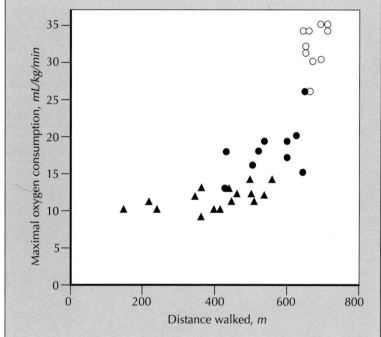

FIGURE 8-17. The most commonly used endpoints to ascertain changes in cardiopulmonary functional status during an exercise tolerance test. Patients exercise on a treadmill or bicycle against a gradually increasing workload until they stop because of dyspnea and fatigue. The most frequently used measure is total exercise time. Peak oxygen consumption is readily determined with equipment to monitor breath-by-breath respiratory gases and air flow. The anaerobic threshold that indicates excess carbon dioxide production from anaerobic metabolism is determined by the examination of several criteria such as a disproportionate increase in carbon dioxide production and ventilatory exchange relative to oxygen uptake, but this threshold is difficult to identify in many patients with heart failure.

Some of the problems with using a peak exercise test to assess the response to treatment include the following: 1) patient's routine daily activities usually do not involve this level of stress; 2) concurrent conditions such as angina, peripheral claudication, and arrhythmias may interfere with an assessment of dyspnea and fatigue; and 3) improvements have often occurred while the patient is taking placebo because of learning effects, training effects, and motivational factors.

FIGURE 8-18. Results of a 6-minute walk test in relation to peak oxygen consumption on a treadmill and New York Heart Association classification [26]. Patients were asked to walk as far as they could in 6 minutes in a level corridor. They could slow down or stop if necessary and were told when 3 and 5 minutes had elapsed. Some encouragement was given (this needs to be standardized to avoid biasing the results of the test). *Closed circles* represent patients whose ordinary physical activity caused symptoms such as dyspnea and fatigue (class II), and *closed triangles* represent patients who became symptomatic during less than ordinary physical activity (class III). *Open circles* represent normal subjects. There were no subjects in this study who were symptomatic with any physical activity or at rest (class IV) or who were not unduly symptomatic during ordinary physical activities (class I). Self-paced walking tests are being evaluated in clinical trials and may serve as a simple measure of the effects of heart failure on daily physical activity (*Adapted from* Lipkin and coworkers [26]; with permission.)

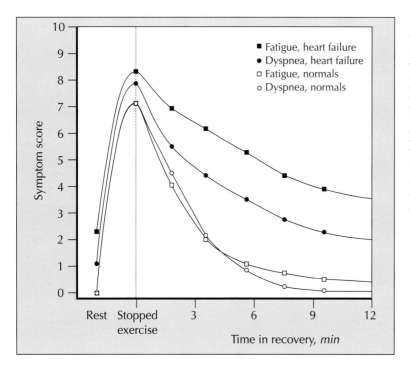

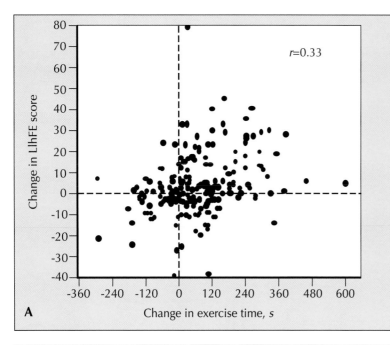

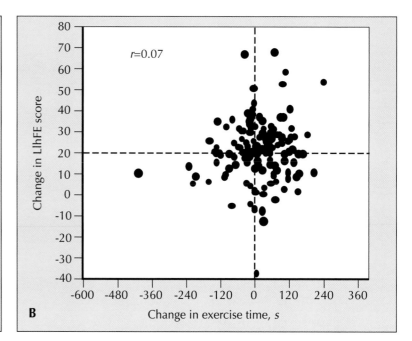

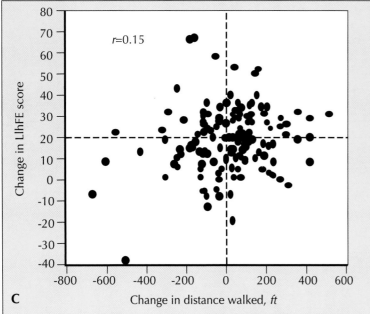

FIGURE 8-19. Prolonged symptoms following exercise in patients with heart failure compared with age-matched normals (Kraemer, unpublished data). Ten subjects in each group exercised on a bicycle until limited by dyspnea and fatigue. Subjects rated their levels of dyspnea and fatigue on a scale from 0 (none) to 10 (worst possible). On average, these patients were more symptomatic at rest and at peak exercise, but the changes in symptoms during exercise were similar in the two groups. In contrast, patients with heart failure had prolonged symptoms during recovery. Ratings of fatigue had not returned to baseline 45 minutes after exercise in the group with heart failure (not shown). Recovery from physical activity may be an important aspect of heart failure that needs to be addressed when evaluating heart failure and responses to therapy.

FIGURE 8-20. Correlations between changes in exercise variables and changes in quality of life as measured by the Minnesota Living with Heart Failure (LIhFE) questionnaire in the pimobendan (**A**) and digoxin withdrawal (**B** and **C**) studies [23,27]. Changes in exercise time for peak exercise tests done according to a modified Naughton protocol are shown in *A* and *B* . Changes in the distance walked for the 6-minute walk test are shown in *C*. The association between these variables was modest at best even though there were significant changes on average in each variable during these studies. These data and similar observations in other studies indicate that exercise tests and quality of life questionnaires provide distinctly different information about a patient's heart failure. Both types of measures are needed for a comprehensive evaluation.

LIVING WITH HEART FAILURE QUESTIONNAIRE

These questions concern how your heart failure (heart condition) has prevented you from living as you wanted during the last month. The items listed below describe different ways some people are affected. If you are sure an item does not apply to you or is not related to your heart failure then circle 0 (No) and go on to the next item. If an item does apply to you, then circle the number rating how much it prevented you from living as you wanted. Remember to think about ONLY THE LAST MONTH.

DID YOUR HEART FAILURE PREVENT YOU FROM LIVING AS YOU WANTED DURING THE LAST MONTH BY:	NO	VERY LITTLE				VERY MUCH
1. causing swelling in your ankles, legs, etc?	0	1	2	3	4	5
2. making you sit or lie down to rest during the day?	0	1	2	3	4	5
3. making your walking about or climbing stairs difficult?	0	1	2	3	4	5
4. making your working around the house or yard difficult?	0	1	2	3	4	5
5. making your going places away from home difficult?	0	1	2	3	4	5
6. making your sleeping well at night difficult?	0	1	2	3	4	5
7. making your relating to or doing things with your friends or family difficult?	0	1	2	3	4	5
8. making your working to earn a living difficult?	0	1	2	3	4	5
9. making your recreational pastimes, sports or hobbies difficult?	0	1	2	3	4	5
10. making your sexual activities difficult?	0	1	2	3	4	5
11. making you eat less of the foods you like?	0	1	2	3	4	5
12. making you short of breath?	0	1	2	3	4	5
13. making you tired, fatigued, or low on energy?	0	1	2	3	4	5
14. making you stay in a hospital?	0	1	2	3	4	5
15. costing you money for medical care?	0	1	2	3	4	5
16. giving you side effects from medications?	0	1	2	3	4	5
17. making you feel you are a burden to your family or friends?	0	1	2	3	4	5
18. making you feel a loss of self-control in your life?	0	1	2	3	4	5
19. making you worry?	0	1	2	3	4	5
20. making it difficult for you to concentrate or remember things?	0	1	2	3	4	5
21. making you feel depressed?	0	1	2	3	4	5

FIGURE 8-21. The Minnesota Living with Heart Failure questionnaire. Improvement in quality of life is one of two primary goals of therapy (prolonged survival being the other). This measure of quality of life, which has been used in many investigations of treatments for heart failure, defines *quality of life* as living as one wants with minimal limitations secondary to heart failure and its treatment. Physical, social, emotional, and economic limitations are included. Patients self-administer the questions after listening to a standard set of instructions. The score is the sum of the responses for all 21 questions. Eight questions including dyspnea and fatigue are highly interrelated and their sum is called the *physical dimension* [27]. Similarly, five interrelated questions comprise an emotional dimension. (*Adapted from* Rector and Cohn [27]; with permission.)

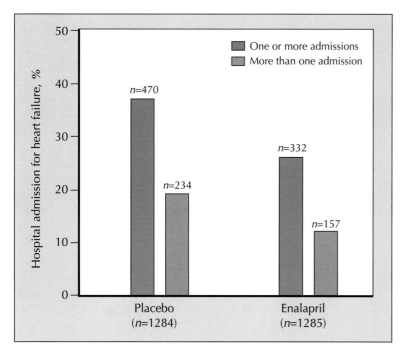

FIGURE 8-22. Percentage of hospital admissions with a primary discharge diagnosis of heart failure during the Studies of Left Ventricular Dysfunction (SOLVD) Treatment Trial [5]. Worsening symptoms of congestive heart failure were treated with diuretics and vasodilators, including an open-label converting enzyme inhibitor if necessary. Approximately 37% of the patients in the placebo group and 26% in the enalapril group were hospitalized for heart failure during an average follow-up of 41 months. There were 288 fewer hospitalizations for heart failure in the enalapril group.

Only about 32% of all hospitalizations in this study were attributed to heart failure, and it is often difficult to assign a primary cause for a hospital admission. Nevertheless, the discharge diagnosis was made without knowledge of the assigned treatment, and the incidence of hospitalizations for heart failure translated into a reduction in total hospitalizations. Reducing the frequency of hospital admissions is clearly a worthwhile therapeutic goal that would be expected to translate into lower costs, better quality of life, and perhaps prolonged life. However, prevention of heart failure may be more cost-effective than maintaining a population with heart failure who are at a high risk for a poor outcome.

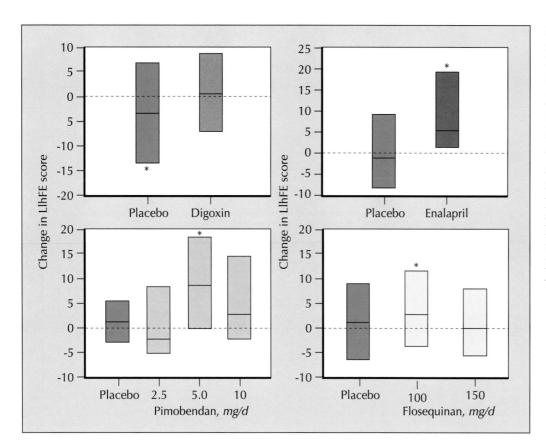

FIGURE 8-23. Responses to different medications as determined by the Minnesota Living with Heart Failure (LIhFE) questionnaire in four randomized, double-blinded clinical trials [23,27–29]. The placebo groups did not exhibit significant changes in any of these trials, and there was a significant difference between the treatment and control arms in each study. The top and bottom of each rectangle represent the 75th and 25th percentiles of the changes in the LIhFE score from baseline, respectively. The horizontal line within each rectangle is the median change score. In the *upper left*, placebo was substituted for digoxin. *Asterisks* indicate $P<0.05$.

References

1. Ho KKL, Anderson KM, Kannel WB, *et al.*: Survival after the onset of congestive heart failure in Framingham Heart Study subjects. *Circulation* 1993, 88:107–115.

2. Brophy JM: Epidemiology of congestive heart failure: Canadian data from 1970 to 1989. *Can J Cardiol* 1992, 8:495–498.

3. Califf RM, Bounous P, Harrell FE, *et al.*: The prognosis in the presence of coronary artery disease. In *Congestive Heart Failure: Current Research and Clinical Applications*. Edited by Braunwald E, Mock MB, Watson JT. New York: Grune & Stratton; 1982:31–40.

4. Kleber FX, Niemoller L, Doering W: Impact of converting enzyme inhibition on progression of chronic heart failure: results of the Munich Mild Heart Failure Trial. *Br Heart J* 1992, 67:289–296.

5. The SOLVD Investigators: Effect of enalapril on survival in patients with reduced left ventricular ejection fractions and congestive heart failure. *N Engl J Med* 1991, 325:293–302.

6. Goldman S, Johnson G, Cohn JN, *et al.*: Mechanism of death in heart failure: the vasodilator-heart failure trials. *Circulation* 1993, 87(suppl VI):24–31.

7. The CONSENSUS Trial Study Group: Effects of enalapril on mortality in severe congestive heart failure: results of the cooperative North Scandinavian enalapril survival study. *N Engl J Med* 1987, 316:1429–1435.

8. Francis GS, Cohn JN, Johnson G, *et al.*: Plasma norepinephrine, plasma renin activity and congestive heart failure: relations to survival and the effects of therapy in V-HeFT II. *Circulation* 1993, 87(suppl VI):40–48.

9. Swedberg K, Eneroth P, Kjekshus J, *et al.*: Hormones regulating cardiovascular function in patients with severe congestive heart failure and their relation to mortality. *Circulation* 1990, 82:1730–1736.

10. Cohn JN, Johnson GR, Shabetai R, *et al.*: Ejection fraction, peak exercise oxygen consumption, cardiothoracic ratio, ventricular arrhythmias, and plasma norepinephrine as determinants of prognosis in heart failure. *Circulation* 1993, 87(suppl VI):5–16.

11. Rector TS, Olivari MT, Levine TB, *et al.*: Predicting survival for an individual with congestive heart failure using the plasma nor-epinephrine concentration. *Am Heart J* 1987, 114:148–152.

12. Cintron G, Johnson G, Francis G, *et al.*: Prognostic significance of serial changes in left ventricular ejection fraction in patients with congestive heart failure. *Circulation* 1993, 87(suppl VI):17–23.

13. Cowie MR, Struthers AD, Wood DA, *et al.*: Value of natriuretic peptides in assessment of patients with possible new heart failure in primary care. *Lancet* 1997, 350:1349–1353.

14. Tsutamoto T, Wade A, Keiko M, *et al.*: Prognostic role of plasma brain natriuretic peptide concentration in patients with chronic symptomatic left ventricular dysfunction. *Circulation* 1997, 96:509–516.

15. Pacher A, Stanek B, HÅlsmann, M, *et al.*: Prognostic impact of big endothelin-1 plasma concentrations compared with invasive hemodynamic evaluation in severe heart failure. *J Am Coll Cardiol* 1996, 27:633–641.

16. Pousset F, Isnard R, Lechat P, *et al.*: Prognostic value of plasma endothelin-1 in patients with chronic heart failure. *Eur Heart J* 1997, 18:254–258.

17. Fu GS, Meissner A, Simon, R: Repolarization dispersion and sudden cardiac death in patients with impaired left ventricular function. *Eur Heart J* 1997, 18:281–289.

18. Barr CS, Naas A, Freeman M, *et al.*: QT dispersion and sudden unexpected death in chronic heart failure. *Lancet* 1994, 327–329.

19. Doval HC, Nul DR, Grancelli HO, *et al.*: Randomised trial of low-dose amiodarone in severe congestive heart failure (GESICA). *Lancet* 1994, 344:493–498.

20. Singh SN, Fletcher RD, Fisher SG, *et al.*: Amiodarone in patients with congestive heart failure and asymptomatic ventricular arrhythmia (CHFSTAT). *N Engl J Med* 1995, 333:77–82.

21. Amiodarone Trial Meta-Analysis Investigators: Effect of prophylactic amiodarone on mortality after acute myocardial infarction and in congestive heart failure: meta-analysis of individual data from 6500 patients in randomised trials. *Lancet* 1997, 350:1417–1424.

22. Moss AJ, Hall WJ, Cannom DS, *et al.*: Improved survival with an implanted defibrillator in patients with coronary disease at high risk for ventricular arrhythmia (MADIT Trial). *N Engl J Med* 1996, 335:1933–1940.

23. Packer M, Gheorghiade M, Young JB, *et al.*: Withdrawal of digoxin from patients with chronic heart failure treated with angiotensin converting enzyme inhibitors. *N Engl J Med* 1993, 329:1–7.

24. Captopril Multicenter Research Group: A placebo-controlled trial of captopril in refractory chronic congestive heart failure. *J Am Coll Cardiol* 1983, 2:755–763.

25. Enalapril Congestive Heart Failure Investigators: Long-term effects of enalapril in patients with congestive heart failure: a multicenter, placebo-controlled trial. *Heart Failure* 1987, 1:102–107.

26. Lipkin DP, Scriven AJ, Crake T, *et al.*: Six minute walking test for assessing exercise capacity in chronic heart failure. *BMJ* 1986, 292:653–655.

27. Rector TS, Cohn JN: Assessment of patient outcome with the Minnesota Living with Heart Failure questionnaire: reliability and validity during a randomized, double-blind, placebo controlled trial of pimobendan. *Am Heart J* 1992, 124:1017–1025.

28. Rector TS, Kubo SH, Cohn JN: Validity of the Minnesota Living with Heart Failure questionnaire as a measure of therapeutic response to enalapril or placebo. *Am J Cardiol* 1993, 71:1106–1107.

29. Massie BM, Berk MR, Brozena SC, *et al.*.: Can further benefit be achieved by adding flosequinan to patients with congestive heart failure who remain symptomatic on diuretic, digoxin and a converting enzyme inhibitor? Results of the Flosequinan-ACE Inhibitor Trial (FACET). *Circulation* 1993, 88:492–501.

Unstable Heart Failure

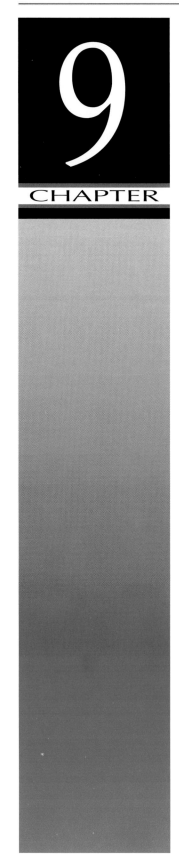

9

CHAPTER

Carl V. Leier

Unstable heart failure represents the clinical state of progressively worsening or decompensated heart failure, which, if not improved within a reasonable time (usually minutes to hours), often evolves into markedly symptomatic heart failure, cardiovascular collapse, and shock or death. The clinical settings include, among others, the patient who arrives in the emergency room in acute pulmonary edema, the patient with postinfarction cardiogenic shock, the patient who cannot be weaned from cardiopulmonary bypass after cardiac surgery, or the chronic heart failure patient who is experiencing a rather abrupt worsening of symptoms. Most patients with unstable heart failure must be approached with a certain sense of urgency.

The management approach to unstable heart failure is directed specifically at improving the tenuous clinical condition and suffering that many of these patients are experiencing, and promptly correcting or reversing the underlying cause of the unstable, decompensated cardiac condition. The 1-year mortality rate for patients who present with acute pulmonary edema and whose underlying lesion or condition is not determined, corrected, or properly treated exceeds 50% and is worse for those who go on to develop cardiogenic shock [1–4]. For many patients, unstable or decompensated cardiac failure cannot be improved without definitive correction of the underlying lesion (*eg*, acute valvular regurgitation, high-grade obstructive disease of the left main coronary artery).

Atherosclerotic coronary artery disease is the most common etiology for acute and chronic heart failure in Western societies. The short- and long-term clinical courses of patients with atherosclerotic heart disease are strongly dependent on the relative amounts of well-perfused viable myocardium, reversibly ischemic myocardium, and infarcted (irreversibly necrotic or fibrotic) myocardium. Methods are now available to save jeopardized, ischemic myocardium from infarction and to bring it back to a viable, functional state; these methods include thrombolysis, interventional coronary catheterization (*eg*, angioplasty), and bypass surgery. For the patient who presents with unstable heart failure secondary to acute myocardial infarction, the concept of "time is muscle" is extremely important. Detection of myocardial infarction, followed by definitive diagnostic and therapeutic interventions (medical or surgical), must take place as soon as possible after patient presentation. A delay in or inefficient delivery of definitive cardiovascular services in this setting unequivocally jeopardizes the immediate and long-term outcome of the patient who presents with symptomatic heart failure caused by occlusive coronary artery disease.

From the standpoint of clinical relevance and application and for the sake of clarity, unstable heart failure is presented here as acute heart failure and decompensated chronic heart failure. The views presented in this chapter are consistent with the heart failure guidelines of the American College of Cardiology/American Heart Association Task Force on Practice Guidelines [5].

ACUTE HEART FAILURE

COMPARISONS OF UNSTABLE VS CHRONIC HEART FAILURE

FEATURE	ACUTE HEART FAILURE	DECOMPENSATED CHRONIC HEART FAILURE	CHRONIC HEART FAILURE
Symptom severity	Marked	Marked	Mild to moderate
Pulmonary edema	Frequent	Frequent	Rare
Peripheral edema	Rare	Frequent	Frequent
Weight gain	None to mild	Frequent	Frequent
Whole-body fluid volume load	No change or mild increase	Markedly increased	Increased
Cardiomegaly	Uncommon	Usual*	Common*
Ventricular systolic function	Hypo-, normo-, or hypercontractile	Reduced*	Reduced*
Wall stress	Elevated	Markedly elevated	Elevated
Activation of sympathetic nervous system	Marked	Marked	Mild to marked
Activation of renin-angiotensin-aldosterone axis	Often increased	Marked	Mild to marked
Reparable, remedial causative lesion(s)	Common	Occasional	Occasional

*Patients with diastolic dysfunction heart failure may have little to no cardiomegaly and normal systolic function.

FIGURE 9-1. Comparisons of unstable versus chronic heart failure. Clinical and pathophysiologic characteristics of the two major categories of unstable heart failure (acute heart failure and decompensated chronic heart failure) are compared with those of chronic heart failure. Chronic heart failure (compensated and decompensated) is accompanied by total volume overload, weight gain, and edema. In contrast, acute heart failure is less characterized by total volume overload but is often accompanied by a shift of intravascular volume centrally to cardiac chambers and pulmonary vasculature. Therefore, diuretics, angiotensin-converting enzyme inhibitors, and digitalis represent rational pharmacotherapy for chronic heart failure. Acute preload and afterload reduction (sublingual and intravenous nitroglycerin or nitroprusside), supplemented by intravenous diuretic administration and occasionally by positive inotropic or vasopressor support (eg, dobutamine, dopamine), represent the proper pharmacotherapeutic approach to most patients with acute heart failure. A combination of these strategies is often necessary to stabilize and improve decompensated chronic heart failure. An important feature that distinguishes the management approach to acute heart failure from that of chronic heart failure is the high incidence of reparable lesions (eg, acute occlusion of a major coronary artery, ruptured chordae tendineae) causing acute heart failure, although an occasional patient with chronic heart failure may also require definitive intervention.

MAJOR CAUSES OF ACUTE HEART FAILURE

Myocardial ischemia-infarction

   Ventricular systolic or diastolic dysfunction

   Mitral valve regurgitation

   Ventricular rupture (septum, free wall)

Disruption of valvular apparatus (aortic, mitral)

Myocarditis or cardiomyopathy

Uncontrolled, severe systemic hypertension

Others, *eg*, cardiac dysrhythmias, pulmonary emboli, pulmonary hypertension, pericardial tamponade

FIGURE 9-2. Major causes of acute heart failure. Acute heart failure is often caused by one or more of these common conditions. It is apparent that many of these disorders and lesions can be definitively treated. Therefore, in addition to clinical and hemodynamic stabilization, the approach to acute heart failure includes an active search and specific intervention for reparable lesions with the dual intent of improving the patient's short- and long-term course and averting a recurrence of acute heart failure and evolution into chronic heart failure.

STEPS IN CLINICAL AND HEMODYNAMIC STABILIZATION OF ACUTE HEART FAILURE

1. Administer oxygen ($\uparrow F_iO_2$)

2. When accompanied by fluid volume overload or a "congestive" component

   Sublingual nitroglycerin

   Intravenous furosemide

   Consider morphine sulfate

   Consider additional preload-afterload reduction

3. Evaluate early for

   Readily reversible causes of acute heart failure (*eg*, cardiac dysrhythmias, pericardial tamponade); if present, initiate appropriate intervention

   Myocardial ischemia-infarction; if present, promptly initiate appropriate interventions (*eg*, thrombolytic therapy, urgent angioplasty)

4. If patient is refractory to above therapies, hypotensive, or in cardiogenic shock

   Intravenous fluid administration if no evidence is found for fluid volume overload

   Consider intravenous inotropic or vasopressor agents

   Consider catheterization (pulmonary and systemic arterial)

   Obtain echocardiogram to assist in diagnosis, evaluation, and reparability of the culprit lesion or condition

   Consider need for mechanical circulatory assistance (intra-aortic balloon counterpulsation)

5. Proceed to definitive diagnostic and interventional procedures

FIGURE 9-3. General management of acute heart failure. Because of the high likelihood of an underlying reparable lesion or condition, the general management approach to acute heart failure emphasizes definitive diagnostic studies. The patient's hemodynamic and clinical status are improved and stabilized to allow safe passage through definitive diagnostic testing (*eg*, echocardiography, cardiac catheterization) and intervention (*eg*, surgery, coronary angioplasty). Major steps in the initial management of acute heart failure [2,5–28] are arranged in the general order of application and according to the general types of acute heart failure encountered:

  1) When possible, it is informative to obtain pulse oximetry or arterial blood for gas analysis before oxygen administration.

  2) Sublingual nitroglycerin can be administered at a dose of 1 tablet (1 or 2 sprays) every 5 minutes three or four times until intravenous nitroglycerin or nitroprusside can take effect. Furosemide is usually administered in a dose range of 20 to 80 mg intravenously. Preload-afterload reduction beyond sublingual nitroglycerin is best achieved by intravenous administration of nitroglycerin or nitroprusside.

  3) The medical history and electrocardiogram are obtained early in the evaluation of the patient with acute heart failure to determine whether myocardial ischemia-infarction is the underlying cause for the acute event and whether the patient is a candidate for acute intervention (*eg*, thrombolytic therapy, coronary angioplasty).

  4) Dobutamine, dopamine, and norepinephrine represent the principal inotropic or vasopressor agents used in this acute care setting.

  5) Once the patient's condition is stabilized, diagnostic and interventional procedures can be performed.

CONSIDERATIONS IN ADMINISTERING MORPHINE SULFATE FOR ACUTE HEART FAILURE

DOSE

2–6 mg intravenously

OPTIONAL THERAPY

Consider in the patient with pulmonary edema who is still dyspneic after admin-istration of sublingual nitroglycerin (× 3–4)

PRECAUTIONS IN PATIENTS WITH HEART FAILURE

Acidosis or marginally compensated acidosis

Chronic lung disease

Inadequate availability of prompt ventilatory support, if needed

FIGURE 9-4. Considerations in administering morphine sulfate for acute heart failure. With the appropriate use of sublingual and intravenous nitroglycerin, morphine sulfate should no longer be viewed as a routine step in the management of acute heart failure, particularly in the presence of the precautions noted.

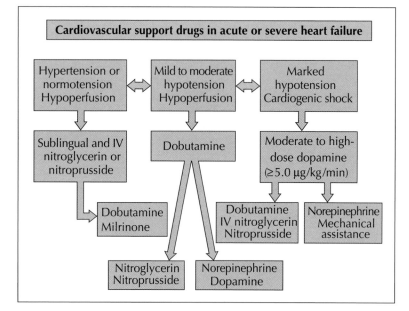

FIGURE 9-5. A practical working diagram of the cardiovascular support drugs commonly employed in the initial short-term management of acute or severe heart failure. It is assumed that patients who require these support drugs have adequate to high left ventricular diastolic filling pressures (≥18 mm Hg) or clinical evidence of fluid volume overload. Systemic hypoperfusion and hypotension in a patient without evidence of volume overload or with filling pressures of less than 18 mm Hg should be approached with a fluid volume challenge as the first step. On the basis of the clinical presentation and the state of systemic perfusion and blood pressure, the initial drug of choice is selected and its dosage is increased until clinical or hemodynamic endpoints are achieved or adverse effects appear. At this point, inadequate improvement of clinical status usually requires either the addition of a second agent as combination therapy or mechanical assistance. IV—intravenous.

PRINCIPAL PRELOAD- AND AFTERLOAD-REDUCING DRUGS FOR ACUTE OR SEVERE HEART FAILURE

DRUG	DOSING	POTENTIAL ADVANTAGE	POTENTIAL DISADVANTAGES
Nitroglycerin	Sublingual: 1 tablet (or 1–2 sprays) × 3–4 at 5-min intervals Intravenous: 0.4 µg/kg/min initially; increase as needed	Favorable effect on coronary vasculature and in myocardial ischemia-infarction	Tolerance during prolonged infusion Fluid retention Inadequate afterload reduction in catastrophic cardio-vascular disorders (eg, acute valvular insufficiency, ventricular rupture)
Nitroprusside	Intravenous: 0.1 µg/kg/min initially; increase as needed	Relatively powerful afterload reduction	Less favorable effect on coronary vasculature and myocardial ischemia; administration must be closely monitored to avoid marked hypotension; thiocyanate or cyanide toxicity during high-dose or prolonged infusions, particularly in patients with renal failure

FIGURE 9-6. Principal preload- and afterload-reducing drugs for acute or severe heart failure. Nitroglycerin and nitroprusside are the primary vasodilators employed to reduce excessive preload and afterload in acute or severe heart failure [6,7]. Nitroglycerin is used most often, particularly in conditions caused by occlusive atherosclerotic coronary artery disease. Nitroprusside is the drug of choice when more aggressive afterload and preload reduction are needed; examples include catastrophic cardiovascular events (eg, acute, severe mitral or aortic regurgitation), hypertensive emergencies (eg, aortic dissection, pulmonary edema), and inadequate response to nitroglycerin. These agents have obviated volume phlebotomy as an intervention for the vast majority of patients who present with acute pulmonary edema.

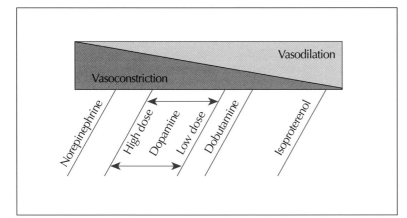

FIGURE 9-7. The comparative systemic vascular response to the major sympathomimetic amines most commonly employed in acute or severe heart failure. Low-dose (<5.0 µg/kg/min) dopamine has significant visceral and renal vasodilatory properties but behaves as a vasoconstrictor at higher doses (>6.0 µg/kg/min) [8–13]. Norepinephrine is used primarily for its vasoconstrictor properties and dobutamine for its positive inotropic and favorable vascular effects (decreasing vascular resistance). Because vasodilatation is more predictably and safely achieved with nitroglycerin and nitroprusside, isoproterenol is at present only infrequently used in the management of acute heart failure.

A. PHARMACOLOGIC PROPERTIES AND THERAPEUTIC CONSIDERATIONS IN USING INOTROPIC AGENTS

PHARMACOLOGIC FEATURE	DOBUTAMINE	DOPAMINE LOW DOSE	DOPAMINE HIGH DOSE	NOREPINEPHRINE
General description	Positive inotrope with balanced peripheral vascular effects	Dopaminergic vasodilator, "renal" dopaminergic dose	Vasopressor with some positive inotropic effects	Vasopressor
Dose, *µg/kg/min*				
Initial	2.0	1.0	5.0	0.03
Usual range	2–20	1–5	5–20	0.02–0.20
Most common adverse effects	Tachycardia Dysrhythmias Angina	Dysrhythmias	Tachycardia Dysrhythmias Intense vasoconstriction Angina	Intense vasoconstriction Dysrhythmias Angina

B. PHARMACOLOGIC PROPERTIES AND THERAPEUTIC CONSIDERATIONS IN USING INOTROPIC AGENTS

PHARMACOLOGIC FEATURE	DOBUTAMINE	MILRINONE	DOPAMINE LOW DOSE	DOPAMINE HIGH DOSE	NOREPINEPHRINE
Receptor agonism					
α	+	0	+	+++	++++
β_1	++++	0	+	++	+
β_2	++	0	0	0	0
Dopaminergic	0	0	+++	++	0
Systemic vascular resistance	↓↓	↓↓↓	↓	↑↑	↑↑↑↑
Stroke volume and cardiac output	↑↑↑↑	↑↑↑↑	↑	↑↑	↑
Ability to increase systemic blood pressure	→ to ↑	→ to ↑	→	↑↑↑	↑↑↑↑
Ventricular filling pressure	↓↓	↓↓↓	↓ to →	→ to ↑↑	→ to ↑↑
Chronotropic	→ to ↑↑	→↓↑	→	→ to ↑↑↑	→ to ↑
Myocardial oxygen demand or supply	→ to ↑	→↓↓	→	→ to ↑↑	→ to ↑↑

Phosphodioesterase inhibitor.

FIGURE 9-8. A and **B,** Principal pharmacologic properties and therapeutic considerations in the use of the major inotropic and vasopressor agents in acute heart failure.

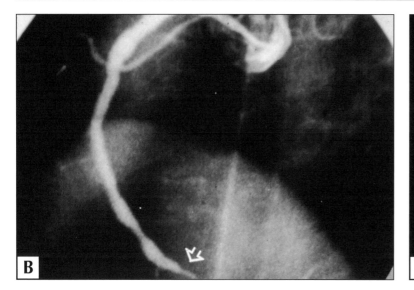

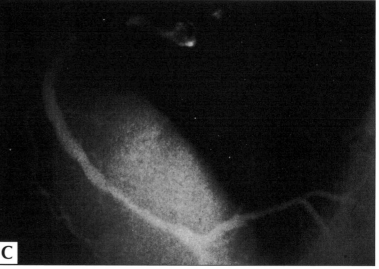

FIGURE 9-9. Electrocardiographic diagnosis of acute myocardial ischemia-infarction as a cause of acute or decompensated heart failure. **A,** Electrocardiographic tracing obtained in the emergency room showing inferoposterior injury in a 61-year-old woman who presented with a 45-minute history of marked dyspnea, chest discomfort, and nausea.

B and **C,** Angioplasty of the acutely thrombosed, high-grade right coronary artery obstruction (*arrow* in *B* depicts point of obstruction) reestablished patency and flow (*C*), and symptoms resolved within 1 hour of presentation.

MANAGEMENT OF ACUTE MYOCARDIAL INJURY–ISCHEMIA–INFARCTION IN THE PRESENTATION OF ACUTE HEART FAILURE

Early detection with successful treatment is crucial for favorable short- and long-term clinical course and prognosis; "time is muscle"

Thrombolytic therapy

    Presentation within 12 h of the onset of angina or angina-equivalent symptoms with ECG changes of injury-ischemia

    Angina or angina-equivalent symptoms and ECG changes of injury-ischemia ± infarction that recur or persist beyond 6 h since the onset of symptoms

Emergent cardiac catheterization ± intervention

    If readily accessible, can be the initial approach to acute myocardial injury-ischemia (catheterization laboratory modalities: angioplasty ± stent placement, assessment for urgent bypass surgery)

    Ischemic symptoms or signs (ECG) that persist or recur beyond initial management and thrombolytic therapy

    Cardiogenic shock or near-shock

    Refractory or recurrent acute heart failure

    Evaluation of clinical events that have a high likelihood of evolving into heart failure (*eg,* new systolic murmur)

FIGURE 9-10. Major issues in the management of myocardial injury- ischemia-infarction in the setting of acute heart failure [2–4,20–28]. The important principles of general management include prompt detection and management of myocardial injury-ischemia- infarction; prompt detection and treatment of the lesions underlying the development of acute heart failure; and vigilance for the complications of ischemia or infarction (*eg,* ruptured myocardium), which can potentially evolve into cardiovascular decompensation and failure. ECG—electrocardiogram.

INDWELLING VASCULAR CATHETERS

A. INDWELLING PULMONARY ARTERY CATHETERS (SWAN-GANZ CATHETER)

APPLICATIONS IN ACUTE HEART FAILURE

Acute heart failure not responsive to standard, initial measures

Cardiogenic shock and near-shock not responsive to initial management

Uncertain status of intravascular volume and ventricular filling pressures

Monitor and guide the administration of fluid volume and cardioactive drugs (*eg*, nitroprusside, dobutamine, dopamine)

Assessment of dyspnea and other potential symptoms of heart failure in patients with other conditions (*eg*, chronic lung disease, marked obesity)

Assist in the determination of whether pulmonary edema is of cardiogenic or noncardiogenic origin

Evaluation of a new systolic murmur when echocardiography is not available or diagnostic

GENERAL REQUIREMENTS

Experienced, proficient operator

Trained personnel to assist in catheter insertion, use, and maintenance

Compatible, accurate amplification-recording equipment

Catheterization laboratory, emergency department, or intensive care unit setting

B. INDWELLING SYSTEMIC ARTERIAL CATHETERS

APPLICATIONS IN ACUTE HEART FAILURE

Continuous monitoring and recording of systemic blood pressure

Conduit for frequent, repeated blood gas determinations

FIGURE 9-11. General indications and other issues of practical application for the pulmonary artery (Swan-Ganz) catheter (**A**) and systemic arterial catheter (**B**). Indwelling vascular catheters may be necessary for the management of acute or severe heart failure. The pulmonary artery catheter can provide useful data to assist in the diagnosis of certain threatening lesions and conditions (*eg*, right ventricular infarction, ruptured ventricular septum) in addition to its use in monitoring fluid and drug therapy.

ECHOCARDIOGRAPHY

GENERAL APPLICATIONS FOR ECHOCARDIOGRAPHY IN ACUTE HEART FAILURE

Part of the overall diagnostic evaluation of acute heart failure

Emergently in

   Cardiogenic shock and near-shock

   Refractory pulmonary edema

When the underlying etiology is not clear or requires confirmation or the differential diagnoses include major, often masked, reparable lesions

In the assessment of the extent of myocardial involvement in acute ischemia and infarction

As part of the cardiac evaluation of unexplained dyspnea and other symptoms of respiratory failure

In the evaluation of a new systolic murmur and its role in the clinical presentation

FIGURE 9-12. Common clinical reasons for the use of echocardiography in acute heart failure. Examples of major, often masked, reparable lesions include clinically silent aortic stenosis, mitral stenosis or regurgitation, pericardial tamponade, and intracardiac tumor. Assessing the extent of myocardial involvement by echocardiography in acute ischemia and infarction is particularly informative in patients with nondiagnostic electrocardiograms (*eg*, left bundle branch block).

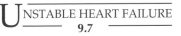

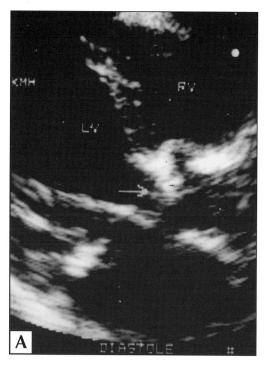

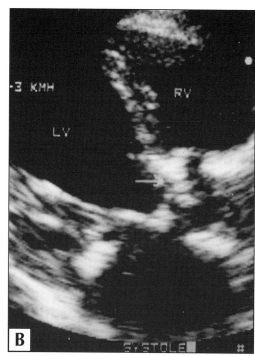

FIGURE 9-13. Echocardiography in the determination of the severity and etiology of ventricular dysfunction and failure. Echocardiograms of a 71-year-old man who presented with acute pulmonary edema after a 4- to 5-month history of dyspnea on exertion. Signs of congestive heart failure were apparent on physical examination. Diastolic (**A**) and systolic (**B**) echocardiograms demonstrated a heavily calcified, poorly mobile, stenotic aortic valve (*arrow*) and consequent ventricular hypertrophy, enlargement, and failure (ejection fraction, 0.24). A systolic murmur was barely audible. This patient represents an example of acute (and chronic) congestive heart failure secondary to silent aortic stenosis. A severely reduced aortic valve area (<0.4 cm^2) was calculated via echo and catheter. Aortic valve replacement dramatically improved the patient's hemodynamic and clinical condition. LV—left ventricle; RV—right ventricle. (*Courtesy of* Dr. Anthony C. Pearson, Columbus, OH.)

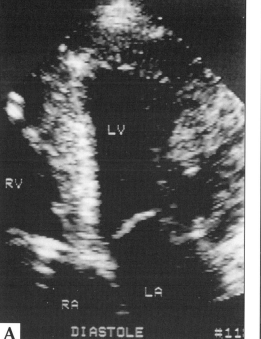

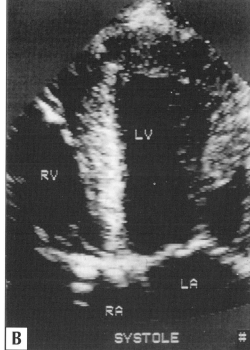

FIGURE 9-14. Echocardiograhy in the diagnosis of occlusive coronary atherosclerosis as a cause of unstable heart failure. A 56-year-old diabetic woman presented with acute dyspnea, mild hypotension, systemic hypoperfusion, and clinical evidence of congestive heart failure. The chronic left bundle branch block seen on electrocardiography precluded additional diagnostic interpretation. Echocardiography demonstrated septal, apical, and anterolateral hypokinesis and probably apical thrombus. Urgent cardiac catheterization and angiography were performed and acute, complete occlusion of the left anterior descending coronary artery was noted. Flow was reestablished by urgent angioplasty, with improvement of her clinical condition over the subsequent 2 days. **A**, Diastole. **B**, Systole. LA—left atrium; LV—left ventricle; RA—right atrium; RV—right ventricle. (*Courtesy of* Dr. Anthony C. Pearson, Columbus, OH.)

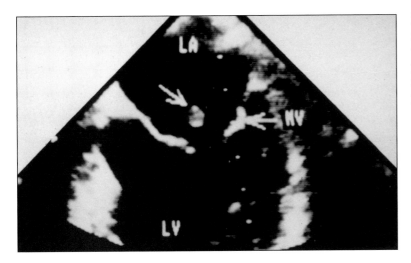

FIGURE 9-15. The pivotal role of echocardiography in acute heart failure. The transesophageal echocardiogram of a 77-year-old woman who developed a new systolic murmur and acute pulmonary edema 2 days after she presented with an anterior myocardial infarction. The *left arrow* depicts the head of a ruptured papillary muscle within the left atrium (LA). Intra-aortic balloon counterpulsation was promptly instituted. The patient was then urgently advanced through coronary angiography into cardiac surgery (mitral valve replacement and coronary artery bypass surgery). After a prolonged postoperative course, she was discharged, clinically improved, to her home. LV—left ventricle; MV—mitral valve. (*Courtesy of* Dr. Anthony C. Pearson, Columbus, OH.)

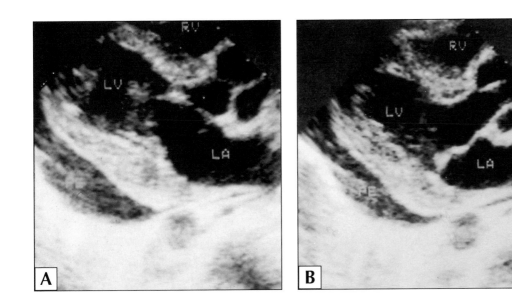

FIGURE 9-16. A 26-year-old man was transferred with a history of 2 days of progressively worsening malaise, generalized weakness, and cardiomegaly on chest radiography. Distended neck veins and hypotension (systemic systolic blood pressure, 70 mm Hg) were noted on physical examination. Echocardiography demonstrated considerable pericardial effusion (PE), with right ventricular collapse (*arrow*) present during diastole (**A**), consistent with tamponade pathophysiology. Rapid intravenous volume administration and pericardiocentesis relieved his symptoms and the near-shock or shock condition. **B,** Systole. LA—left atrium; LV—left ventricle; RV—right ventricle. (*Courtesy of* Dr. Anthony C. Pearson, Columbus, OH.)

INTRA-AORTIC BALLOON COUNTERPULSATION

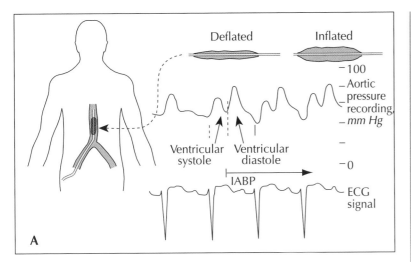

FIGURE 9-17. Intra-aortic balloon counterpulsation. **A,** Mechanical support in acute heart failure via intra-aortic balloon counterpulsation (IABP). By inflating a balloon within the blood-filled aorta during diastole, intra-aortic counterpulsation improves hemodynamics by augmenting coronary or myocardial and peripheral tissue perfusion. Myocardial oxygen consumption and ventricular afterload are reduced as well [15–20]. **B,** General applications in acute heart failure. ECG—electrocardiogram.

B. GENERAL APPLICATIONS FOR INTRA-AORTIC BALLOON COUNTERPULSATION

Cardiogenic shock

Cardiogenic near-shock not responsive to standard therapy

Acute pulmonary edema and other forms of acute cardiac failure not responsive to standard initial therapy

Acute heart failure accompanied by refractory angina or an obstructive lesion of the left main coronary artery

For clinical and hemodynamic stabilization through definitive diagnostic and therapeutic procedures

Relative contraindications in acute heart failure

Significant aortic insufficiency

Aortic dissection, aneurysm

THE MAJOR, DEFINITIVE DIAGNOSTIC, AND INTERVENTIONAL PROCEDURES MOST COMMONLY USED IN THE MANAGEMENT OF ACUTE HEART FAILURE

DIAGNOSTIC	INTERVENTIONAL
Electrocardiography	Thrombolysis
Chest radiography	Coronary angioplasty ± stent placement
Echocardiography (transthoracic, transesophageal)	Coronary artery bypass surgery
Cardiac catheterization	Valvular repair or replacement
Coronary arteriography	Repair of ventricular rupture (septal, papillary, free wall)
Contrast ventriculography	Others (eg, pericardiocentesis for tamponade, aortic surgery of acute dissection)

FIGURE 9-18. Procedures most commonly used in the management of acute heart failure. Echocardiography and catheterization are the major diagnostic modalities used to define the presence and reversibility of the causative lesion in acute heart failure. Other methods, such as nuclear magnetic resonance imaging, may also be useful in certain clinical conditions. Based on the findings of these diagnostic studies, a variety of interventions may be used to reverse and treat the culprit lesion. A crucial component in management of acute heart failure is clinical and hemodynamic stabilization of the patient to allow performance of definitive diagnostic studies and interventional procedures. The short- and long-term outcomes of patients with acute heart failure are directly related to the proficient management of acute heart failure, clinical and hemodynamic stabilization, and definitive diagnosis and intervention.

CAVEATS AND PITFALLS IN THE MANAGEMENT OF ACUTE HEART FAILURE

Misdiagnosis

Delay in the diagnosis and treatment of myocardial ischemia-infarction

Overtreatment

Unattended or unmonitored "gap" in management

FIGURE 9-19. The most common major caveats and pitfalls in the overall management of acute heart failure. A number of other conditions, many readily treatable, can present with symptoms and signs very similar to those of acute heart failure. These include pulmonary embolization, acute asthma, pneumonia, and septicemia, among others. A good medical history and physical examination, selection of key diagnostic studies, and clinical judgment are the best tools available to obviate misdiagnosis.

As noted in Figure 9-10, an immediate effort must be made to exclude or detect the presence of myocardial ischemia or infarction as the underlying cause of acute heart failure. Any delay in this process allows ischemic myocardium to convert to infarction, and thus threatens the short- and long-term clinical course and prognosis. Overtreatment of acute heart failure, particularly acute pulmonary edema, is not uncommon in critical care medicine. The apparent urgency of the clinical presentation creates a sense that the patient has to be treated "fast and hard." Sublingual and intravenous nitroglycerin, high or repeated doses of diuretics, and morphine sulfate usually provide symptomatic relief but occasionally lead to overdiuresis, hypotension, and impaired peripheral perfusion. Good judgment in clinical therapeutics is the best means of prevention. It is not uncommon for the treated acute heart failure patient to pass through an unattended and unmonitored management "gap." This usually occurs after the initial management and before the patient's continued care is assumed by the inpatient medical team. This period represents a vulnerable time in a patient's early course, and is often further complicated by unfavorable logistic situations, such as an interhospital transfer or the transport or transfer from the emergency department to the intensive or coronary care unit. The consequences of misdiagnosis or overtreatment often appear at this time.

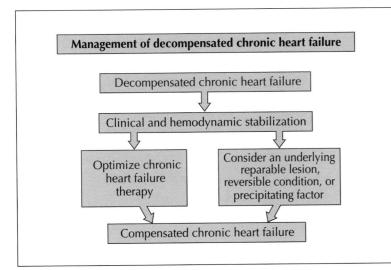

Management of decompensated chronic heart failure

Decompensated chronic heart failure

Clinical and hemodynamic stabilization

Optimize chronic heart failure therapy

Consider an underlying reparable lesion, reversible condition, or precipitating factor

Compensated chronic heart failure

FIGURE 9-20. Management of decompensated chronic heart failure. The majority of patients with chronic heart failure who experience a period of decompensation respond clinically to temporary hemodynamic stabilization or optimization of chronic heart failure therapy (*see* Fig. 9-25). An occasional patient decompensates because of a superimposed lesion or condition, which may be reparable or reversible (*eg*, new-onset atrial fibrillation or flutter, myocardial ischemia, pulmonary embolization).

MAJOR PRECIPITATING FACTORS FOR DECOMPENSATION OF CHRONIC HEART FAILURE

Inadequate therapy or noncompliance

Drug resistance or tolerance

Adverse drug effects

Negative inotropic properties

Salt and water retention

Drug cancellation of a therapeutic effect

Deterioration of underlying cardiac disease

Excessive salt intake

Complicating conditions

Myocardial ischemia-infarction

Uncontrolled systemic hypertension

Dysrhythmias

Development or exacerbation of valvular dysfunction

Pulmonary embolization

Others

FIGURE 9-21. Major precipitating factors for decompensation of chronic heart failure. Several reparable lesions, reversible conditions, and precipitating factors should be considered when a patient with heart failure presents with decompensation. Complicating conditions include atrial flutter or fibrillation with or without rapid ventricular response, mitral regurgitation, or renal dysfunction that could lead to renal failure. Among adverse drug effects, certain calcium channel blockers (*eg*, verapamil) and antiarrhythmic drugs (*eg*, disopyramide) may have negative inotropic properties, and nonsteroidal anti-inflammatory drugs can cause salt and water retention. While the patient's decompensated heart failure is being improved and stabilized, the physician should evaluate via medical history and physical examination whether any of these conditions may have led to the decompen-sation and, when appropriate, obtain specifically directed laboratory tests (*eg*, echocardiography-Doppler studies to assess severity of valvular regurgitation).

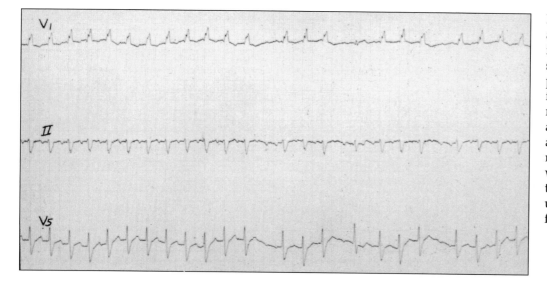

FIGURE 9-22. Electrocardiograpy in assessing decompensated chronic heart failure. A 70-year-old man with chronic, stable systolic and diastolic heart failure presented with increasing dyspnea, fatigue, malaise, and weakness. The rhythm strip of his electrocardiogram on admission showed a rapidly conducting atrial flutter. The dysrhythmia was of recent onset. Slowing the ventricular rate with digitalis and subsequent conversion to sinus rhythm resulted in a return to his usual state of well-compensated heart failure.

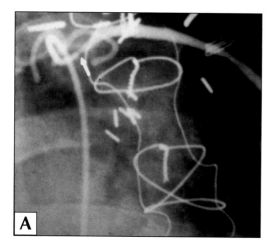
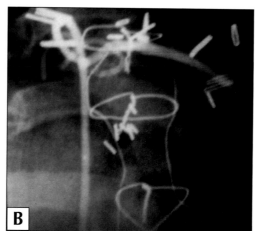

FIGURE 9-23. Coronary arteriography in the evaluation of unstable heart failure. A 39-year-old man with chronic heart failure presented with increasing angina, dyspnea at rest, and two recent episodes of acute pulmonary edema. **A,** Coronary arteriography demonstrated a high-grade occlusive lesion (*arrow*) of the very proximal portion of a previous saphenous vein graft to the left anterior descending coronary artery. **B,** Laser-assisted angioplasty reestablished good patency and flow to the graft, with resolution of the angina and the symptoms of acute decompensated heart failure.

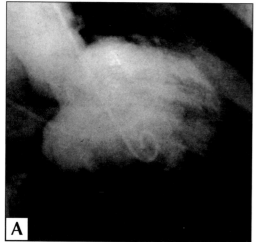
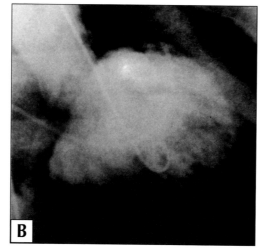

FIGURE 9-24. The diastolic (**A**) and systolic (**B**) frames of a contrast ventriculogram performed on a 47-year-old woman with long-standing systemic hypertension and a 3-year history of chronic heart failure. Discontinuation of her antihypertensive therapy and dietary indiscretion (excessive salt intake during the first week of her new job as a waitress) led to severe decompensated heart failure. After the initial management of decompensated heart failure, reestablishment of her antihypertensive therapy, optimization of her chronic heart failure medication, and dietary measures returned her to a state of stable compensation.

A. THERAPEUTICS FOR CHRONIC HEART FAILURE

STANDARD MAINTENANCE THERAPY

Angiotensin-converting enzyme inhibitors

Diuretics

Digoxin

Consider β-blockers with vasodilating properties

SUPPLEMENTAL AGENTS

Hydralazine-nitrate combination*

Nitrates*

Anticoagulation, antithrombotic agents

Calcium-channel blockers (second- and third-generation dihydropyridines)*

B. THERAPEUTICS FOR CHRONIC HEART FAILURE

SUPPORT DRUGS USED DURING PERIODS OF
DECOMPENSATION IN CHRONIC HEART FAILURE

Diuretics (intravenously administered or ↑ dose)

Positive inotropic agents (± vasodilating properties)

  Dobutamine (see Fig. 9-29)

  Dopamine (low to moderate dose)

  Phosphodiesterase inhibitors (eg, milrinone)
    Under active investigation
      Levosimendan
      Toborinone

Vasodilators

  IV nitroglycerin

  Nitroprusside

  Under active investigation

  Endothelin blockers

  β-Natriuretic peptide

Vasopressors

  Dopamine (moderate to high dose)

  Norepinephrine

FIGURE 9-25. Therapeutics for chronic heart failure. **A,** In patients with chronic congestive heart failure, optimization of standard therapy with angiotensin-converting enzyme inhibitors, diuretics, digoxin, third-generation β-blockers (with vasodilating properties, *eg,* carvediol), and the judicious use of supplemental agents are often effective in averting clinical decompensation. *Asterisks* indicate drugs that are not yet approved for a heart failure indication by the Food and Drug Administration.

  B, Once decompensation has occurred, parenteral agents are frequently necessary to regain clinical stability. Shown are the agents most commonly used to improve and stabilize severely decompensated chronic heart failure. Dobutamine and dopamine (low to moderate dose) are particularly effective in acutely improving clinical and hemodynamic status and stabilizing the status during a period of diuresis and readjustment of chronic therapy. Vasodilators are employed to improve hemodynamics and systemic perfusion in chronic heart failure patients with adequate to high systemic blood pressure, and vasopressors are used in conditions of marked hypotension or shock. The clinical application of these agents is similar to that discussed previously for the treatment of acute heart failure. IV—intravenous.

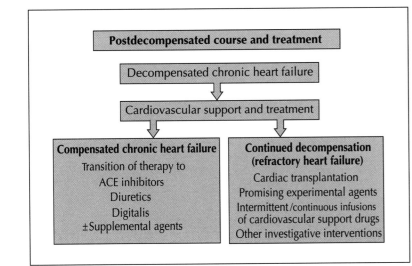

FIGURE 9-26. Course and treatment for postdecompensated chronic heart failure. With appropriate cardiovascular support and management, most patients with decompensated chronic heart failure can be converted to a state of clinical compensation. Other than cardiac transplantation, the management choices for patients who continue to have decompensated (refractory) chronic heart failure are limited to investigative approaches including experimental drugs or procedures (*eg,* ventricular reduction surgery) and intermittent or continuous infusion of a cardiovascular support drug (*eg,* dobutamine, milrinone). ACE—angiotensin-converting enzyme.

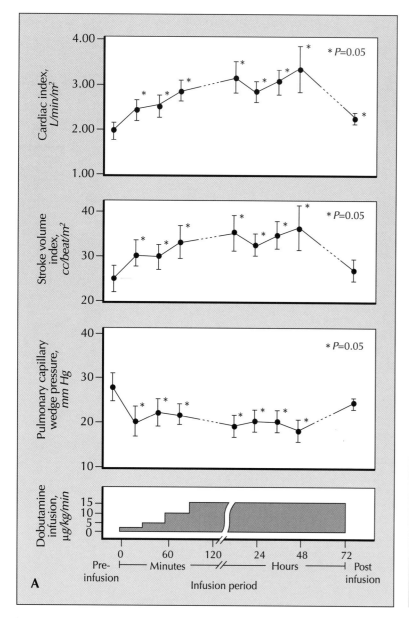

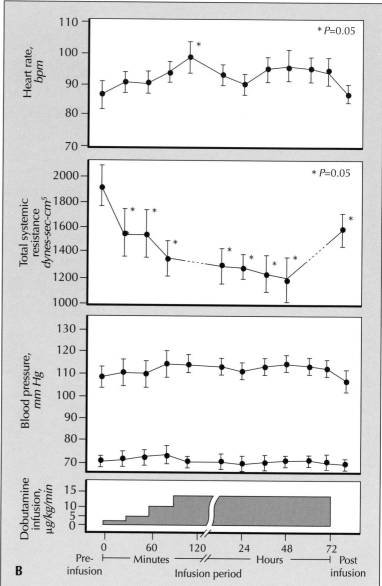

FIGURE 9-27. Hemodynamic dose-response (**A**) and continuous-infusion curves (**B**) for dobutamine in 25 patients with severe chronic congestive heart failure. Data are presented as ± SEM with *P*<0.05 versus baseline preinfusion value. (*Adapted from* Leier and coworkers [11]; with permission.)

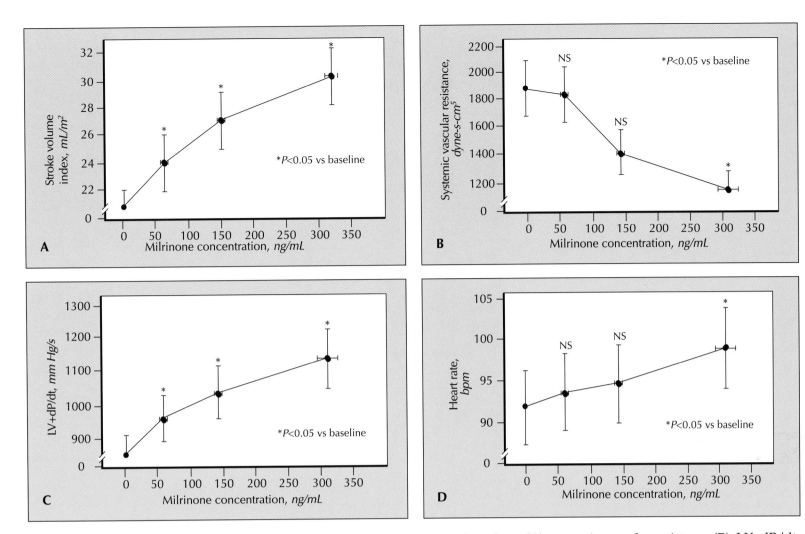

FIGURE 9-28. Dose-response of the hemodynamic effects to three doses (12.5, 25, and 50 µg/kg) of milrinone administered as an intravenous bolus over 15 to 60 seconds in 11 patients with moderate to severe congestive heart failure. Shown are the effects on stroke volume (**A**), systemic vascular resistance (**B**), LV+dP/dt (**C**), and heart rate (**D**). NS—not significant. (*Adapted from* Jaski and coworkers [14]; with permission.)

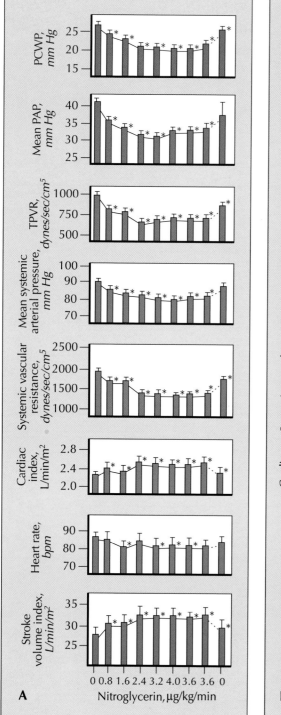

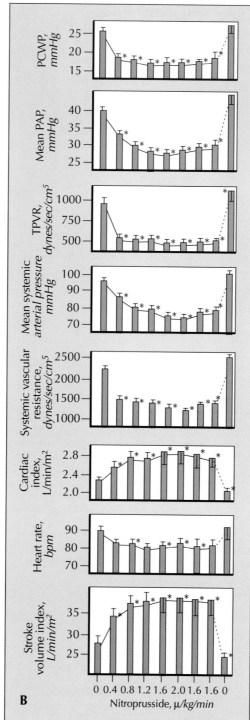

FIGURE 9-29. Hemodynamic responses to intravenously administered nitroglycerin (**A**) and nitroprusside (**B**) in patients with severe chronic congestive heart failure. Each drug was administered in five dose increments (30 minutes at each level) followed by the determined optimal maintenance dose. PAP —pulmonary artery pressure; PCWP —pulmonary capillary wedge pressure; TPVR —total pulmonary vascular resistance. (*Adapted from* Leier and coworkers [7]; with permission.)

REFERENCES

1. Goldberger JJ, Peled HB, Stroh JA, *et al*.: Prognostic factors in acute pulmonary edema. *Arch Intern Med* 1986, 146:489–493.

2. Forrester JS, Diamond G, Chatterjee K, *et al*.: Medical therapy of acute myocardial infarction by application of hemodynamic subsets. *N Engl J Med* 1976, 295:1356–1362, 1404–1413.

3. Hands ME, Rutherford JD, Muller JE, *et al*.: The in-hospital development of cardiogenic shock after myocardial infarction: incidence, predictors of occurrence, outcome and prognostic factors. *J Am Coll Cardiol* 1989, 14:40–46.

4. Goldberg RJ, Gore JM, Alpert JS, *et al*.: Cardiogenic shock after acute myocardial infarction. *N Engl J Med* 1991, 325:1117–1122.

5. Heart Failure Guidelines Committed of the American College of Cardiology/American Heart Association: Guidelines for the evaluation and management of heart failure. *J Am Coll Cardiol* 1995, 26:1376–1398.

6. Franciosa JA, Guiha NH, Limas CL, *et al*.: Improved left ventricular function during nitroprusside infusion in acute myocardial infarction. *Lancet* 1972, 1:650–654.

7. Leier CV, Bambach D, Thompson MJ, *et al*.: Central and regional hemodynamic effects of intravenous isosorbide dinitrate, nitroglycerin, and nitroprusside in patients with congestive heart failure. *Am J Cardiol* 1981, 48:1115–1123.

8. Leier CV: Acute inotropic support: intravenously administered positive inotropic drugs. In *Cardiotonic Drugs*, ed 2. Edited by Leier CV. New York: Marcel Dekker; 1991:63–106.

9. Loeb HS, Winslow EBJ, Rahimtoola SH, *et al*.: Acute hemodynamic effects of dopamine in patients with shock. *Circulation* 1971, 44:163–173.

10. Holzer J, Karliner JS, O'Rourke RA, *et al*.: Effectiveness of dopamine in patients with cardiogenic shock. *Am J Cardiol* 1973, 32:79–84.

11. Leier CV, Webel J, Bush CA: The cardiovascular effects of the continuous infusion of dobutamine in patients with severe cardiac failure. *Circulation* 1977, 56:468–472.

12. Leier CV, Heban PT, Huss P, *et al*.: Comparative systemic and regional hemodynamic effects of dopamine and dobutamine in patients with heart failure. *Circulation* 1978, 58:466–475.

13. Francis GS, Sharma B, Hodges M: Comparative hemodynamic effects of dopamine and dobutamine in patients with acute cardiogenic circulatory collapse. *Am Heart J* 1982, 103:995–1000.

14. Jaski B, Fifer MA, Wright RF, *et al*.: Positive inotropic and vasodilator actions of milrinone in patients with severe congestive heart failure. *J Clin Invest* 1985, 75:643–649.

15. Sander CA, Buckley MJ, Leinbach RC, *et al*.: Mechanical circulatory assistance: current status and experience with combining circulatory assistance, emergency coronary angiography, and acute myocardial revascularization. *Circulation* 1972, 45:1291–1313.

16. Bardet J, Masquet C, Kahn J-C, *et al*.: Clinical and hemodynamic results of intra-aortic balloon counterpulsation and surgery for cardiogenic shock. *Am Heart J* 1977, 93:280–288.

17. Johnson SA, Scanlon PJ, Loeb HS, *et al*.: Treatment of cardiogenic shock in myocardial infarction by intra-aortic balloon counterpulsation and surgery. *Am J Med* 1977, 62:687–692.

18. O'Rourke MF, Sammel N, Chang VP: Arterial counterpulsation in severe refractory heart failure complicating acute myocardial infarction. *Br Heart J* 1979, 41:308–316.

19. DeWood MA, Notski RN, Hensely GR, *et al*.: Intra-aortic balloon counterpulsation with and without reperfusion for myocardial infarction shock. *Circulation* 1980, 61:1105–1112.

20. Kovack PJ, Rasak MA, Bates ER, *et al*.: Thrombolysis plus aortic counterpulsation with and without reperfusion for myocardial infarction shock. *Circulation* 1980, 61:1105–1112.

21. Rothbaum DA, Linnemeier TJ, Landin RJ, *et al*.: Emergency percutaneous transluminal coronary angioplasty in acute myocardial infarction: a 3 year experience. *J Am Coll Cardiol* 1987, 10:264–272.

22. Lee L, Bates ER, Pitt B, *et al*.: Percutaneous transluminal coronary angioplasty improves survival in acute myocardial infarction complicated by cardiogenic shock. *Circulation* 1988, 78:1345–1351.

23. Ellis SG, O'Neill WW, Bates ER, *et al*.: Implications of patient triage from survival and left ventricular functional recovery analyses in 500 patients treated with coronary angioplasty for acute myocardial infarction. *J Am Coll Cardiol* 1989, 13:1251–1259.

24. Lee L, Erbel R, Brown TM, *et al*.: Multicenter registry of angioplasty therapy of cardiogenic shock: initial and long-term survival. *J Am Coll Cardiol* 1991, 17:599–603.

25. Hochman JS, Boland J, Sleeper LA, *et al*.: Current spectrum of cardiogenic shock and effect of early revascularization on mortality. *Circulation* 1995, 91:873–881.

26. Lamas GA, Glaker GA, Mitchell G, *et al*.: Effect of infarct artery patency on prognosis after acute myocardial infarction. *Circulation* 1995, 92:1101–1109.

27. Holmes DR Jr, Bates ER, Kleiman NS, *et al*.: Contemporary reperfusion therapy for cardiogenic shock: the Gusto-1 trial experience. *J Am Coll Cardiol* 1995, 26:668–674.

28. Berger PB, Holmes DR, Stebbins AL, *et al*. for the Gusto-1 Investigators: Impact of an aggressive invasive catheterization and revascularization strategy on mortality in patients with cardiogenic shock in the Gusto-1 trial. *Circulation* 1997, 96:122–127.

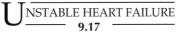

STANDARD THERAPY OF HEART FAILURE

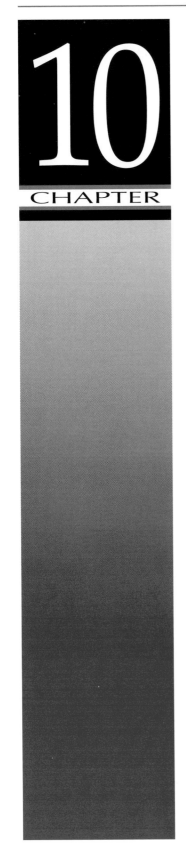

CHAPTER 10

Robert J. Cody

Digitalis plays an important role in the treatment of patients in whom systolic dysfunction is a major component. Although its therapeutic benefits were demonstrated more than two centuries ago, the efficacy of digitalis in the treatment of patients in normal sinus rhythm with heart failure has remained controversial. Furthermore, beneficial effects beyond a direct inotropic or hemodynamic benefit may account for much of the clinical outcome in humans. The absence of a significant reduction in mortality in a large prospective trial (Digitalis Investigation Group [DIG] trial) is balanced against the clinical benefit demonstrated in two independent digoxin withdrawal studies.

Diuretics are an effective and essential component of therapy for edema management in heart failure. In addition to their predictable effects on fluid and electrolyte balance, diuretics have a number of metabolic side effects. The value of diuretic therapy is enhanced by the thoughtful utilization of these agents. Earlier use of combined diuretic regimens, avoidance of excessive loop diuretic dosage, and identification of early stages of decompensation permit effective reduction of "congestive" symptoms and minimizes the requirement for hospitalization.

The use of vasodilators for the treatment of heart failure developed from the observation that these agents were effective in the management of patients with cardiogenic shock or severe mitral regurgitation after myocardial infarction. This acute hemodynamic concept was subsequently extended to the longer-term use of oral vasodilators for the treatment of ambulatory patients with heart failure. However, many of the initial trials of prototype vasodilators failed to demonstrate clinical efficacy during long-term use. It is now apparent that functional improvement and increased survival are also relevant clinical therapeutic goals, and these endpoints have now become the benchmarks for the evaluation of new vasodilators.

In the early 1980s, angiotensin-converting enzyme (ACE) inhibitors showed promising results for the management of refractory hypertension and were found to have favorable acute hemodynamic effects in patients with heart failure. On the basis of these observations, orally active ACE inhibitors were applied to the management of such patients. During the past 15 years, a compelling body of data has shown that these agents exert beneficial effects on clinical status, functional capacity, and survival in patients with congestive heart failure.

Compared with direct-acting agents such as hydralazine, ACE inhibitors are rather weak vasodilators. This observation, combined with the clinical success of ACE inhibitors, has played an important role in development of the hypothesis that nonhemodynamic actions confer long-term clinical benefit and mortality reduction. Among possible mechanisms, correction of neurohormonal abnormalities and reversal of myocardial and vascular cellular abnormalities have been demonstrated. Recent clinical observations and pharmacologic advances have demonstrated that the renin-angiotensin-aldosterone pathway can be effectively inhibited at several sites by both traditional and newer pharmacologic agents.

The combination of hydralazine and isosorbide dinitrate has also provided improved survival (albeit to a lesser degree than ACE inhibitors) and improved exercise capacity with long-term administration. However, to date, direct-acting vasodilators have been less successful than ACE inhibitors. Flosequinan, a newer direct-acting vasodilator, produced a greater mortality than placebo.

Initial studies with calcium channel antagonists frequently resulted in adverse hemodynamic outcomes and failed to show chronic clinical efficacy. Recent controlled clinical trials suggest a neutral overall mortality effect.

The triad of digoxin-diuretic-"vasodilator" therapy for heart failure was first established more than 25 years ago. This older, somewhat arbitrary, triad was subsequently challenged by the results of ACE inhibitor trials. As we enter the 21st century, a more rational algorithm for heart failure therapy must continue to evolve, encompassing primary disease management, targeted modification of secondary maladaptation, and more effective distribution of proven drug therapy.

Mechanism of Action of Cardiac Glycosides in Heart Failure

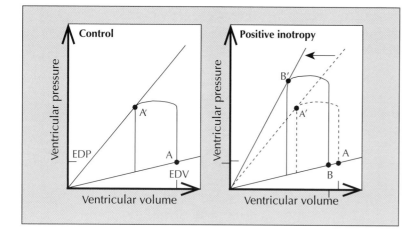

FIGURE 10-1. The positive inotropic effect of cardiac glycosides. Not until the 1920s was it understood that cardiac glycosides increase the force of contraction of cardiac muscle (*ie*, a positive inotropic effect), resulting in a shift upward and to the left of the ventricular function curve. The effect in the intact heart is illustrated by the two pressure-volume loops shown here, in which an increase in contractility due to digoxin results in a shift upward and to the left of the pressure-volume relation at the end of systole (A'-B'). When stroke volume remains constant, as shown here, or increases, as is often the case clinically in patients with heart failure, the end-diastolic pressure (EDP) and volume (EDV) also decline (A-B). This results in decreased congestive symptoms and increased cardiac output. As predicted by the Laplace relationship, the resulting decrease in ventricular chamber dimensions also reduces wall tension, a major determinant in myocardial oxygen consumption. Therefore, although the initial increase in myocardial contractility necessarily results in an increase in cardiac muscle cell ATP (and oxygen) consumption, the final net effect of the drug may be to lower cardiac oxygen consumption [4].

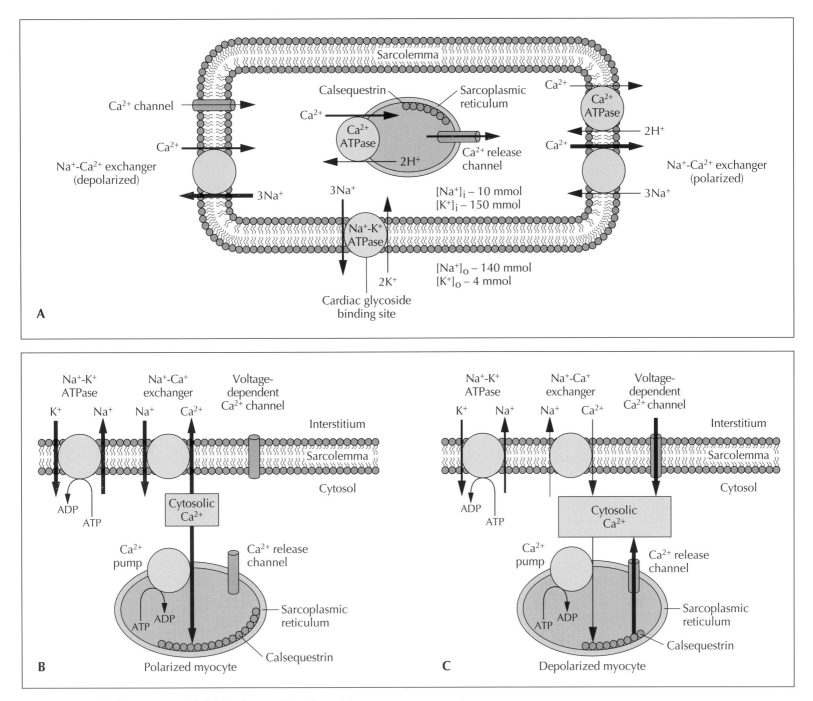

FIGURE 10-2. Sodium pump inhibition by cardiac glycosides. The present understanding of the mechanism by which the cardiac glycosides induce a positive inotropic effect in cardiac muscle is based on the specificity of these drugs for Na^+K^+-ATPase (or the "sodium pump"), a cell membrane protein responsible for the active (ie, ATP-consuming) transport of the monovalent cations Na^+ and K^+.

A, Both Na^+ and Ca^{2+} ions enter cardiac muscle cells during each cycle of depolarization, contraction, and repolarization. Ca^{2+} is also released from internal stores in an intracellular compartment called the sarcoplasmic reticulum (SR), where it is bound to the protein calsequestrin. During cellular repolarization, Na^+ is actively extruded by Na^+K^+-ATPase, while Ca^{2+} is either pumped back into the SR

by a Ca^{2+}-ATPase or is removed from the cell by a cell membrane transport protein that exchanges Na^+ for Ca^{2+}. This Na^+ for Ca^{2+} exchanger transports three Na^+ ions in for every Ca^{2+} ion out when the cell is polarized, using the favorable chemical and electrical potential of Na^+ to drive the exchange reaction. **B,** The direction and magnitude of Na^+ and Ca^{2+} transport during diastole (polarized myocyte).

C, The direction and magnitude of Na^+ and Ca^{2+} transport during systole (depolarized myocyte). Note that the exchanger may briefly run in reverse during cell depolarization when the electrical gradient across the plasma membrane is transiently reversed. The capacity of the exchanger to extrude Ca^{2+} from the cell depends critically on the intracellular Na^+ concentrations [4].

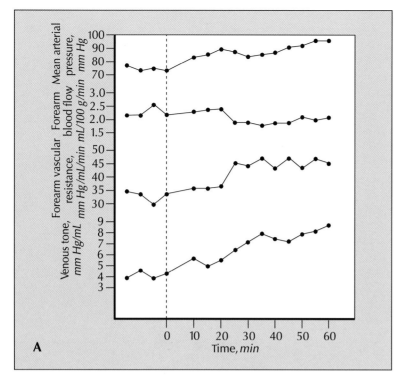

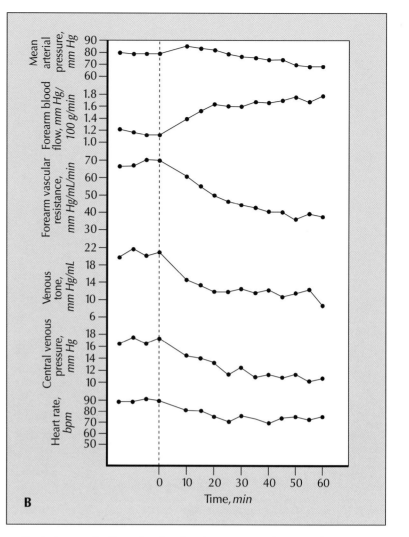

FIGURE 10-3. Cardiac glycosides and peripheral vascular resistance in heart failure. Cardiac glycosides have been known for over 30 years to affect peripheral venous and arterial tone.

A, In a series of pioneering studies, Mason *et al.* [5] noted that a 10-minute intravenous infusion of 8.5 µg/kg ouabain in normal subjects increased mean arterial pressure as well as forearm vascular resistance and venous tone .

B, In marked contrast, forearm vascular resistance and venous tone decreased in patients with NYHA class III or IV heart failure symptoms after an intravenous dose of ouabain, as shown by the data from a representative patient. Whereas the response in normal subjects is due in part to a direct effect of cardiac glycosides on peripheral vascular tone, the opposite and rapid hemodynamic response to ouabain observed in heart failure

patients is now believed to be due in part to a decrease in sympathetic nervous system activity mediated by enhanced sensitivity of the baroreflex response. (*Adapted from* Mason and coworkers [5]; with permission.)

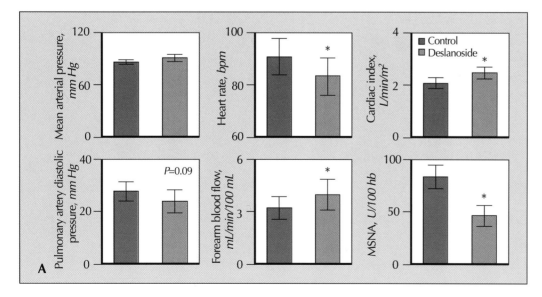

FIGURE 10-4. Sympathetic nervous system activity in heart failure: response to digitalis versus dobutamine. **A,** Ferguson *et al.* [6] noted that although infusion of the cardiac glycoside deslanoside was associated with increased forearm blood flow and cardiac index was increased, muscle sympathetic nerve activity (MSNA) was markedly decreased in patients with NYHA class III and IV heart failure (*n*=8; mean±SEM).

(continued)

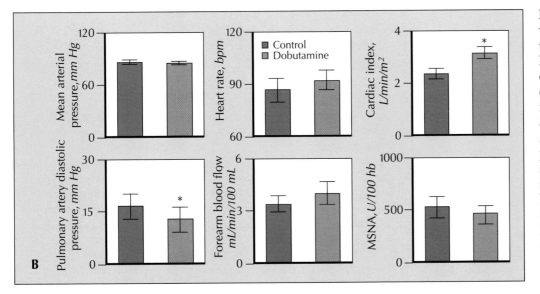

FIGURE 10-4. *(continued)* **B,** To determine whether these changes could be ascribed to an increase in cardiac output per se, Ferguson *et al.* also examined the response of a similar group of heart failure patients to dobutamine, titrated to achieve the same increase in pulmonary artery O_2 saturation as was achieved by infusion of deslanoside. Although cardiac index increased and pulmonary artery pressure declined significantly, as expected, there were no significant changes in heart rate, forearm blood flow, or MSNA in these patients (*n*=8). *Asterisk* indicates $P<0.05$. hb— heartbeat. (*Adapted from* Ferguson and coworkers [6]; with permission.)

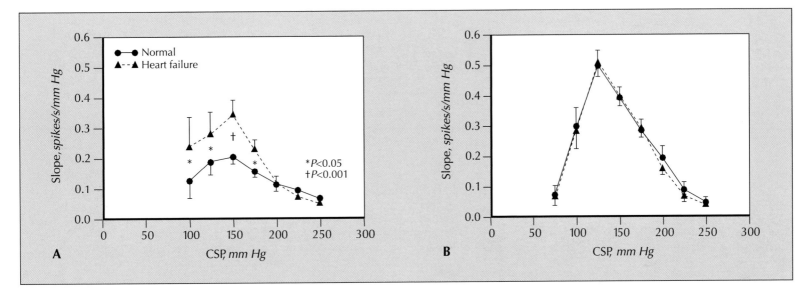

FIGURE 10-5. Improved carotid baroreflex responsiveness after cardiac glycosides. **A,** Direct infusions of ouabain into the arterial supply of isolated carotid sinus preparations (CSP) from a dog model of heart failure with a documented desensitization of the baroreflex response restored the responsiveness of the isolated baroreceptor to increases in CSP toward normal. **B,** No change was observed after ouabain in isolated CSPs from normal dogs. These and other experimental data reinforce data from patients that cardiac glycosides act directly to reset arterial baroreflex sensitivity in heart failure. (*Adapted from* Wang and coworkers [7]; with permission.)

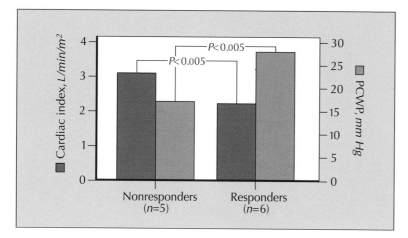

FIGURE 10-6. Digoxin in hospitalized heart failure patients. Gheorghiade *et al.* [8] carried out a small, prospective trial of intravenous digoxin administration to hospitalized patients who had severe (NYHA class IV) symptoms and who had been medically stabilized with diuretics and vasodilators. Approximately half of the patients (six of 11) experienced a significant hemodynamic improvement after receiving 1.0 mg of intravenous digoxin, as judged by a decrease in pulmonary capillary wedge pressure (PCWP) of 5 mm Hg and/or an increase in cardiac index of 0.5 L/min/m^2. There were important baseline hemodynamic differences between digoxin responders and nonresponders, as shown in this figure, although reportedly there were no other significant differences in the etiology of the heart failure in each patient's heart failure score or in left ventricular ejection fraction. Although all patients had class IV symptoms on admission to hospital, those with markedly abnormal hemodynamics after initiation of optimal medical management with diuretics and vasodilators were more likely to exhibit a favorable hemodynamic response. (*Adapted from* Gheorghiade and coworkers [8]; with permission.)

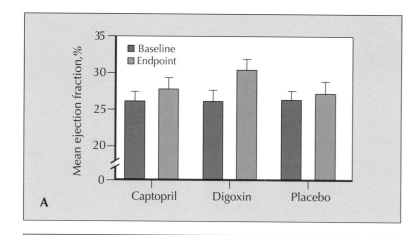

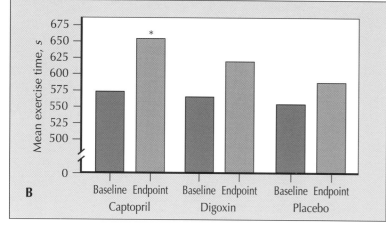

FIGURE 10-7. Captopril-Digoxin Multicenter Research Group trial. **A,** In the Captopril-Digoxin Multicenter Research Group trials [9], 300 patients with generally mild to moderate (NYHA classes II and III) heart failure symptoms were randomized to receive captopril, digoxin, or placebo, with diuretics administered as necessary. Both captopril and digoxin significantly reduced morbidity, as judged by the need for increasing doses of diuretics, emergency room visits, or hospitalization, compared with placebo. This figure illustrates the change in left ventricular ejection fraction from baseline for patients assigned to captopril, digoxin, or placebo. Only patients who received digoxin exhibited a significant increase in ejection fraction ($P<0.05$) during the trial. An important caveat in interpreting the results of this trial is that during the pretrial patient evaluation period, any patient who did not tolerate withdrawal from standard (*ie,* digoxin) therapy was not randomized or entered into the study, thereby excluding a number of patients who, by definition, would probably have been digoxin responders. **B,** All patients in this study were receiving background diuretic therapy. Captopril was associated with a significant increase in exercise performance compared with placebo. The digoxin treatment group showed a small trend toward improvement of exercise tolerance. The digoxin group demonstrated a small but significant increase of ejection fraction. *Asterisk* indicates a significantly greater increase of exercise duration from baseline compared with the placebo response ($P<0.05$). There were greater requirements for diuretic supplementation, more frequent emergency room visits, and a greater need for hospitalization in the placebo group, who were receiving only diuretic therapy. (*Adapted from* Captopril-Digoxin Multicenter Research Group [9]; with permission.)

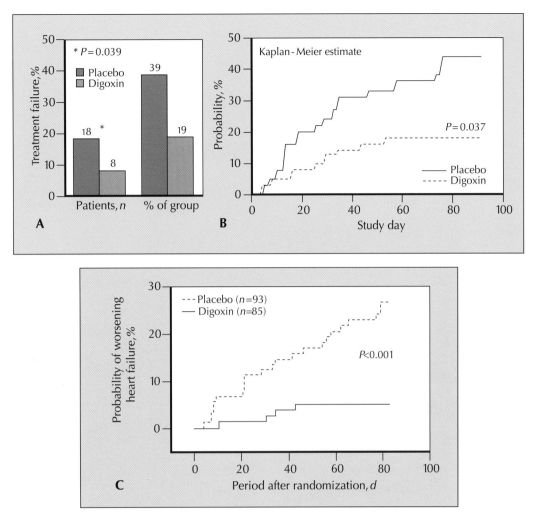

FIGURE 10-8. Digoxin in heart failure: the PROVED (Prospective Randomized Study of Ventricular Failure and the Efficacy of Digoxin) trial. To evaluate prospectively whether patients with well-compensated heart failure symptoms in sinus rhythm who were already receiving digoxin, with or without a diuretic, would tolerate withdrawal from the cardiac glycoside, 88 patients with mild to moderate heart failure (NYHA class II predominantly), who were not receiving a vasodilator, were randomized either to continue on active drug or to receive a placebo in the PROVED trial [10]. **A,** Treatment failure, defined as number of patients and percentage of treatment group demonstrating a statistically greater occurence of failure in patients withdrawn from dioxin treatment. **B,** The time to treatment failure, or a hospital evaluation or admission for heart failure symptoms, was significantly higher in the placebo group compared with the digoxin-treated group. **C,** Digoxin in heart failure: the RADIANCE (Randomized Assessment [of the effect of] Digoxin and Inhibitors of the Angiotensin Converting Enzyme [ACE]) trial. The RADIANCE trial design was essentially identical to that shown in Fig. 10-8A for the PROVED trial, except that patients were receiving either captopril or enalapril, in addition to digoxin and diuretics, before randomization [11]. Study investigators were asked to achieve optimal fluid balance on diuretics during the stabilization period, and a captopril or enalapril dose of at least 25 mg or 5 mg/d, respectively (average dose 73 mg/d and 13 mg/d in the placebo group, 77 mg/d and 17 mg/d in the digoxin group). As in PROVED, the target serum digoxin concentration was between 0.9 and 2.0 ng/mL, and the average serum concentration of digoxin was about 1.2 ng/mL on an average dose of 0.38 mg/d. Of the 178 patients randomized, all were in NYHA class II or III. No patients with severe heart failure (NYHA class IV) were studied, largely because digoxin's efficacy was already considered established for this group of patients. Nevertheless, the proportion of patients in class III heart failure was somewhat higher (about 35% of the total) than in PROVED (about 19%).

There were highly significant differences in both primary and secondary endpoints between patients receiving optimal ACE inhibitor and diuretic therapy who were randomized to continue receiving digoxin compared with those who were switched to placebo. There was a significant increase in the cumulative probability of worsening heart failure (defined as in PROVED) in this Kaplan-Meier analysis over the duration of the study. This amounts to a 20% absolute risk reduction for patients who continued to receive digoxin. (Parts A and B *adapted from* Uretsky and coworkers [10]; part C *adapted from* Packer and coworkers [11]; with permission.)

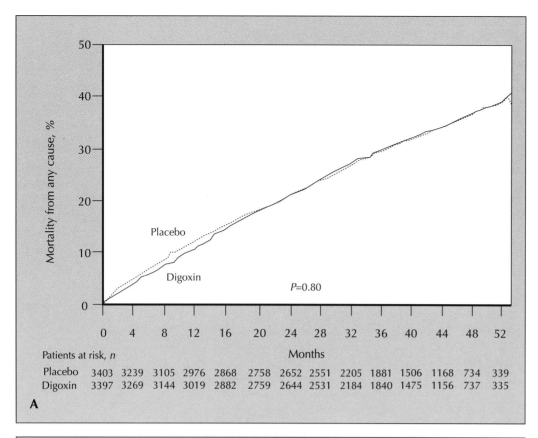

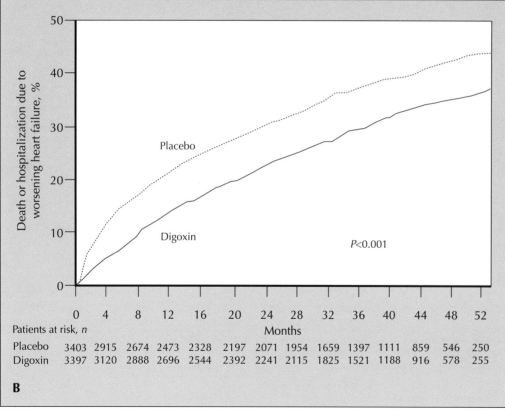

FIGURE 10-9. The Digitalis Investigation Group (DIG) trial evaluated the effects of digoxin on survival in 6800 patients. The average follow-up was 37 months. Digoxin did not increase or decrease overall mortality (**A**). However, digoxin-treated patients had a reduction in the overall rate of hospitalization and also the rate of hospitalization for worsening heart failure (**B**). There was no increased risk of ventricular arrhythmias in the digoxin-treated group. (*Adapted from* Digitalis Investigation Report [12].)

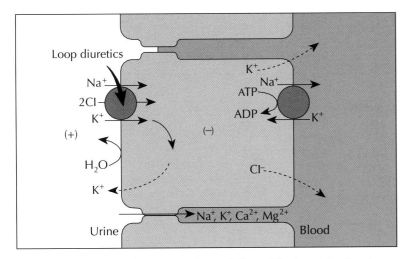

FIGURE 10-10. Loop diuretics in heart failure. The introduction in the 1960s of diuretics that act within the loop of Henle, so-called "high-ceiling" or "loop" diuretics, dramatically affected the ability of clinicians to improve symptoms of congestive heart failure with minimum toxicity and predictable efficacy compared with other drugs available at that time. These diuretics act on a specific

transport protein, the $Na^+K^+/2Cl^-$ cotransporter, located on the apical membrane of renal epithelial cells in the ascending limb of Henle's loop. Ions transported into the cell are then transferred out of the cell by Na^+K^+-ATPase (the "sodium pump") on the basolateral membranes of these cells. Loop diuretics also decrease the absorption of Ca^{2+} and Mg^{2+} in this portion of the nephron, cations whose absorption is indirectly linked to NaCl uptake. Thus, hypocalcemia and hypomagnesia, as well as hypokalemia and volume depletion, may result from prolonged use of these drugs.

Loop diuretics also reduce the tonicity of the medullary interstitium by preventing the normal uptake of solute in the absence of water in the thick ascending limb of Henle's loop. This limits the kidney's ability to concentrate the urine and may contribute to the development of hyponatremia. The loop diuretics are clearly the most useful diuretics as single agents for patients with decompensated congestive failure, in large part because of the magnitude of the natriuresis that can be achieved over a short period, which can reach as high as 20% of the filtered load of sodium. Typically, the fraction of NaCl filtered at the glomerulus and reabsorbed in the ascending limb of the loop of Henle declines from about 20% to 13% with a loop diuretic, resulting in a 1% to 2% increase in the fractional excretion of sodium over 24 hours. [4]

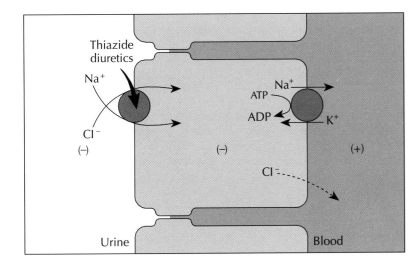

FIGURE 10-11. Thiazide diuretics. In general, the thiazide diuretics are not useful as single drugs for the therapy of volume retention in heart failure patients, largely because their site of action in the distal convoluted tubule permits rapid adjustment of water and solute absorption in other more proximal nephron segments. Interestingly, the target renal tubular protein of the thiazide class of diuretics, the electroneutral Na^+Cl^- cotransporter, has recently been cloned and sequenced. This is the last of the known diuretic-responsive renal epithelial cell transport proteins to be identified. Many other tissues also express this transport protein, which may have important implications for understanding the effectiveness of these drugs in the treatment of hypertension as well as their less desirable metabolic effects on lipid and glucose metabolism. Unlike loop diuretics, thiazides enhance calcium reabsorption but not that of magnesium, although magnesium wasting is much more pronounced with loop diuretics [4].

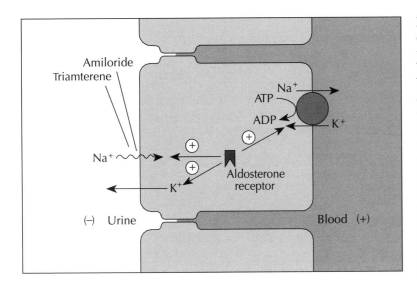

FIGURE 10-12. Potassium-sparing diuretics. The potassium-sparing diuretics fall into two categories: agents such as amiloride and triamterene, which reduce Na^+ conductance through an apical membrane sodium channel; and aldosterone antagonists, which, by inhibiting the actions of aldosterone at its intracellular receptor in renal epithelial cells of the distal collecting duct, reduce Na^+ uptake from the tubular lumen and decrease K^+ secretion by several mechanisms. Aldosterone antagonists also limit the kidney's ability to acidify the urine by inhibiting the action of aldosterone on a renal tubular proton pump. Although none of these diuretics is effective as a single agent in the treatment of heart failure, they play a useful role in diminishing renal K^+ wasting. When combined with loop or thiazide diuretics, the aldosterone antagonists also prevent Mg^{2+} depletion. Because ACE inhibitors increase the serum K^+ concentration, an effect that may be magnified by β-blockers and NSAIDS, potassium-sparing diuretics should be prescribed cautiously for patients who are already receiving vasodilators of this class [4].

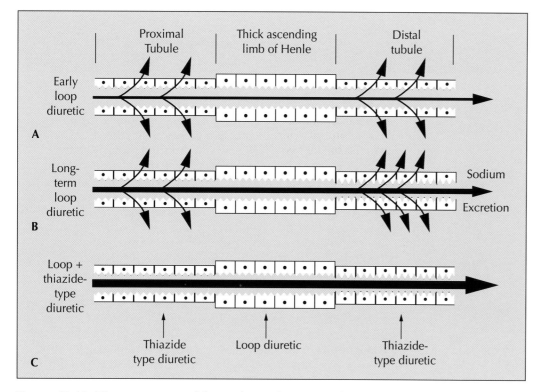

FIGURE 10-13. Three segments of the nephron: the proximal tubule, thick ascending loop of Henle, and distal tubule. Under normal conditions, sodium is reabsorbed along all three segments. This figure represents the condition in congestive heart failure in which many

patients have a reduction in glomerular filtration rate and, therefore, increased proximal tubular sodium reabsorption. **A,** Early loop diuretic. Blockade of sodium reabsorption at the thick ascending loop of Henle is represented, also demonstrating that the loop diuretic has no appreciable effect on proximal or distal sodium reabsorption. **B,** Long-term loop diuretic. The adverse effect of distal tubular hypertrophy. Thus, an increased load of sodium continues to be avidly reabsorbed proximally. The loop diuretic blocks reabsorption at the thick ascending loop of Henle. However, in the presence of distal tubular hypertrophy, due to uncontrolled sodium intake and the effects of enhanced sodium delivery during loop diuretic therapy, there is additional avid sodium reabsorption in the distal tubule, resulting in a reduction of sodium excretion compared with earlier stages of loop diuretic therapy. **C,** Loop plus thiazide-type diuretic. Blockade of sodium reabsorption at both the proximal and distal tubule, combined with the effect of the loop diuretic, reestablishes enhanced sodium excretion. (*Adapted from* Cody and Pickworth [13]; with permission.)

Importance of Dietary Sodium Restriction

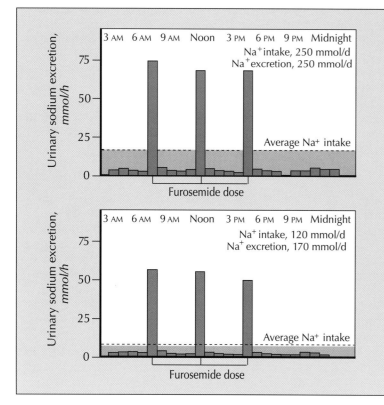

FIGURE 10-14. Importance of dietary salt intake on the renal response to loop diuretics. Because most loop diuretics are short-acting drugs, it is always more effective to give multiple daily doses rather than the same total amount as a single daily dose.

Avid sodium retention during the remainder of the day after a single dose tends to minimize the daily net loss of NaCl (*ie*, a negative sodium balance). Even multiple daily doses of a loop diuretic are ineffective unless the NaCl content in the diet is reduced concomitantly. The effect of three daily intravenous doses of furosemide (40 mg) on daily sodium balance is illustrated in patients on chronic diuretic therapy at two different levels of dietary sodium intake. In each panel, hourly sodium excretion is shown on the vertical axis of these histograms, and the result of the three daily doses is illustrated.

The *dashed horizontal lines* represent the daily sodium intake on each diet averaged over 24 hours. Negative Na^+ balance is shown above the dashed line, in *upper bars,* and positive balance (*ie*, sodium retention) appears below the dashed line. The small *lower bars* between furosemide doses reflect sodium excretion during each urinary collection period. Only urinary sodium excretion that represents a net negative sodium balance (*ie*, sodium loss greater than intake) is shown. For a daily net negative sodium balance to occur, the volume of all the bars must exceed the total area below the *dashed line* for a given diuretic and dietary sodium regimen. There was no net loss of sodium in these subjects on a high-sodium intake (250 mmol Na^+/d), whereas a moderate reduction in sodium intake to 120 mmol/d (equivalent to a "no added salt" diet) resulted in a moderate negative sodium balance in each 24-hour period. A more severe dietary restriction (*eg*, to 20 mmol/d) will lead to a marked negative sodium balance and weight loss but may be complicated by the development of excess volume depletion, hyponatremia and hypokalemia, and a hypochloremic metabolic alkalosis, unless the patient is carefully monitored. (*Adapted from* Wilcox and coworkers [14]; with permission.)

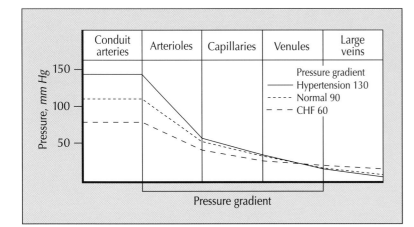

FIGURE 10-15. In addition to the absolute blood pressure within the artery at any given time, there is a change in pressure gradient from the conduit arteries to the large veins, and theoretical normal values can be derived from population studies. In hypertension, for example, the gradient from the aorta to the level of the venae cavae is quite high. In contrast, patients with congestive heart failure (CHF) have a relatively low mean pressure in the conduit arteries and relatively high pressure in the venous system. Therefore, the reduction of this pressure gradient or circulatory pressure adversely influences the perfusion pressure of important regional vascular beds, such as those of the brain, kidneys, and skeletal muscle.

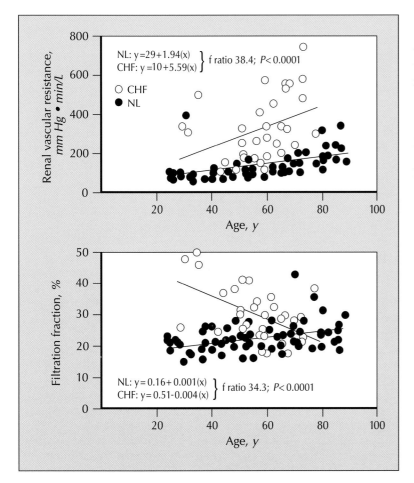

FIGURE 10-16. Renal blood flow and function are impaired in congestive heart failure (CHF), where superimposed, age-dependent vasoconstriction can also readily be seen. Here, renal function and vascular resistance in CHF patients are compared with those in normal (NL) subjects. Although normal subjects exhibit a gradual increase in renal resistance as a function of age, renal vascular resistance is much higher for the CHF population in all age groups and exhibits an accelerated, age-dependent increase. The highest filtration fraction occurs in the younger CHF patients and paradoxically demonstrates an age-dependent decrease in heart failure. However, the filtration fraction remains relatively increased in the latter patients. (*Adapted from* Cody and coworkers [15]; with permission.)

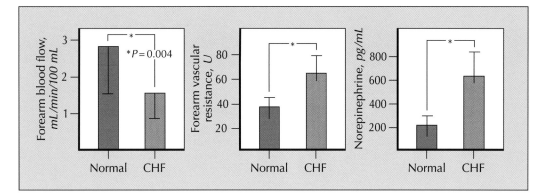

FIGURE 10-17. An example of altered regional flow in congestive heart failure (CHF) is that which involves the limb, comprising skin, muscle, and bone tissues. Compared with normal subjects, a significant reduction in forearm blood flow and an increase in forearm vascular resistance are associated with the characteristic increase of plasma norepinephrine in patients with CHF. The reduction of blood flow to the forearm is largely brought about by a decrease in cutaneous blood flow. This reduction of limb flow impairs exercise performance and thermal equilibrium. Values represent mean ± SD. (*Adapted from* Cody and coworkers) [16].

VASODILATOR THERAPY OF HEART FAILURE

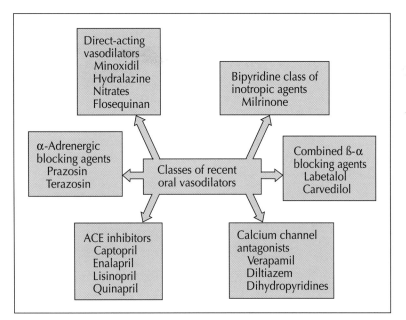

FIGURE 10-18. Classification of newer oral vasodilators, according to their presumed mechanism of action, reveals that, although most of these compounds are effective for reversal of vasoconstriction in hypertension, many have been problematic in the treatment of congestive heart failure (CHF). Of the direct-acting vasodilators, only hydralazine and nitrates (administered in combination) have been effective in CHF. Early studies with α-adrenergic blocking agents demonstrated tachyphylaxis. β-Blocking agents with combined α-blocking vasodilator properties have been and continue to be evaluated in the treatment of CHF. Although labetalol did not demonstrate long-term benefit, early studies with carvedilol demonstrate improved clinical status. Angiotensin-converting enzyme (ACE) inhibitors evoke vasodilating effects by inhibition of angiotensin II production. Calcium antagonists are represented here by the prototypes verapamil and diltiazem, as well as by the general dihydropyridine class. The prototype dihydropyridine is nifedipine. Although newer calcium antagonists are spoken of as either "second" or "third generation," this class of drugs has in fact undergone continuous development. Newer agents in this class are relatively more vasoselective and include nicardipine, nitrendipine, isradipine, and amlodipine. The bipyridine class of peak III phosphodiesterase inhibitors is represented here by milrinone. This class of compounds demonstrated positive inotropic activity and direct vasodilator properties. Although studies with oral milrinone have ceased and the compound is no longer in development, it remains a prototype for this class of "inodilators" and is used for short-term intravenous therapy of CHF.

DIRECT-ACTING VASODILATORS

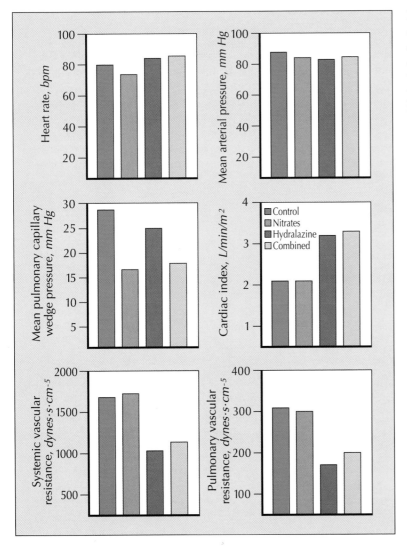

FIGURE 10-19. The concept of combined vasodilator therapy is evident from these early studies demonstrating the hemodynamic efficacy of hydralazine and nitrates [17]. The rationale for this combination was derived from the presumed benefit of combined venous dilatation produced by nitrates and arterial dilatation produced by hydralazine. Hydralazine increased cardiac index and reduced systemic vascular resistance. In combination, reduction in cardiac filling pressures was achieved, with increase of cardiac index and reversal of vasoconstriction. It is notable that these changes occurred without significant reduction in mean arterial pressure or heart rate. These acute responses have been paralleled by short-term hemodynamic studies. The survival benefit of combined therapy has been attributed to a direct hemodynamic effect [17].

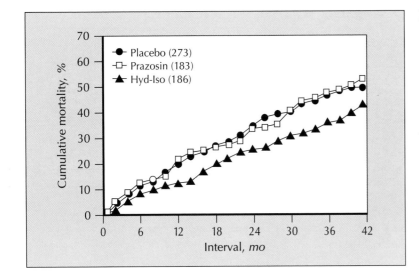

FIGURE 10-20. Mortality outcome of vasodilator therapy. In addition to short-term hemodynamic improvement, the VHeFT (Veterans Administration Vasodilator in Heart Failure Trial) I study demonstrated a favorable effect on survival with the combination of hydralazine and isosorbide dinitrate (Hyd-Iso). As shown here, the α-adrenergic blocking agent prazosin did not significantly reduce mortality. In fact, the VHeFT I study provided the final data that led to the discontinuation of α-adrenergic blocking agents for treatment of heart failure. In contrast, the combination of hydralazine and isosorbide dinitrate significantly reduced mortality. This was the first published, prospective, placebo-controlled, randomized survival study in heart failure to demonstrate an improved survival outcome for the pharmacologic treatment of congestive heart failure. (*Adapted from* Cohn and coworkers [18].)

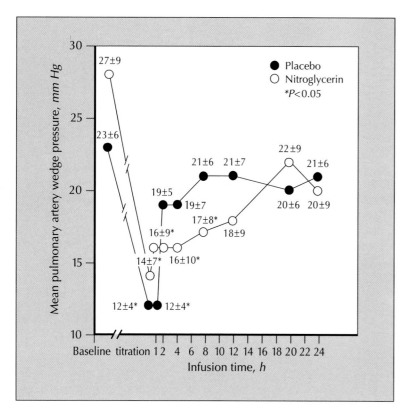

Figure 10-21. Tolerance to intravenous nitroglycerin. The difficulty with nitrate preparations is the development of hemodynamic tolerance, which is evident with even short-term administration, as demonstrated in this figure. Patients with moderate to severe heart failure were randomized to placebo or continuous intravenous nitroglycerin infusion for 24 hours; both groups initially were titrated to a normal pulmonary artery wedge pressure with nitroglycerin. Patients then were divided into those switched to placebo and those maintained on nitroglycerin. The placebo group demonstrated an immediate increase of pulmonary capillary wedge pressure, which returned to baseline over the ensuing 24 hours. In the nitroglycerin group, pulmonary capillary wedge pressure progressively increased, so that at 20 and 24 hours there was no significant difference between the placebo and nitroglycerin groups. This demonstrates the rapid development of hemodynamic tolerance to nitroglycerin. (*Adapted from* Elkayam and coworkers [19].)

ACE INHIBITORS IN CONGESTIVE HEART FAILURE

OVERVIEW

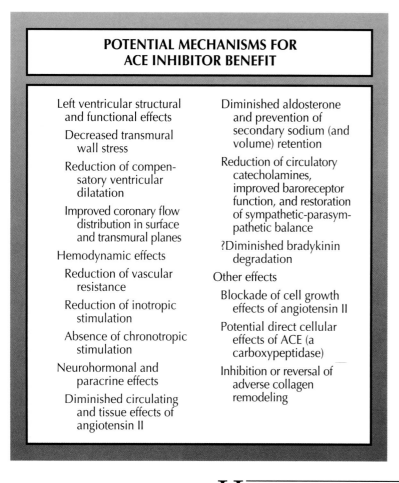

POTENTIAL MECHANISMS FOR ACE INHIBITOR BENEFIT

Left ventricular structural and functional effects

Decreased transmural wall stress

Reduction of compensatory ventricular dilatation

Improved coronary flow distribution in surface and transmural planes

Hemodynamic effects

Reduction of vascular resistance

Reduction of inotropic stimulation

Absence of chronotropic stimulation

Neurohormonal and paracrine effects

Diminished circulating and tissue effects of angiotensin II

Diminished aldosterone and prevention of secondary sodium (and volume) retention

Reduction of circulatory catecholamines, improved baroreceptor function, and restoration of sympathetic-parasympathetic balance

?Diminished bradykinin degradation

Other effects

Blockade of cell growth effects of angiotensin II

Potential direct cellular effects of ACE (a carboxypeptidase)

Inhibition or reversal of adverse collagen remodeling

Figure 10-22. Angiotensin-converting enzyme (ACE) inhibitors have demonstrated clinical benefit in all stages of heart failure. It is now apparent from many studies that the short- and long-term benefits of ACE inhibitors go beyond their vasodilating properties. The primary mechanism of action for this class of agents is blockade of angiotensin II formation, which inhibits the endocrine, paracrine, and cellular growth effects of angiotensin II. Among the beneficial outcomes are reversal of vasoconstriction and suppression of aldosterone synthesis, which thereby limits aldosterone-mediated sodium retention and potassium loss. Cellular effects include inhibition of angiotensin II–mediated hypertrophy, and it has been proposed that reversal of collagen matrix deposition, mediated by angiotensin II or aldosterone, is of clinical relevance.

Additional contributing effects that are difficult to quantify clinically include inhibition of bradykinin degradation and promotion of prostaglandin synthesis. The former may be important at a cellular level by enhancing the vasorelaxant effects of endothelium-derived relaxing factor, and the latter may be important in terms of improving regional blood flow, particularly within the kidney. Finally, a purely hemodynamic effect, regardless of the mechanisms that produce it, could contribute to the beneficial effects of ACE inhibitors. However, on the basis of findings with other pure vasodilators, it is unlikely to be the only mechanism. (*Adapted from* Cody [20].)

EARLY TRIALS IN CONGESTIVE HEART FAILURE

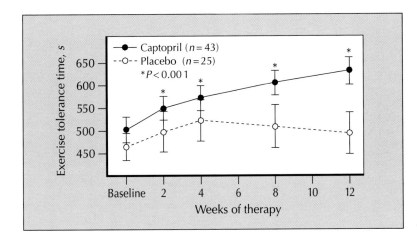

FIGURE 10-23. The Captopril Multicenter Research Group conducted the first placebo-controlled exercise study in heart failure patients, evaluating the response to captopril versus placebo. This figure demonstrates the importance of frequent baseline exercise tests and the need for longer-term follow-up evaluation in clinical drug trials. An increase of exercise performance in the placebo group was evident in the first 4 weeks of the study and paralleled the improvement in the captopril group. However, whereas after 4 weeks the captopril-treated group continued to demonstrate a progressive increase in exercise time, the placebo group reached a plateau and then exhibited a decrease in exercise performance. This study demonstrated the clinical efficacy of captopril in improving functional performance. (*Adapted from* Captopril Multicenter Research Group [21].)

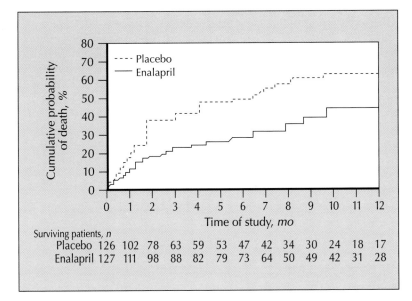

FIGURE 10-24. The CONSENSUS (Cooperative North Scandinavian Enalapril Survival Study) trial, the first mortality study of an angiotensin-converting enzyme (ACE) inhibitor in patients with congestive heart failure, demonstrated that an ACE inhibitor improved mortality compared with placebo. A lesser-known aspect of the study was that the mean age of the patients at randomization was 70 years. In addition, the majority of patients were elderly and belonged to New York Heart Association functional class IV despite digoxin and diuretic therapy. Approximately 25% of the patients in this trial were also receiving other vasodilators, such as nitrates, before randomization. Early diagnosis of the placebo and enalapril treatment groups prompted early termination of the study. The mean dose of enalapril was just under 20 mg/d. Careful dose titration obviated the excess hypotension observed in early stages of the study. (*Adapted from* CONSENSUS Trial Study Group [22].)

TRIALS IN MILD TO MODERATE CONGESTIVE HEART FAILURE

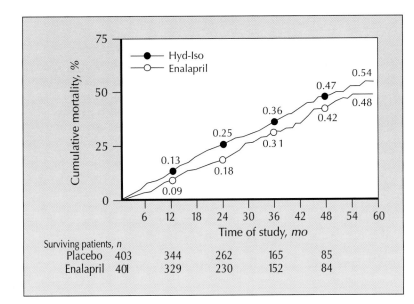

FIGURE 10-25. Following early pivotal trials of angiotensin-converting enzyme (ACE) inhibitors, their use in milder cases of heart failure was further explored. The VHeFT (Veterans Administration Cooperative Vasodilator Heart Failure Trial) II study compared the combination of hydralazine/isosorbide dinitrate (Hyd-Iso), which previously demonstrated improved mortality in the VHeFT I study (compared with placebo and prazosin) to the ACE inhibitor enalapril. Compared with Hyd-Iso, enalapril demonstrated a further significant improvement in survival. Of note in this study was that the Hyd-Iso group demonstrated a significant increase in exercise tolerance and ejection fraction compared with the enalapril group. This suggests that different "vasodilator" groups may produce independent functional or survival benefit in heart failure and provides support for combined vasodilator therapy in heart failure, adding newer vasodilator groups against ACE inhibitor background. (*Adapted from* Cohn and coworkers [23].)

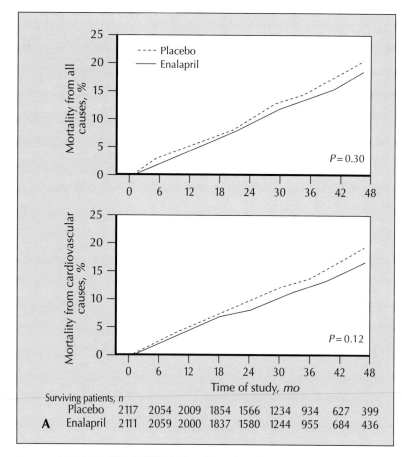

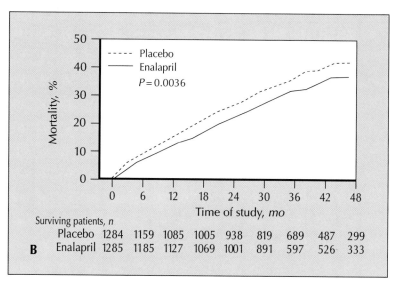

Surviving patients, n									
Placebo	1284	1159	1085	1005	938	819	689	487	299
B Enalapril	1285	1185	1127	1069	1001	891	597	526	333

Surviving patients, n									
Placebo	2117	2054	2009	1854	1566	1234	934	627	399
A Enalapril	2111	2059	2000	1837	1580	1244	955	684	436

FIGURE 10-26. **A,** The SOLVD (Studies of Left Ventricular Dysfunction) study. The prevention subgroup of the SOLVD study extended the assessment of angiotensin-converting enzyme (ACE) inhibitors to patients with asymptomatic left ventricular dysfunction. Patients in this study were New York Heart Association (NYHA) functional class I (two thirds of patients) or NYHA functional class II

(one third of patients). The results of all-cause mortality and cardio-vascular mortality are shown. Despite the relatively long follow-up of patients (approximately 4 years), there was no significant reduction of mortality in enalapril-treated patients compared with placebo. **B,** The SOLVD treatment subgroup demonstrated mortality benefit in moderate heart failure. The treatment subgroup included patients who already had symptomatic congestive heart failure and were randomized to either placebo or enalapril therapy. Criteria for randomization were a baseline ejection fraction of 35% or less and symptomatic heart failure. The majority of patients in this study had functional class II congestive heart failure. Enalapril was associated with a significant reduction in mortality compared with placebo in these patients. This mortality benefit was primarily the result of reducing mortality due to congestive heart failure. Mortality due to presumed arrhythmic death was not significantly different from placebo. (Part A *adapted from* the SOLVD Investigators [24]; part B *adapted from* the SOLVD Investigators [25].)

POSTINFARCTION LEFT VENTRICULAR DYSFUNCTION

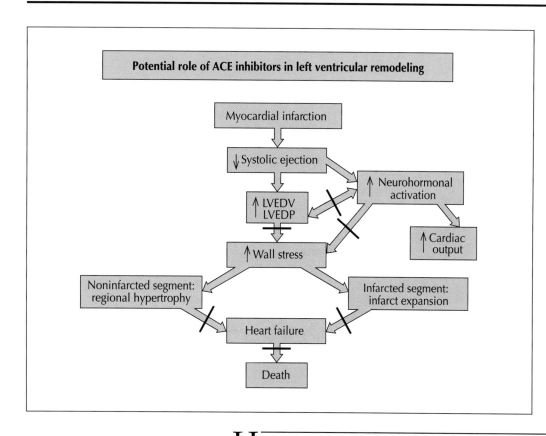

FIGURE 10-27. Although the patho-physiology of infarct healing is complex, there are several potential mechanisms by which an angiotensin-converting enzyme (ACE) inhibitor may favorably improve left ventricular remodeling. Shown with *intersecting bars* are sites at which an ACE inhibitor may interrupt an adverse consequence of myocardial infarction that would contribute to heart failure or death. LVEDP—left ventricular end-diastolic pressure; LVEDV—left ventricular end-diastolic volume. (*Adapted from* McKay and coworkers [26]; with permission.)

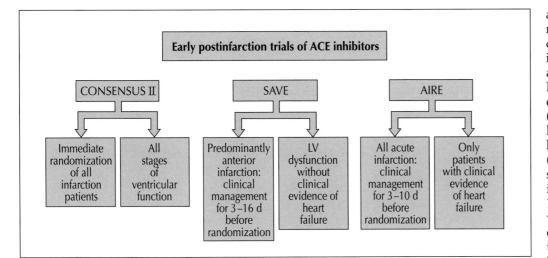

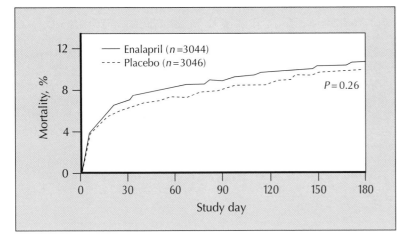

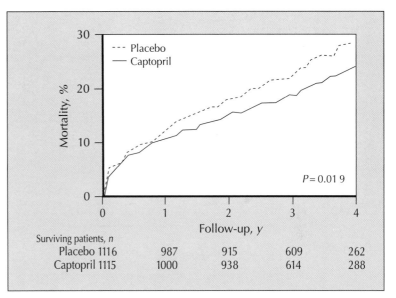

FIGURE 10-28. Three postinfarction trials of angiotensin-converting enzyme (ACE) inhibitors evaluated various populations and degrees of ventricular dysfunction. In CONSENSUS II (Cooperative New Scandinavian Enalapril Survival Study), there was immediate randomization of all infarct patients, irrespective of the stage of ventricular function, to either placebo or the intravenous ACE inhibitor enalaprilat. The latter was then followed by oral enalapril. In SAVE (Survival and Ventricular Enlargement), patients with

acute myocardial infarction who had been managed clinically in the interval of 3 to 16 days before randomization were included in the study. This population primarily had anterior wall myocardial infarctions. Patients were included in randomization only if they had evidence of left ventricular (LV) dysfunction with an ejection fraction of less than 40% without clinical evidence of heart failure, such as rales. In the AIRE (Acute Infarction Ramipril Evaluation) study, patients with acute myocardial infarction were managed clinically for 3 to 10 days before randomization. Patients were randomized only if they had clinical evidence of heart failure. This is in contrast to the asymptomatic LV dysfunction of the SAVE study. In the AIRE study, however, patients with severe heart failure or cardiogenic shock were excluded. No ejection fraction cutoff was utilized in this study, and the clinical diagnosis of heart failure was made by the attending physician.

FIGURE 10-29. It should be noted that mortality benefit has not been demonstrated in all postinfarction trials. In the CONSENSUS (Cooperative Scandinavian Enalapril Survival Study) II study, enalapril did not significantly reduce short-term myocardial infarction mortality. Follow-up was for 180 days, with a mortality endpoint consistent with myocardial infarction rather than congestive heart failure, which typically requires longer follow-up. There was a relatively low overall mortality rate as this study included patients without heart failure. This study was terminated early, and it was postulated that excessive hypotension with intravenous administration of enalapril obscured clinical benefit. (*Adapted from* Swedberg and coworkers [27].)

FIGURE 10-30. In contrast to CONSENSUS (Cooperative Scandinavian Enalapril Survival Study) II, the results of the SAVE (Survival and Ventricular Enlargement) study demonstrated that an angiotensin-converting enzyme (ACE) inhibitor given to the high-risk anterior myocardial infarction subgroup was associated with a 19% reduction in all-cause mortality. There was no effect of captopril compared with placebo on short-term mortality during the first year of follow-up. After 1 year of follow-up, mortality reduction was evident in the captopril group. This suggested that the reduction may be due to a decrease in deaths related to the development of heart failure. (*Adapted from* Pfeffer and coworkers [28].)

EFFECT OF CAPTOPRIL ON CUMULATIVE CARDIOVASCULAR EVENTS

EVENT	RISK REDUCTION WITH CAPTOPRIL, %	P VALUE
Cardiovascular deaths	21	0.014
CHF requiring ACE inhibitor	37	0.001
CHF requiring hospitalization	22	0.019
Recurrent MI	25	0.015
Death		
CV/recurrent MI	22	0.003
CV/CHF/MI	24	0.001

FIGURE 10-31. The effect of captopril on fatal and nonfatal cardio-vascular (CV) endpoints in the SAVE (Survival and Ventricular Enlargement) trial. The relative risk reduction for captopril compared with placebo, and the level of significance are shown. Although some of these factors may have been predictable, such as the reduction of risk of congestive heart failure (CHF) requiring hospitalization, the 25% reduction of recurrent myocardial infarction (MI) was unexpected. This finding suggests a secondary prevention benefit of angiotensin-converting enzyme (ACE) inhibitors, a potential that is being actively investigated. (*Adapted from* Pfeffer and coworkers [28].)

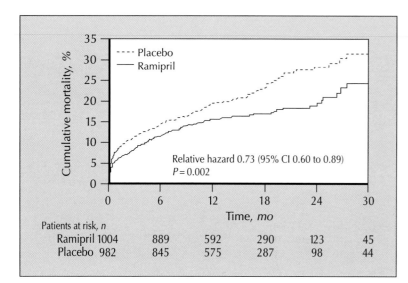

Patients at risk, n					
Ramipril 1004	889	592	290	123	45
Placebo 982	845	575	287	98	44

FIGURE 10-32. The outcome of the all-cause mortality primary endpoint in the AIRE (Acute Infarction Ramipril Evaluation) trial, based on intention to treat. It is instructive to compare this figure with the results of the SAVE (Survival and Ventricular Enlargement) trial in Fig. 10-30. In AIRE there is an early divergence of survival benefit for ramipril, which is not apparent in SAVE. Many believe that this reflects the greater clinical severity of heart failure in AIRE, whereas patients in SAVE had asymptomatic left ventricular dysfunction. In fact, clinical evidence of heart failure excluded patients from SAVE. In AIRE, this early survival benefit persisted throughout follow-up, as the survival curves continue to diverge. This suggests that, in contrast to SAVE, early survival benefit results from reduction of mortality related to heart failure, which continues through follow-up. CI—confidence interval. (*Adapted from* AIRE Study Investigators [29].)

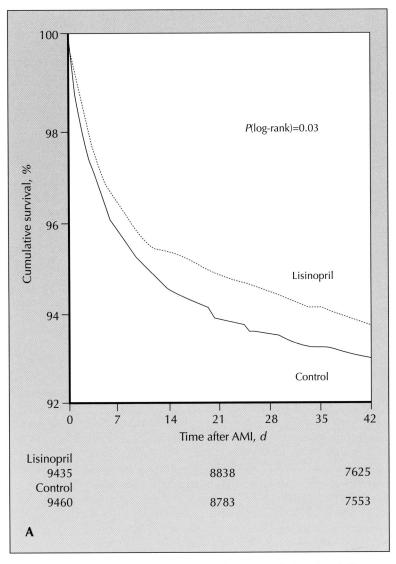

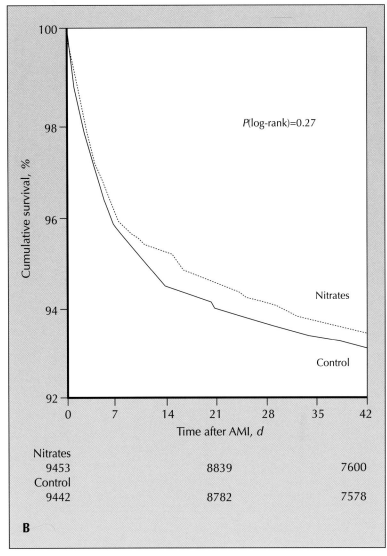

FIGURE 10-33. The GISI-3 (Gruppo Italiano per lo Studio della Sopravvevenza nell' Infarto Miocardio) study. In this study, a factorial design permitted analysis of the effects of the angiotensin-converting enzyme inhibitor lisinopril and transdermal glyceryl trinitrate on survival in 19,394 patients randomized to therapy within 24 hours of acute myocardial infarction (AMI) symptoms. **A,** Lisinopril therapy was associated with a significant increase in survival compared with the control group. **B,** Although nitrate therapy was associated with a trend for improvement, this did not achieve significance. It should be noted that the patients randomized in this study were not stratified according to the magnitude of ventricular dysfunction. The favorable effect of lisinopril achieved significance, despite the treatment of a large number of low-risk patients. A similar observation was made in the ISIS-4 (International Study of Infarct Survival) trial. This study evaluated more than 58,000 patients and demonstrated a favorable reduction in mortality in captopril-treated patients. Nitroglycerin therapy (oral controlled-release mononitrate) did not produce a significant improvement in survival (Part A *adapted from* Gruppo Italiano per lo Studio della Sopravvevenza nell' Infarto Miocardio [31]; part B *adapted from* ISIS 4 [32].)

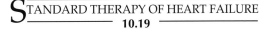

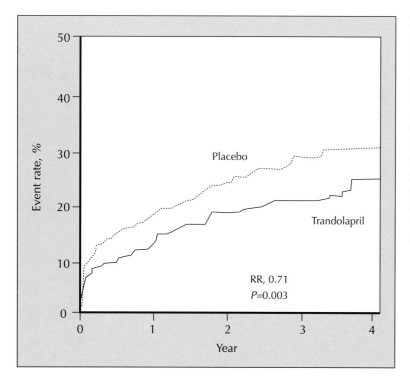

FIGURE 10-34. The Trandolapril Cardiac Evaluation (TRACE) study. In contrast to the GISI-3 (Gruppo Italiano per lo Studio della Sopravvevenza nell' Infarto Miocardio) and ISIS-4 (International Study of Infarct Survival) studies, the TRACE study focused on the high-risk patient population with left ventricular (LV) dysfunction immediately following myocardial infarction. This trial demonstrated immediate benefit of the angiotensin-converting enzyme (ACE) inhibitor in the high-risk LV dysfunction group, and the benefit continued to improve during 4 years of follow-up. Thus, in a group of patients at high risk for mortality following acute myocardial infarction, the ACE-inhibitor benefit was more pronounced than in the larger population studies such as GISI-3 and ISIS-4, which included large segments of patients at low-risk with normal or near-normal ventricular function. RR—relative risk. (*Adapted from* Kober and coworkers [30].)

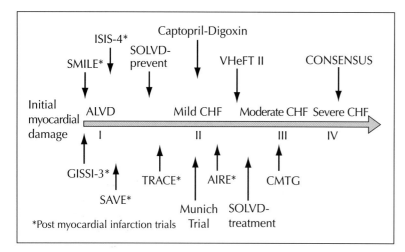

FIGURE 10-35. The relationship of positive or favorable clinical trials with angiotensin-converting enzyme (ACE) inhibitors can be shown in relation to the severity of congestive heart failure (CHF). *Vertical arrows* indicate the approximate mean value of the New York Heart Association (NYHA) functional class for all patients enrolled in each of the studies. The initial myocardial damage (*left*) may result from myocardial infarction or coronary ischemia, hypertension, idiopathic cardiomyopathy, or valvular heart disease. The *horizontal arrow* shows progression from asymptomatic left ventricular dysfunction (ALVD) to severe CHF with the corre-

sponding NYHA functional classification below the symptomatic groupings (Roman numerals I to IV). In actuality, the chronologic development of ACE inhibitor trials would be more closely represented by a grouping of these studies from right to left.

Both the SAVE study and the AIRE study were conducted in patients after myocardial infarction (*asterisks*). In SAVE, patients had ALVD. In AIRE, only patients with symptomatic left ventricular dysfunction were enrolled. These studies covered the range of ventricular dysfunction after myocardial infarction. Not shown is CONSENSUS II, which was a true postmyocardial infarction study conducted in all patients with acute myocardial infarction, irrespective of left ventricular function. This study did not demonstrate a short-term mortality benefit, in contrast to the long-term benefit in SAVE and the short- and long-term benefit in AIRE. Additional trials (*ie*, GISSI-3, ISIS-4, SMILE, TRACE) have demonstrated ACE-inhibitor benefit in the postinfarction population. AIRE—Acute Infarction Ramipril Evaluation; CRMG—Captopril Multicenter Research Group exercise study; CONSENSUS—Cooperative North Scandinavian Enalapril Survival Study; GISSI—Gruppo Italiano per lo Studio della Sopravvevenza nell' Infarto Miocardio; ISIS—International Study of Infarct Survival; SAVE—Survival and Ventricular Enlargement; SMILE—Survival of Myocardial Infarction Long-Term Evaluation; SOLVD—Studies of Left Ventricular Dysfunction prevention study; TRACE—Trandolapril Cardiac Evaluation; V-HeFT II—Veterans Administration Cooperative Vasodilator Heart Failure Trial.

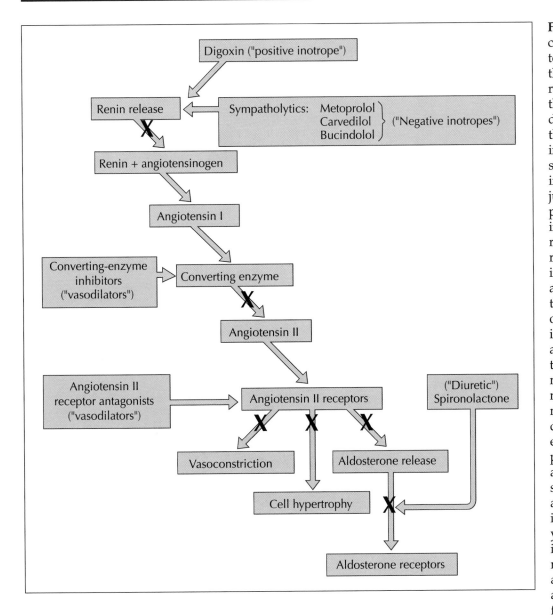

FIGURE 10-36. Although angiotensin-converting enzyme inhibitors are considered to be the standard approach for inhibition of the renin-angiotensin-aldosterone system, a review of the literature clearly demonstrates that many pharmacologic therapeutic classes, despite a broad diversity in their putative therapeutic effects, have been shown to inhibit the renin-angiotensin-aldosterone system in varying degrees. Digoxin ("positive inotrope") blocks release of renin from the juxtaglomerular cells of the kidney. Sympatholytic agents ("negative inotropes") inhibit the sympathetic stimulus for renin release, which is a prominent feature for renin release in heart failure. Both converting inhibitors and angiotensin receptor antagonists have hemodynamic properties that would be considered "vasodilator" in overall action. Whereas converting enzyme inhibitors prevent the generation of angiotensin II, the receptor antagonists block the effects of circulating angiotensin II at multiple target organ sites. These distinct mechanisms of action have currently evoked many studies comparing the similarities and differences for these two groups as well as evaluation of the combination of the two pharmacologic groups for the potentiation of angiotensin II inhibition. Finally, although spironolactone is considered a "diuretic," it is actually a specific antagonist of aldosterone at its receptor site, and data from the last several years suggest that spironolactone may exert its effects in many locations, including the myocardium, blocking the adverse effects of aldosterone. Newer, more specific aldosterone antagonists are currently being evaluated to further clarify the specific role of aldosterone independent of angiotensin II.

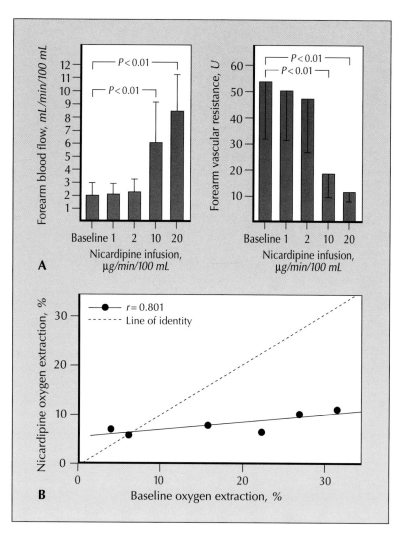

A

B

FIGURE 10-37. The direct vasodilator effects of the dihdropyridine group of calcium antagonists as shown by the regional administration of aqueous nicardipine.

A, In the absence of myocardial influences or reflex control, infusion of nicardipine directly into the brachial artery at progressive dose increments produced a significant increase in forearm blood flow (*left*), and reduction of forearm vascular resistance (*right*). This achieved statistical significance at an infusion rate of 10 μg/min/100 mL of forearm volume.

B, The effect of nicardipine on six patients in whom simultaneous brachial artery and basilic vein oxygen samples permitted calculation of oxygen extraction. If there was no metabolic response to vasodilation, oxygen extraction would be unchanged and would fall upon the line of identity. However, in response to the vasodilation with nicardipine, there was reduction of oxygen extraction with improved flow. This effect was greatest in those patients with the highest baseline oxygen extraction. (*Adapted from* Cody [33]; with permission.)

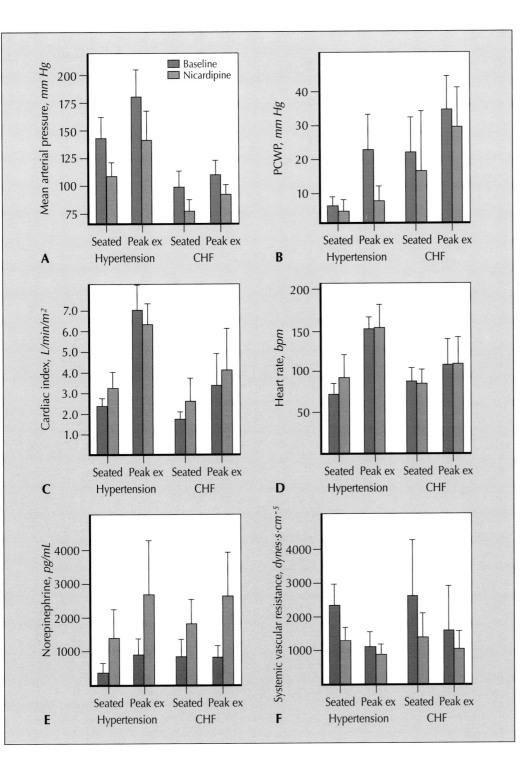

FIGURE 10-38. The hemodynamic response to newer dihydropyridines may be greater than the response to earlier calcium antagonists. This is exemplified by nicardipine. Short-term hemodynamic efforts of the calcium antagonist nicardipine were compared in patients with hypertension (*n*=10) and congestive heart failure (CHF; *n*=10). Both resting (seated) and maximal exercise (peak ex) values are given. The same methodology was used in each patient group. Both hypertensive and CHF patients were characterized by vasoconstriction, which was reversed by the oral administration of nicardipine through the course of 1 week. This was associated with a reduction in mean arterial pressure (*panel A*) and pulmonary capillary wedge pressure (PCWP; *panel B*). The reduction in PCWP at rest and maximal exercise in the presence of vasoconstriction reversal is consistent with the relative vasoselectivity of nicardipine in this population, particularly because cardiac index (*panel C*) was not adversely affected. In fact, cardiac index was actually increased at rest and with maximal exercise in the CHF population, the group in whom the greatest adverse outcome would be anticipated from a negative inotropic effect. In the hypertensive population, both resting and maximal exercise heart rates tended to increase, this was not observed in the CHF population (*panel D*). This was evidence against a direct positive chronotropic effect of nicardipine. Nevertheless, plasma norepinephrine was increased at rest and at maximal exercise in both populations (*panel E*). This increase of norepinephrine has not been reported with other newer dihydropyridines, such as amlodipine. In both cardiovascular disorders, nicardipine produced comparable reductions of systemic vascular resistance (*panel F*) at rest and at peak exercise. (*Adapted from* Cody [33]; with permission.)

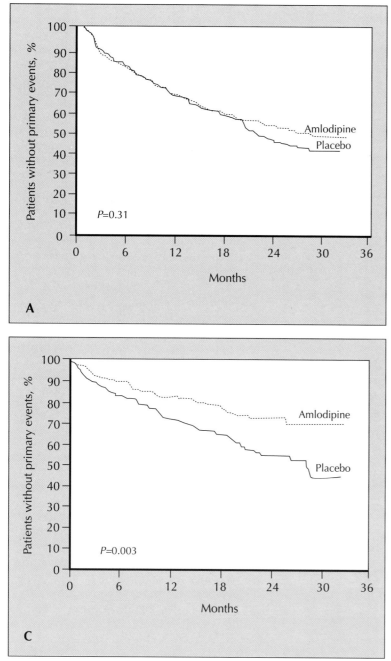

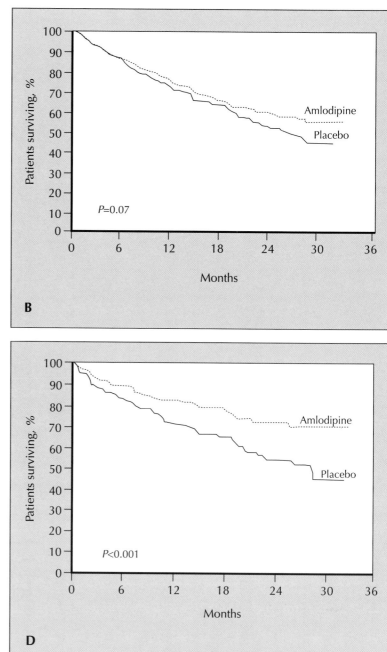

FIGURE 10-39. The Prospective Randomized Amlodipine Survival Evaluation (PRAISE) study. The calcium channel antagonist amlodipine was evaluated in a large prospective study to determine the effects on overall mortality, as this particular calcium channel antagonist was reported to have less adverse effects on cardiac and clinical status than its predecessors. In the PRAISE study, 1153 patients receiving digoxin, diuretic, and angiotensin-converting enzyme inhibitor therapy were randomized to placebo or amlodipine. **A** to **D**, Amlodipine had no significant effect on mortality compared with the placebo-treated group. In a subanalysis, patients whose heart failure was not ischemic in origin showed a significant mortality benefit compared with those in the placebo group. This unanticipated finding has raised questions regarding possible mechanism of benefit in the nonischemic group compared with the ischemic group. Therefore, PRAISE-II is currently being conducted to determine the effects of amlodipine on survival in a patient population that is exclusively composed of patients with nonischemic etiology of heart failure. (*Adapted from* Packer and coworkers [34].)

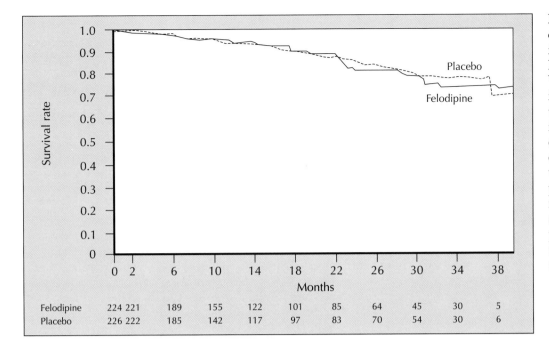

Felodipine	224	221	189	155	122	101	85	64	45	30	5
Placebo	226	222	185	142	117	97	83	70	54	30	6

FIGURE 10-40. In a second large study of a calcium channel antagonist, the effects of felodipine were evaluated in the V-HeFT III (Veterans Administration Cooperative Vasodilator Heart Failure Trial). Although felodipine produced a vasodilator effect, there was no mortality benefit when felodipine was added to standard therapy of enalapril and diuretics. The study evaluated exercise tolerance, left ventricular function, quality of life, and plasma neurohormones in addition to the mortality effect. Plasma norepinephrine and quality-of-life measures at most time points were not significantly different in the treatment groups. (*Adapted from* Cohn and coworkers [35].)

SUMMARY

TRADITIONAL CLASSIFICATION OF HEART FAILURE THERAPY

Digoxin (inotrope)
Diuretic
Vasodilator

FIGURE 10-41. Traditional classification of heart failure therapy. The traditional classification of heart failure therapy was based upon observations of acute interventions more than 20 years ago. These observations were extrapolated to chronic therapy when digoxin was thought to be a "positive inotropic" agent. Diuretics were assumed to be a foundation of therapy in all patients, and it was assumed that oral vasodilator therapy would produce a long-term benefit similar to that observed in the acute setting.

NEW CLASSIFICATION OF HEART FAILURE THERAPY

Improve myocardial function
  Limit or reverse ischemia
  Normalize blood pressure
  Control lipids
  Reduction of market obesity

Management of sodium and water retention
  Dietary Na$^+$ control
  Diuretic
    ↓AVP
    ↓RAAS
    ↑Natriuretic peptides
    ↑GFR?

Modulate adverse myocardial, vascular, and cell-growth
  maladaptation
  Reset autonomic and reflex abnormalities
  Reduce angiotensin II levels
  Reduce aldosterone levels
  Reduce endothelin levels
  Increase nitric oxide activity
  Emerging cellular approaches

FIGURE 10-42. New classification of heart failure therapy. Since the initial observations regarding the traditional classification of heart failure therapy, particularly observations in the past 10 years, it is evident that effective therapeutic agents such as angiotensin-converting enzyme inhibitors and β-adrenergic blockade cross the boundaries of the older classification. In addition, many of the effects that are currently thought to confer a long-term clinical and mortality benefit do not fit within the old treatment paradigm. Evolution toward a more rational approach to therapy should be based on the information generated in the past two decades. This includes efforts to improve myocardial function by treating the underlying etiology of heart failure. In many cases, this is either a primary or secondary prevention approach. The presence of edema due to sodium and water retention has traditionally been a clinical hallmark of heart failure. With more aggressive management of asymptomatic left ventricular dysfunction and mild heart failure, edema may not necessarily be a prominent feature. Control of dietary sodium intake (2 to 3 g/d of sodium) is important, regardless of the presence or absence of edema. Although diuretics remain the current approach to treating sodium and water retention, therapies that inhibit arginine vasopressin, the renin-angiotensin-aldosterone system, and potentially, amplification of the response to natriuretic peptides, form a more logical treatment for edema. Ultimately, any drug therapy or management system that would improve glomerular filtration rate (GFR) would be a much more direct approach to therapy. Finally, the basis for the progression of heart failure is the abnormal myocardial, vascular, and cell-growth control mechanisms as the disease evolves. Many of these functions are mediated by vasoactive substances and neurohormonal factors. Appropriate modulation of these factors is therefore mandatory. Emerging approaches toward evaluating abnormal cellular function and the basis for tissue necrosis and apoptosis, together with the potential of gene-guided therapy, offer great promise as we enter the 21st century.

ACKNOWLEDGEMENT

The author and editors acknowledge the contributions of Ralph A. Kelly, MD, and Thomas W. Smith, MD, to the first edition.

REFERENCES

1 Smith TW, Braunwald E, Kelly RA: The management of heart failure. In *Heart Disease, A Textbook of Cardiovascular Medicine*, edn 4. Edited by Braunwald E. Philadelphia: WB Saunders; 1992:464-519

2. Cohn JW: Drugs used to control vascular resistance and capacitance. In *The Heart*. Edited by Schlant RC, Alexander RW. New York: McGraw-Hill; 1994:611–620.

3. Cody RJ: Diuretic therapy of congestive heart failure. In *Heart Failure: Scientific Principles and Clinical Practice*. Edited by Poole-Wilson P, Colucci W, Chatterjee K, *et al.* New York: Churchill Livingstone; 1997:635–648.

4. Kelly RA, Smith TW: Treatment of stable heart failure: digitalis and diuretics. In *Atlas of Heart Diseases: Hypertension: Mechanisms and Therapy*. Edited by Braunwald E, Colucci WS. Philadelphia; Current Medicine; 1995:10.1–10.16.

5. Mason DT, Braunwald E, Karsh RB, *et al.*: Studies on Digitalis: X. Effects of ouabain on forearm vascular resistance and venous tone in normal subjects and in patients in heart failure. *J Clin Invest* 1964, 43:532–543.

6. Ferguson DW, Berg WJ, Sanders JS, *et al.*: Sympathoinhibitory responses to digitalis glycosides in heart failure patients: direct evidence from sympathetic neural recordings. *Circulation* 1989, 80:65–77.

7. Wang W, Chen J-S, Zucker IH: Carotid sinus baroreceptor sensitivity in experimental heart failure. *Circulation* 1990, 81:1959–1966.

8. Gheorghiade M, St Clair J, St Clair C, *et al.*: Hemodynamic effects of intravenous digoxin in patients with severe heart failure initially treated with diuretics and vasodilators. *J Am Coll Cardiol* 1987, 9:849–857.

9. Captopril-Digoxin Multicenter Research Group: Comparative effects of therapy with captopril and digoxin in patients with mild to moderate heart failure. *JAMA* 1988, 259:539–544.

10. Uretsky BF, Young JB, Shahidi FE, *et al.*: Randomized study assessing the effect of digoxin withdrawal in patients with mild to moderate chronic congestive heart failure: results of the PROVED trial. *J Am Coll Cardiol* 1993, 22:955–962.

11. Packer M, Gheorghiade M, Young JB, *et al.*: Withdrawal of digoxin from patients with chronic heart failure treated with angiotensin-converting-enzyme inhibitors. *N Engl J Med* 1993, 329:1–7.

12. Digitalis Investigation Group: The effect of digoxin on mortality and morbidity in patients with heart failure. The Digitalis Investigation Group (DIG) Trial. *N Engl J Med* 1997, 336:525–533.

13. Cody RJ, Pickworth KK: Approaches to diuretic therapy and electrolyte imbalance in congestive heart failure. In *Update in Congestive Heart Failure: Cardiology Clinics*, vol 12. Edited by Deedwania PC. Philadelphia: WB Saunders; 1994:37–50.

14. Wilcox CS, Mitch WE, Kelly RA, *et al.*: Response to furosemide: I. Effect of salt intake and renal compensation. *J Lab Clin Med* 1983, 102:450–458.

15. Cody RJ, Ljungman S, Covit AB, *et al.*: Regulation of glomerular filtration rate in chronic congestive heart failure patients. *Kidney Int* 1988, 34:361–367.

16. Cody RJ, Riew KD, Kubo SH: Reversal of a calcium-mediated vasoconstrictor component in patients with congestive heart failure. *Clin Pharmacol Ther* 1989, 46:291–296.

17. Chatterjee K, Brundage BH, Ports TA: Nonparenteral vasodilator therapy for chronic congestive heart failure. *Compr Ther* 1979, 5:48–55.

18. Cohn JN, Archibald DG, Ziesche S, *et al.*: Effect of vasodilator therapy on mortality in chronic congestive heart failure: results of a Veterans Administration Cooperative Study. *N Engl J Med* 1986, 314:1547–1552.

19. Elkayam U, Kulick D, McIntosh N, *et al.*: Incidence of early tolerance to hemodynamic effects of continuous infusion of nitro-glycerin in patients with coronary artery disease and heart failure. *Circulation* 1987, 76:577–584.

20. Cody RJ: Angiotensin-converting enzyme inhibitors: mechanisms, pharmacodynamics, and clinical trials in heart failure. *Cardiol Rev* 1994, 2:145–156.

21. Captopril Multicenter Research Group: A placebo-controlled trial of captopril in refractory heart failure. *J Am Coll Cardiol* 1983, 2:755–763.

22. CONSENSUS Trial Study Group: Effects of enalapril on mortality in severe congestive heart failure. *N Engl J Med* 1987, 316:1429–1435.

23. Cohn JN, Johnson G, Ziesche S, *et al.*: A comparison of enalapril with hydralazine-isosorbide dinitrate in the treatment of chronic congestive heart failure. *N Engl J Med* 1991, 325:303–310.

24. SOLVD Investigators: Effect of enalapril on mortality and the development of CHF in asymptomatic patients with reduced left ventricular ejection fractions. *N Engl J Med* 1992, 327:685–691.

25. The SOLVD Investigators: Effect of enalapril on survival in patients with reduced left ventricular ejection fractions and congestive heart failure. *N Engl J Med* 1991, 325:293–302.

26. McKay RG, Pfeffer MA, Pasternal RC, *et al.*: Left ventricular remodeling after myocardial infarction: a corollary to infarct expansion. *Circulation* 1986, 74:693–702.

27. Swedberg K, Held P, Kek-hu J, *et al.*: Effect of the early administration of enalapril on mortality in patients with acute-myocardial infarction. Results of the Cooperative New Scandinavian Enalapril Survival Study II (CONSENSUS II). *N Engl J Med* 1992, 327:678–684.

28. Pfeffer MA, Braunwald E, Moy LA, *et al.* on behalf of the SAVE Investigators: Effect of captopril on mortality and morbidity in patients with left ventricular dysfunction after myocardial infarction: results of the Survival and Ventricular Enlargement Trial. *N Engl J Med* 1992, 327:669–677.

29. Acute Infarction Ramipril Efficacy (AIRE) Study Investigators: Effect of ramipril on mortality and morbidity of survivors of acute myocardial infarction with clinical evidence of CHF. *Lancet* 1993, 342:821–827.

30. Kober L, Torp-Pedersen C, Carsen JE, *et al.* for the Trandolapril Cardiac Evaluation (TRACE) Study Group: A clinical trial of the angiotensin-converting-enzyme inhibitor trandolapril in patients with left ventricular dysfunction after myocardial infarction. *N Engl J Med* 1995, 333:1670–1676.

31. Gruppo Italiano per lo Studio della Sopravvevenza nell' Infarto Miocardico: GISSI-3: effects of lisinopril and transdermal glyceryl trinitrate singly and together on 6-week mortality and ventricular function after acute myocardial infarction. *Lancet* 1994, 343:1115–1122.

32. ISIS-4 Collaborative Group: ISIS-4: a randomized factorial trial assessing early oral captopril, oral mononitrate, and intravenous magnesium sulphate in 58,050 patients with suspected acute myocardial infarction. *Lancet* 1995, 345:669–685.

33. Cody RJ: Vascular and myocardial responses to calcium antagonists: implications for hypertension and congestive heart failure. In *Calcium Antagonists in Clinical Medicine*. Edited by Epstein M. Philadelphia: Hanley & Belfus; 1992:105–135.

34. Packer M, O'Connor CM, Ghali JK, *et al.*: Effect of amlodipine on morbidity and mortality in severe chronic heart failure. Prospective Randomized Amlodipine Survival Evaluation (PRAISE) Study Group. *N Engl J Med* 1996, 335:1107–1114.

35. Cohn JN, Ziesche S, Smith R, *et al.* for the Vasodilator-Heart Failure Trial (V-HeFT) Study Group: Effect of the calcium antagonist felodipine as supplementary vasodilator therapy in patients with chronic heart failure treated with enalapril. VHeFT III. *Circulation* 1997, 96:856–863.

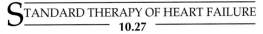

Treatment of Heart Failure: New Approaches

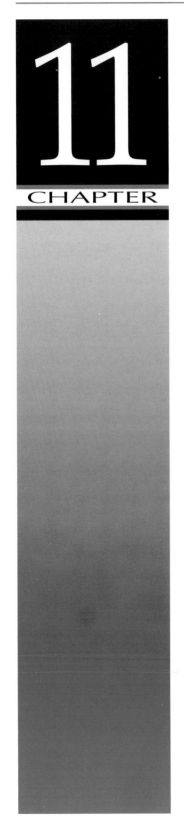

11

CHAPTER

Michael M. Givertz and Wilson S. Colucci

Major goals in the therapy of systolic heart failure include the amelioration of symptoms and the reduction of mortality. As discussed in Chapter 10, there is now compelling evidence that angiotensin-converting enzyme (ACE) inhibitors achieve both of these goals and therefore are first-line therapy. The clinical utility of digitalis has also been established. Digitalis consistently improves symptoms and exercise capacity and reduces hospitalizations for heart failure. Because digitalis is neutral with regard to survival, it is a second-line agent behind ACE inhibitors. Despite the appropriate use of ACE inhibitors and digitalis, many patients remain symptomatic and have a reduced survival. Fortunately, the past few years have witnessed an unprecedented number of new therapeutic approaches to heart failure. Of these, the most extensively studied new agents have been the β-adrenergic antagonists. A rapidly growing body of evidence suggests that these agents can improve symptoms, morbidity, and survival, and recently, the β-adrenergic antagonist carvedilol has been approved for the treatment of heart failure in several countries, including the United States.

The demonstration that β-adrenergic antagonists can also slow the progression of myocardial dysfunction has highlighted the importance of this as a goal of therapy. As discussed in Chapter 4, the progressive nature of myocardial dysfunction is due primarily to the process of myocardial "remodeling." Remodeling is the result of a composite of molecular and cellular events, including hypertrophy, apoptosis and fetal gene expression of myocytes, and changes in the extracellular matrix, which taken together adversely affect the structure and function of the myocardium. It is increasingly apparent that agents that alleviate myocardial wall stress or block the actions of angiotensin or norepinephrine (*eg*, vasodilators, ACE inhibitors, and β-adrenergic antagonists) can slow the progression of myocardial dysfunction. As a result, new strategies for inhibiting the sympathetic nervous system (*eg*, centrally acting sympatholytic agents) and the renin-angiotensin system (*eg*, angiotensin receptor antagonists) are being evaluated in patients with heart failure. It now appears likely that additional factors contribute to myocardial remodeling, including endothelin, inflammatory cytokines, and reactive oxygen species. This appreciation has led to the development of novel agents and strategies that are now being subjected to clinical testing. These include agents that inhibit endothelin receptors or that reduce the levels of inflammatory cytokines and oxidative stress.

Three new classes of intravenously active agents are undergoing extensive clinical testing and have the potential to be available commercially in the near future. OPC-18790 is a quinolinone derivative related to vesnarinone that exerts both direct inotropic and vasodilating actions. Levosimendan increases the sensitivity of the myocardium to calcium, is a mild phosphodiesterase inhibitor, and activates adenosine triphosphate–dependent potassium channels. Because of its ability to augment contractility without increasing intracellular calcium concentration, levosimendan may be less prone to causing arrhythmias than conventional positive inotropic agents. Brain natriuretic peptide is a recombinant human protein that exerts potent vasodilator and natriuretic actions when administered to patients with heart failure. These agents show the potential to improve the efficacy and safety of the short-term treatment of decompensated heart failure.

β-BLOCKERS

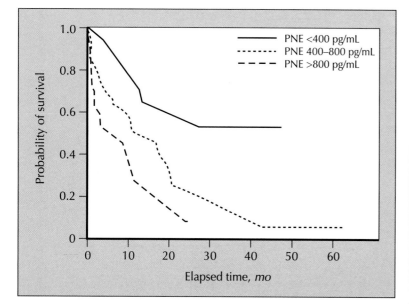 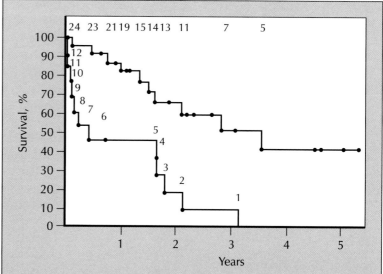

FIGURE 11-1. The level of activation of the sympathetic nervous system predicts survival in patients with chronic systolic heart failure. Cohn *et al.* [1] measured plasma norepinephrine (PNE) levels in 106 patients with functional class III to IV heart failure and followed them prospectively for a mean of 27 months. As shown by the survival curves, patients in the highest tercile (*dashed line*; plasma norepinephrine levels greater than 800 pg/mL) had significantly decreased long-term survival when compared with patients in either the middle (*dotted line*) or lowest terciles (*solid line*). Neurohormonal data from the Studies of Left Ventricular Dysfunction (SOLVD) [2] further demonstrated that norepinephrine levels are also increased in patients with asymptomatic left ventricular dysfunction. These and other studies have raised the possibility that chronic overactivity of the sympathetic nervous system could contribute to mortality in patients with heart failure, and might contribute to disease progression even in patients with early, asymptomatic disease. (*Adapted from* Cohn and coworkers [1]; with permission.)

FIGURE 11-2. β-Adrenergic antagonists for treatment of dilated cardiomyopathy. In the 1970s, Swedberg *et al.* [3] in Goteberg, Sweden, published a series of pioneering studies that suggested that β-adrenergic antagonists could be of clinical value in the treatment of patients with dilated cardiomyopathy. In these open-label studies, the addition of a β-adrenergic antagonist to standard treatment with digitalis and diuretics was associated with improvements in symptoms and ventricular function and, as shown here, improved survival. In 24 patients treated with β-adrenergic antagonists (*upper curve*), the 3-year survival was improved when compared with a group of 12 historical controls (*lower curve*). (*Adapted from* Swedberg and coworkers [3]; with permission.)

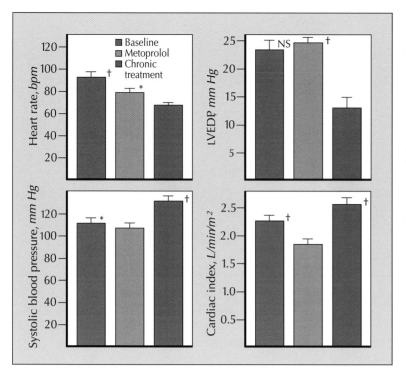

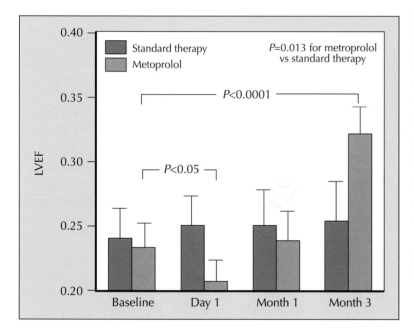

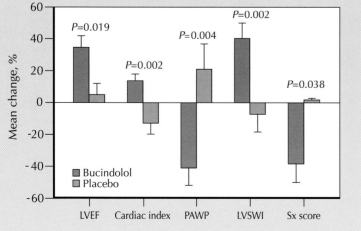

FIGURE 11-3. Acute and chronic hemodynamic effects of β-blockers in patients with heart failure. Role of sympathetic nervous system in heart failure. The sympathetic nervous system, acting via stimulation of myocardial β-adrenergic receptors, plays an important role in supporting cardiac pump function for patients with myocardial failure. Not surprisingly, in such patients the immediate effect of a β-blocker is deterioration in hemodynamic performance. Intravenous administration of a low dose of the β-adrenergic antagonist metoprolol to patients with heart failure decreased heart rate and cardiac index and caused a small increase in left ventricular end-diastolic pressure (LVEDP). Although the acute vascular effect of β-blockade is to increase systemic vascular resistance, systolic blood pressure decreased, reflecting a decrease in cardiac output. In striking contrast, long-term administration of oral metoprolol to the same patients was associated with a decrease in LVEDP and an increase in cardiac index despite a further decrease in heart rate indicative of more complete β-blockade. Data such as these indicate that although the acute hemodynamic effect of β-adrenergic blockade is to worsen hemodynamics, long-term treatment is associated with improvement in ventricular function. (*Adapted from* Hjalmarson and Waagstein [4].)

FIGURE 11-4. Time course of the increase in left ventricular ejection fraction (LVEF) with chronic β-blocker therapy in patients with heart failure. One of the most consistent findings in controlled trials of chronic β-blocker therapy in patients with heart failure has been an increase LVEF. The increase in ejection fraction is time-dependent. Hall *et al.* [5] demonstrated that after 1 day of therapy with metoprolol, patients demonstrated a significant reduction in LVEF that was associated with an increase in end-systolic volume. However, with continued therapy, and despite up-titration to higher doses of metoprolol, LVEF returned to baseline by 1 month and was significantly increased over baseline by 3 months. Overall, LVEF increased from 23% to 32% (*P*=0.001). In the placebo group, there were no significant changes in ejection fraction or left ventricular volumes. Data from this and other studies (*eg, see* Fig. 11-6) demonstrate that long-term improvements in LVEF are associated with improved left ventricular function. (*Adapted from* Hall and coworkers [5]; with permission.)

FIGURE 11-5. Bucindolol therapy for idiopathic dilated cardiomyopathy. Bucindolol, a nonselective β-adrenergic antagonist with direct vasodilator properties, has received intense scrutiny in a number of small trials. In one study (shown here), 24 patients with idiopathic dilated cardiomyopathy were challenged with bucindolol. Of these, 23 patients tolerated the drug and were subsequently randomized to bucindolol (*n*=14) or placebo (*n*=9) for a total treatment duration of 3 months. During randomized therapy, use of bucindolol caused significant improvements in left ventricular ejection fraction (LVEF), cardiac index, pulmonary artery wedge pressure (PAWP), left ventricular stroke work index (LVSWI), and symptom (Sx) score. (*Adapted from* Gilbert and coworkers [6].)

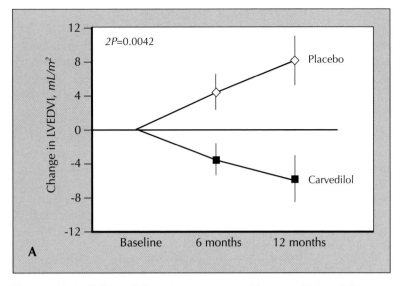

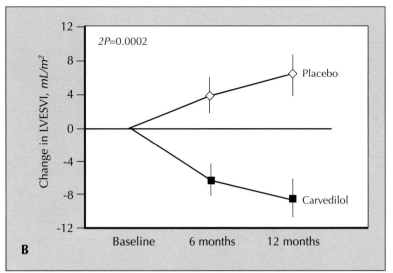

FIGURE 11-6. Effect of chronic treatment with carvediol on left ventricular volumes. The Australia–New Zealand Heart Failure Research Collaborative Group randomized patients with ischemic heart failure and a left ventricular ejection fraction (LVEF) of less than 45% to carvedilol or placebo. An echocardiographic substudy was performed on 123 patients to determine the effects of treatment on left ventricular (LV) size and function at 6 and 12 months. After

6 months of therapy, LVEF had increased by 4.9% in the carvedilol group compared with the placebo group (2P<0.001). As shown, the LV end-diastolic (**A**) and end-systolic (**B**) volume indices (LVEDVI and LVESVI, respectively) increased in the placebo group at 1 year but were reduced in the carvedilol-treated patients. These data suggest that carvedilol exerted a beneficial "reverse" remodeling effect. (*Adapted from* Doughty and coworkers [7]; with permission.)

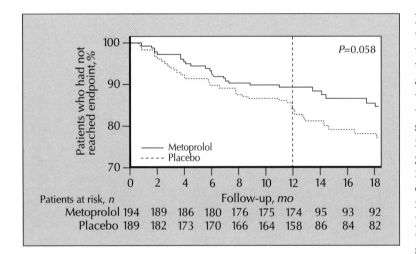

FIGURE 11-7. The Metoprolol in Dilated Cardiomyopathy (MDC) trial was the first large controlled trial of β-adrenergic antagonists in the treatment of congestive heart failure. In this study, 383 patients with heart failure secondary to idiopathic dilated cardiomyopathy and an ejection fraction less of less than 40% were randomized to therapy with placebo or metoprolol in addition to conventional therapy. The majority of patients had functional class II and III symptoms. Metoprolol, initiated at a dose of 5 mg twice a day, was increased to 50 to 75 mg twice a day. The metoprolol treatment group had a 34% reduction in the primary endpoint of clinical deterioration, which was defined as the need for cardiac transplantation or death. This improvement was due entirely to a reduction in the need for transplantation (two metoprolol patients, 19 placebo patients), with no difference in the number of deaths in each group (23 metoprolol, 19 placebo). In a subgroup of 41 patients, there was significant improvement in exercise duration and the hemodynamic response to exercise, with increases in cardiac index, stroke work, arterial pressure, and oxygen consumption [8]. (*Adapted from* Waagstein and coworkers [9]; with permission.)

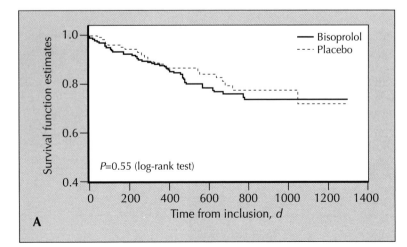

FIGURE 11-8. The Cardiac Insufficiency Bisoprolol Study (CIBIS) randomized 641 patients with heart failure of ischemic or non-ischemic etiology and a left ventricular ejection fraction of less than 40% to treatment with the β_1- selective antagonist bisoprolol or placebo. Essentially all of the patients (95%) were in New York Heart Association functional class III, and the rest were in class IV. All patients received diuretics, and 90% received angiotensin-converting enzyme inhibitors. After a mean follow-up of 1.9 years, there was no significant difference in mortality between the groups (relative risk for bisoprolol, 0.80; 95% confidence interval, 0.56 to 1.15; P=0.22). In a subgroup analysis of patients with (**A**) and (*continued*)

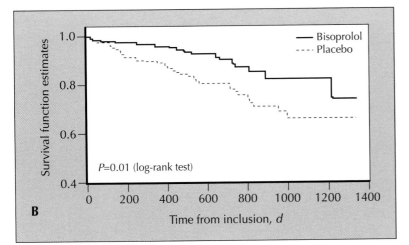

B

FIGURE 11-8. *(continued)* without (**B**) a history of myocardial infarction, bisoprolol appeared to reduce mortality in the patients with non-ischemic cardiomyopathy (*P*=0.01 by log-rank test). (*Adapted from* the CIBIS Investigators [10]; with permission.)

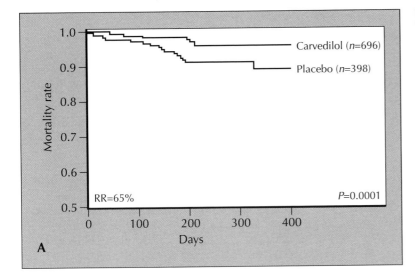

A

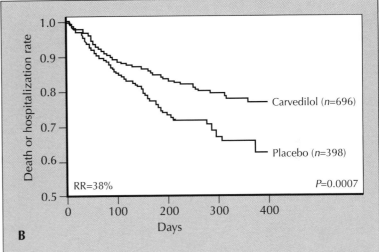

B

FIGURE 11-9. US Carvedilol Heart Failure Trials Program: effect on major clinical events. In 1997, the US Food and Drug Administration approved carvedilol, a nonselective β-adrenergic antagonist with α₁-adrenergic receptor blocking and antioxidant properties, as adjunctive therapy for patients with mild to moderate heart failure. This decision was based in large part on the results of the US Carvedilol Heart Failure Trials Program, which randomized 1094 patients with chronic heart failure and a left ventricular ejection fraction of 35% or less to placebo or carvedilol in addition to conventional therapy with digoxin, diuretics, and an angiotensin-

converting enzyme inhibitor. Patients were assigned to one of four treatment protocols based on exercise capacity as assessed by a 6-minute walk test. After a mean follow-up of 7 months, the overall mortality rate was 7.8% in the placebo group versus 3.2% in the carvedilol group (risk reduction [RR], 65%; 95% confidence interval, 39% to 80%; *P*<0.001) (**A**). In addition, carvedilol resulted in a 27% reduction in the risk of cardiovascular hospitalization (*P*=0.036) and a 38% reduction in the combined endpoint of death or cardio-vascular hospitalization (**B**; *P*=0.007). (*Adapted from* Packer and coworkers [11]; with permission.)

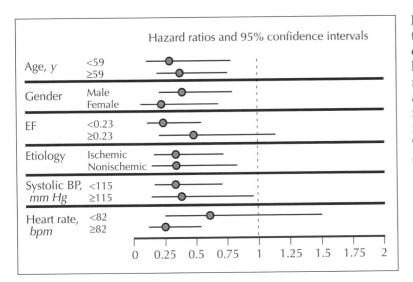

FIGURE 11-10. In the US Carvedilol Heart Failure Trials Program, the reduction in mortality with carvedilol was similar regardless of age, gender, left ventricular ejection fraction (EF), the etiology of heart failure, resting systolic blood pressure (BP), or heart rate. A recent meta-analysis of randomized clinical trials of β-adrenergic antagonists in heart failure [12] observed similar reductions in mortality for patients with ischemic (OR, 0.69; 95% confidence interval, 0.45 to 0.98) and non-ischemic cardiomyopathy (OR, 0.69; 95% confidence interval, 0.47 to 0.99). (*Adapted from* Packer and coworkers [11]; with permission.)

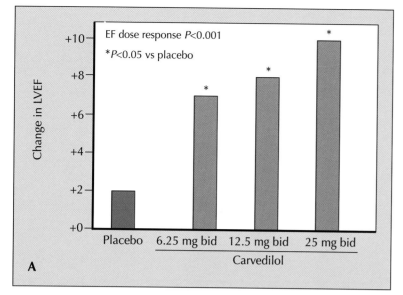

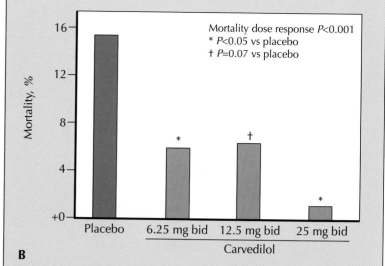

FIGURE 11-11. Effect of carvedilol on ejection fraction and mortality in the Multicenter Oral Carvediol Heart Failure Assesment (MOCHA) trial. The MOCHA trial, a component of the US Carvedilol Heart Failure Trials Program, tested whether the effects of carvedilol were dose-related. Patients (*n*=345) with mild to moderate heart failure were randomly assigned to treatment with placebo or carvedilol in one of three target doses: 6.25 mg twice a day (low-dose group), 12.5 mg twice a day (medium-dose group), or 25 mg twice a day (high-dose group). Although carvedilol had no effect on the primary end-point of submaximal exercise, there were significant dose-related improvements in left ventricular function (**A**) and all-cause mortality (**B**). In this study, carvedilol also lowered the hospitalization rate by approximately 60%. bid—twice a day. (*Adapted from* Bristow and coworkers [13]; with permission.)

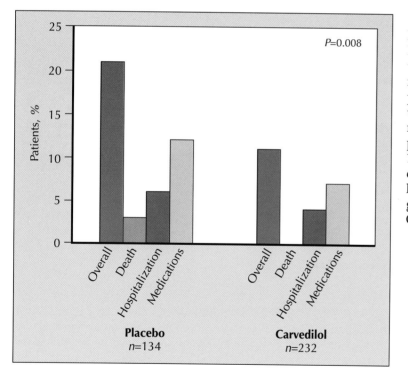

FIGURE 11-12. Effect of carvedilol on the clinical progression of heart failure. Another stratified trial within the US Carvedilol Heart Failure Trials Program examined the effect of carvedilol on the clinical progression of heart failure in 366 patients with only mild functional impairment. The primary endpoint of clinical progression was defined as death due to heart failure, hospitalization for heart failure or a sustained increase in heart failure medications for more than 30 days. As shown, heart failure progression occurred in 21% of placebo patients compared with 11% of carvedilol patients (48% risk reduction, *P*=0.008). The effect of carvedilol was not influenced by gender, age, or the etiology of heart failure. Carvedilol also improved both physician and patient global assessments and reduced all-cause mortality. (*Adapted from* Colucci and coworkers [14]; with permission.)

β-BLOCKER TRIALS IN PROGRESS

STUDY	NYHA	LVEF	PLANNED ENROLLMENT, N	TREATMENT
MERIT-HF	II to IV	<0.40	3200	Metoprolol XL vs placebo
BEST	III to IV	≤0.35	2800	Bucindolol vs placebo
COMET	II to IV	≤0.35	2800	Carvedilol vs Metoprolol
CAPRICORN	I to IV Post-AMI	≤0.40	2600	Carvedilol vs placebo
COPERNICUS	IIIB to IV	<0.25	1800	Carvedilol vs placebo

FIGURE 11-13. β-Blocker trials in progress. Many issues remain regarding the use of β-blockers for the treatment of left ventricular failure, and these are being addressed by several large trials that are currently underway. The Metoprolol Randomized Intervention Trial in Heart Failure (MERIT-HF) and β-Blocker Evaluation Survival Trial (BEST) are examining the effects of metoprolol and bucindolol, respectively, on survival. COMET is comparing the effects of carvedilol and metoprolol in patients with functional class II to IV heart failure. COPERNICUS is a trial of carvedilol in 1800 patients with severe heart failure. CAPRICORN is examining the effects of carvedilol on mortality in patients with left ventricular dysfunction after myocardial infarction.

CLINICAL PHARMACOLOGY OF β-ADRENERGIC ANTAGONISTS

	β_1/β_2 ADRENERGIC RECEPTORS, RELATIVE SELECTIVITY	VASODILATOR MECHANISMS	INTRINSIC SYMPATHOMIMETIC ACTIVITY
Nebivolol	300	Direct	0
Bisoprolol	120	0	0
Metoprolol	75	0	0
Celiprolol	70	β_2 Agonist	+
Atenotol	40	0	0
Carvedilol	10	α_1 Antagonist	0
Propranolol	1	0	0
Pindolol	1	β_2 Agonist	+
Bucindolol	1	Direct	0
Labetalol	1	α_1 Antagonist	0

FIGURE 11-14. Clinical pharmacology of β-adrenergic antagonists. The pharmacology of β-adrenergic antagonists differs substantially with regard to properties such as the relative selectivity for β_1- versus β_2-adrenergic receptors and the presence or absence of various vasodilator mechanisms and intrinsic sympathomimetic activity. Shown are the major pharmacologic properties of several β-blockers. *Zero* indicates no activity; *plus signs* indicate activity; *direct* indicates a direct vasodilator action. In addition to these properties, carvedilol and its metabolite have been shown to exert potent antioxidant effects *in vitro*. Whether the non–β-blocking properties of these agents contribute to their clinical efficacy remains to be determined.

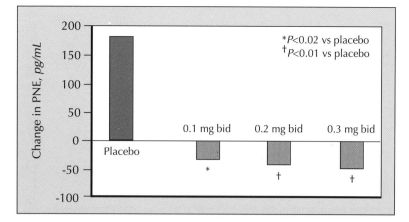

FIGURE 11-15. Central-acting sympathetic inhibitors as treatment for heart failure. Chronic overactivity of the sympathetic nervous system appears to contribute to the progression of myocardial failure (*see* Fig. 11-1). Agents acting via the central nervous system

to inhibit sympathetic outflow might therefore provide another means of therapy in patients. In short-term studies, the central α_2-adrenergic agonist clonidine has been shown to reduce preload, heart rate, and mean arterial pressure in heart failure patients. However, chronic clonidine use may be limited by side effects (*eg*, dry mouth and fatigue). Moxonidine is a central sympatholytic agent whose actions are mediated by imidazoline receptors. Moxonidine is currently approved in Europe for the treatment of hypertension, and preliminary data suggests that moxonidine causes dose-related reductions in plasma norepinephrine (PNE), blood pressure, and heart rate in patients with heart failure. Shown are changes in PNE in patients with class II to III heart failure after chronic oral therapy with placebo or 1 of 3 doses of moxonidine. Moxonidine for Congestive Heart Failure (MOXCON) is a phase III clinical trial that will test the effect of sustained-release moxonidine on mortality in approximately 4500 patients with symptomatic left ventricular dysfunction. The study began in mid-1998. bid—twice a day. (*Adapted from* Swedberg and coworkers [15]; with permission.)

ANGIOTENSIN RECEPTOR BLOCKERS

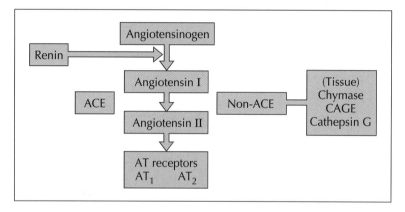

FIGURE 11-16. Several non-enzymatic pathways independent of angiotensin-converting enzyme (ACE) exist for the conversion of angiotensin I to angiotensin II and may contribute to persistent availability of both circulating and tissue angiotensin despite treatment with ACE inhibitors. Direct antagonism of angiotensin II receptors is an alternative strategy for inhibiting the effects of angiotensin.

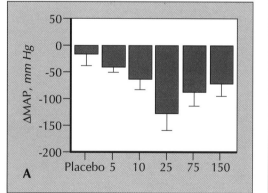

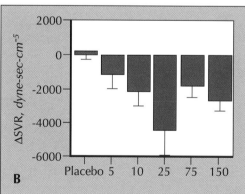

FIGURE 11-17. The hemodynamic effects of a single oral dose (5 to 150 mg) of losartan, a non-peptide angiotensin II receptor antagonist, were evaluated in 66 patients with class II to IV heart failure and left ventricular ejection fraction less than 40%. Losartan decreased the mean arterial pressure (MAP; **A**) and systemic vascular resistance (SVR; **B**) with maximal effects at a dose of 25 mg ($P<0.05$ compared with placebo). (*continued*)

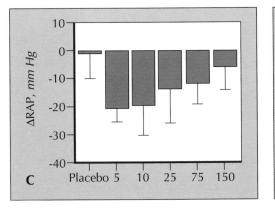

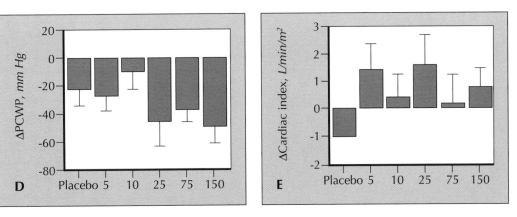

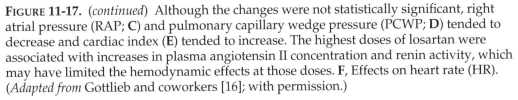

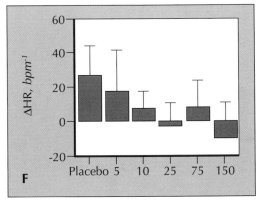

FIGURE 11-17. (*continued*) Although the changes were not statistically significant, right atrial pressure (RAP; **C**) and pulmonary capillary wedge pressure (PCWP; **D**) tended to decrease and cardiac index (**E**) tended to increase. The highest doses of losartan were associated with increases in plasma angiotensin II concentration and renin activity, which may have limited the hemodynamic effects at those doses. **F**, Effects on heart rate (HR). (*Adapted from* Gottlieb and coworkers [16]; with permission.)

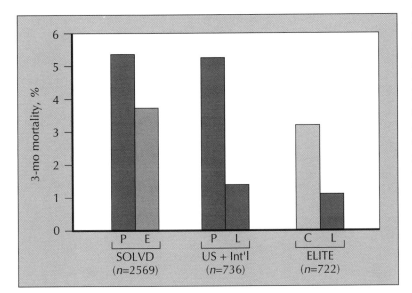

FIGURE 11-18. The Evaluation of Losartan in the Elderly (ELITE) study randomly assigned 722 patients 65 years of age or older with symptomatic left ventricular failure to receive losartan (titrated to 50 mg once daily) or captopril (titrated to 50 mg three times daily) for 48 weeks. Although there was no difference between the drugs with regard to the primary endpoint of the study (an increase in serum creatinine of ≥0.3 mg/dL), there was an unexpected 46% decrease in all-cause mortality (95% confidence interval, 5% to 69%; $P=0.035$). Similar reductions in mortality were observed in two placebo-controlled 12-week exercise studies (US+Int'l) involving 736 patients with symptomatic heart failure. In these studies, losartan had no effect on the primary endpoint of exercise time. The figure combines mortality rates from the enalapril (E) arm of the SOLVD treatment trial, the captopril (C) arm of ELITE, the losartan (L) arms of ELITE and the losartan exercise study, and for the placebo arms of SOLVD and the losartan exercise study. (*Adapted from* Pitt and coworkers [17]; with permission.)

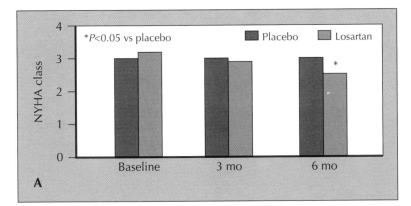

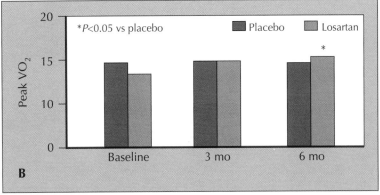

FIGURE 11-19. Although there is theoretical reason to suggest that combined therapy with an angiotensin II receptor antagonist and an angiotensin-converting enzyme inhibitor would be more clinically effective than therapy with either alone, this thesis has not been fully tested. In one small study, 32 patients with functional class III to IV heart failure on conventional doses of angiotensin-converting enzyme inhibitors were randomized to receive adjunctive therapy with placebo or losartan 50 mg once daily for 6 months (**A**). At 6 months, the addition of losartan was associated with a lower New York Heart Association (NYHA) functional class and a higher peak VO$_2$ (**B**). (*Adapted from* Hamroff and coworkers [18]; with permission.)

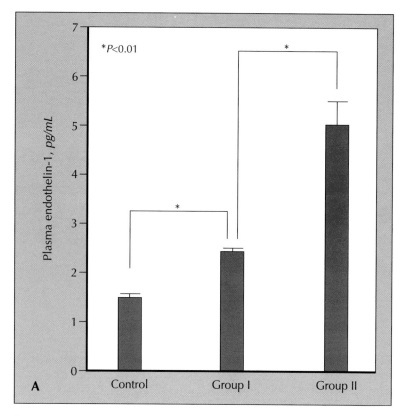

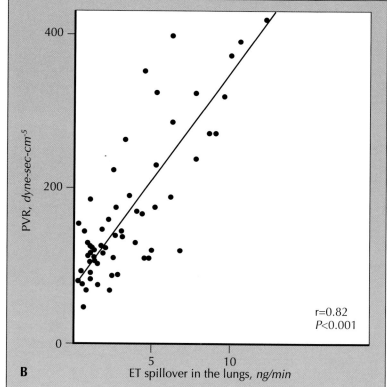

FIGURE 11-20. Endothelin (ET) is a potent vasoconstrictor peptide which can exert long-term effects on myocardial growth and phenotype. Plasma ET levels are elevated in patients with congestive heart failure and correlate in general with disease severity. **A,** The relationship between plasma ET-1 levels and the severity of disease. Control subjects consisted of 20 age-matched normal subjects. Groups I and II consisted of 33 patients in New York Heart Association (NYHA) class II and 29 patients in NYHA class III or IV, respectively. **B,** The correlation between resting pulmonary vascular resistance (PVR) and ET spillover in the lungs in the 62 patients in *A*. ET-1 spillover correlated strongly with PVR, suggesting that the pulmonary vascular bed is an important source of ET-1, which appears to be a key mediator of secondary pulmonary hypertension. (*Adapted from* Tsutamoto and coworkers [19].)

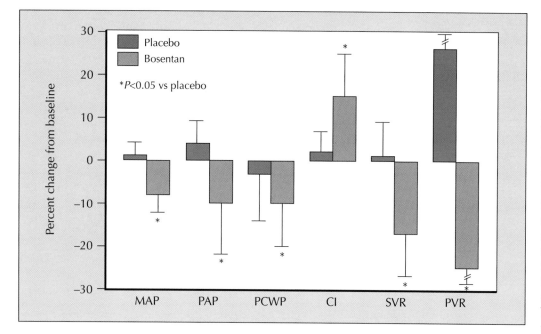

FIGURE 11-21. Understanding the actions of endothelin has been greatly aided by the development of several nonpeptide molecules that block endothelin receptors. Whereas some of these antagonists are subtype selective (*eg*, BQ-123, ET_A selective), others are nonselective

(*eg*, bosentan). Encouraged by results in animal models of heart failure showing beneficial effects of endothelin receptor antagonists on left ventricular remodeling and survival, clinical investigators have begun to address the role of these agents in patients with heart failure. Kiowski *et al.* [20] randomized 24 patients with functional class III heart failure to intravenous bosentan or placebo. Shown here is the change in hemodynamics 60 minutes after drug administration, expressed as the percent change from baseline. Bosentan decreased mean arterial pressure (MAP), mean pulmonary artery pressure (PAP), and mean pulmonary capillary wedge pressure (PCWP) and increased cardiac index (CI). Consistent with the strong relationship between plasma endothelin and pulmonary hypertension, bosentan caused a greater decrease in pulmonary vascular resistance (PVR) than systemic vascular resistance (SVR). (*Adapted from* Kiowski and coworkers [20]; with permission.)

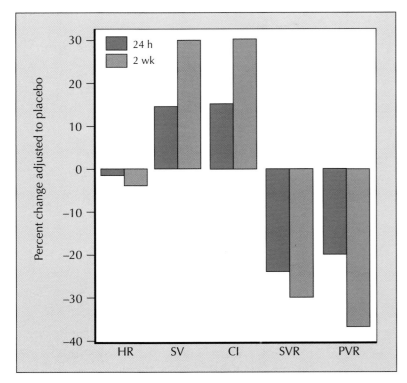

FIGURE 11-22. The hemodynamic effects of bosentan administered orally for 2 weeks were determined in 36 patients with functional class III heart failure and left ventricular ejection fraction less than 30% despite therapy with an angiotensin-converting enzyme inhibitor, digoxin, and diuretics. Hemodynamics were measured during the first 24 hours of treatment and again after 2 weeks. Shown are the changes at 24 hours and 2 weeks normalized to placebo. Interestingly, the magnitude of the hemodynamic effects increased between days 1 and 14. Congestive heart failure symptoms were improved, and bosentan was well tolerated, except for symptomatic hypotension in six patients. Plasma endothelin levels increased with bosentan use. CI—cardiac index; HR—heart rate; PVR—pulmonary vascular resistance; SV—stroke volume; SVR—systemic vascular resistance. (*Adapted from* Sutsch and coworkers [21]; with permission.)

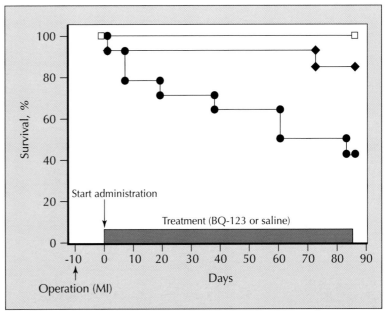

FIGURE 11-23. The pathophysiologic role of endothelin in the progression of heart failure. The observation that endothelin levels are elevated in patients with heart failure, taken together with the known actions of endothelin on cardiovascular tissues, has raised the possibility that endothelin plays a pathophysiologic role in the progression of myocardial failure. Support for this thesis comes from studies in animal models of heart failure in which beneficial long-term effects of endothelin receptor blockade have been demonstrated. Sakai *et al.* [22] studied the effects of the ET_A receptor antagonist BQ-123 on survival in rats after experimental myocardial infarction. Addition of BQ-123 to the drinking water beginning 10 days after coronary artery ligation (*closed diamonds*) resulted in a significant improvement in survival over animals treated with saline (*closed circles*). The *open squares* represent sham-operated animals treated with saline. The effects of chronic endothelin receptor blockade on survival and disease progression have not yet been studied in humans. (*Adapted from* Sakai and coworkers [22]; with permission.)

CYTOKINE ANTAGONISTS

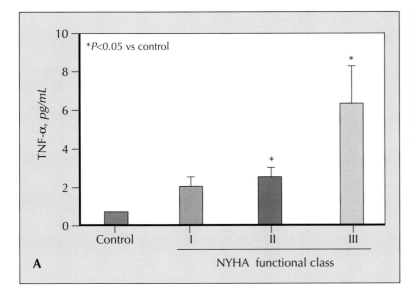

FIGURE 11-24. Proinflammatory cytokines such as tumor necrosis factor-α (TNF-α), interleukin-1β (IL-1β) and interleukin-6 (IL-6) may play an important pathophysiologic role in the progression of myocardial failure. The circulating levels of TNF-α and IL-6 were analyzed in randomly selected plasma samples from 63 patients in functional classes I to III enrolled in the neurohormonal substudies of the SOLVD trial. Compared with age-matched controls, patients with left ventricular dysfunction had elevated TNF-α levels (**A**) in direct proportion to functional class. (*continued*)

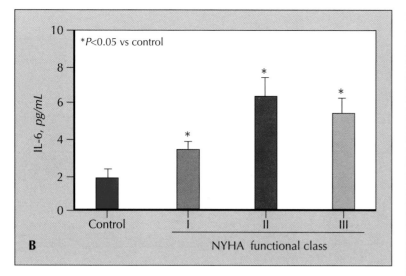

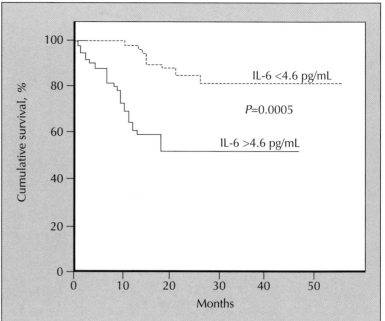

FIGURE 11-24. (*continued*) IL-6 levels (**B**) were also elevated in patients, although the levels did not correlate with functional class. (*Adapted from* Torre-Amione and coworkers [23]; with permission.)

FIGURE 11-25. To examine the prognostic role of circulating cytokines in patients, plasma interleukin-6 (IL-6) levels were measured in 100 patients with chronic heart failure who were followed for a mean of 28 months (range, 3 to 54). During the follow-up period, 31 patients had a cardiovascular death. When patients were stratified based on median plasma concentration (4.6 pg/mL) of IL-6, Kaplan-Meier analysis demonstrated reduced survival in patients with higher IL-6 levels (*solid line*). In a multivariate analysis, plasma levels of IL-6 ($P<0.0001$) and norepinephrine ($P=0.0004$) and left ventricular ejection fraction ($P=0.015$) were independent predictors of mortality. (*Adapted from* Tsutamoto and coworkers [24].)

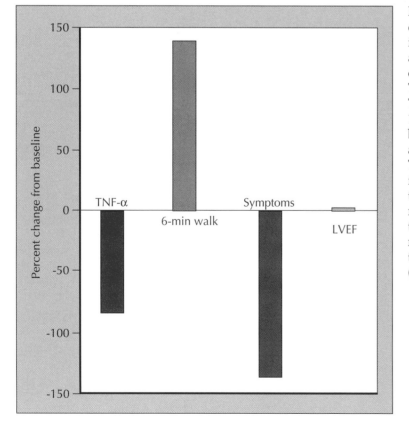

FIGURE 11-26. The recognition that tumor necrosis factor-α (TNF-α) may contribute to disease progression in heart failure and other inflammatory disease states has led to the development of anti–TNF-α therapies. Chimeric monoclonal antibodies to TNF-α can induce remission in patients with refractory Crohn's disease. TNFR:Fc is a recombinant fusion protein consisting of a soluble TNF receptor linked to the Fc portion of human immunoglobulin 1. Soluble TNF-α receptors bind to and inactivate TNF-α and have been shown to reduce disease activity in patients with rheumatoid arthritis. Shown are preliminary data from a phase I pilot study of TNFR:Fc (1 to 4 mg/m^2) in patients with functional class III heart failure. In this study, circulating levels of TNF-α were reduced on the first day of intravenous administration of TNFR:Fc and remained reduced for 2 weeks. TNFR:Fc treatment was well tolerated in all patients. In this small, uncontrolled trial, the 6-minute walk distance and symptoms were improved although there was no change in left ventricular ejection fraction (LVEF). (*Adapted from* Deswal and coworkers [25].)

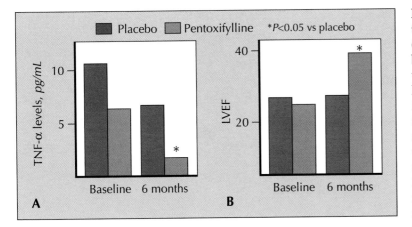

FIGURE 11-27. Pentoxifylline, a xanthine derivative used for the treatment of claudication, suppresses tumor necrosis factor–α (TNF-α) production *in vitro* and *in vivo*. Improved outcomes have been reported in patients with rheumatoid arthritis and graft-versus-host disease. This single-center, controlled study tested the hypothesis that pentoxifylline would improve left ventricular function in patients with idiopathic dilated cardiomyopathy. A total of 28 men in functional class II to III heart failure treated with angiotensin-converting enzyme inhibitors, digitalis, and diuretics were randomized to receive pentoxifylline (400 mg three times daily) or placebo for 6 months. Pentoxifylline reduced TNF-α levels (**A**) and increased left ventricular ejection fraction (LVEF) from 22% to 39% (**B**). This marked effect on ventricular function may have been due, in part, to other pharmacologic properties of pentoxifylline, including phosphodiesterase III inhibition. (*Adapted from* Sliwa and coworkers [26].)

ANTIOXIDANTS

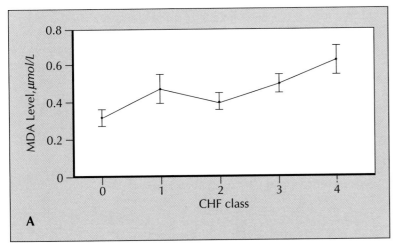

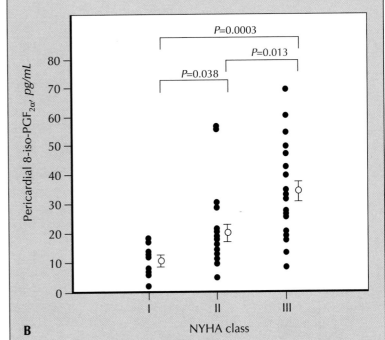

FIGURE 11-28. Reduced myocardial antioxidant activity and increased oxidant damage have been demonstrated in animal models of heart failure, and markers of oxidative stress are increased in patients with chronic heart failure (CHF), leading to the thesis that reactive oxygen species may contribute to the progression of myocardial dysfunction in patients. Plasma concentrations of malondialdehyde (MDA) and vitamins E and C were measured in 58 patients with functional class I to III heart failure and 19 control subjects. MDA levels were significantly elevated in patients vs. controls ($P<0.005$). **A,** The degree of elevation correlated with functional class ($P<0.01$). Although vitamin E levels did not differ between heart failure patients and control subjects, vitamin C levels were lower in patients with heart failure. A more specific technique for assessing oxidant stress *in vivo* involves measuring stable endproducts of lipid peroxidation, called F_2-*isoprostanes* [27]. 8-iso-prostaglandin $F_{2\alpha}$ levels were measured in the pericardial fluid of 51 consecutive patients with ischemic or valvular heart disease referred for cardiac surgery. **B,** Pericardial levels of 8-iso-$PGF_{2\alpha}$ increased with the severity of heart failure. In a subgroup of patients who underwent preoperative echocardiography, pericardial levels of 8-iso-$PGF_{2\alpha}$ correlated with left ventricular end-diastolic dimension. NYHA—New York Heart Association. (Part A *adapted from* Keith and coworkers [28]; part B *adapted from* Mallat and coworkers [29]; with permission.)

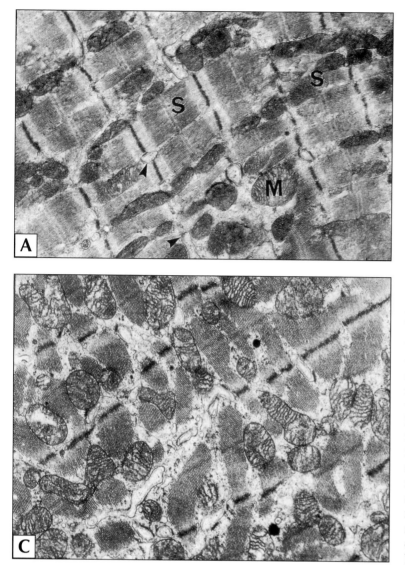

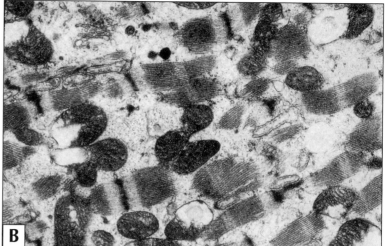

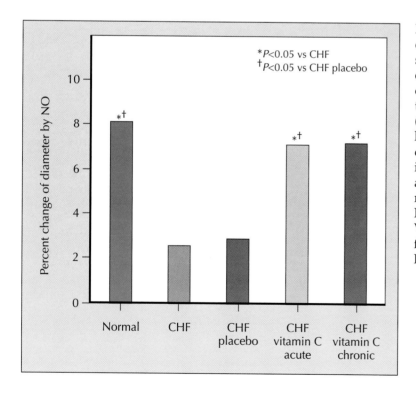

FIGURE 11-29. In animal models of ischemia-reperfusion, antioxidants have been shown to reduce free radical generation, prevent myocyte damage, and improve ventricular function. In this study, Dhalla *et al.* [30] examined the effects of vitamin E therapy in aortic-banded guinea pigs, a model of pressure overload–induced failure. **A,** An electron micrograph of a sham-operated guinea pig heart demonstrating normal ultrastructure, including myofibrils, sarcomeres (S), mitochondria (M), and T tubules (*arrowheads*). **B,** A micrograph from a guinea pig that was banded for 20 weeks and did not receive subcutaneous vitamin E implants. There is ultrastructural damage characterized by increased vacuolization, loss of contractile elements, and mito-chondrial injury with dropout of christae membranes. **C,** A micrograph from a guinea pig with banding for 20 weeks and chronic treatment with vitamin E. There is less vacuolization, mitochondrial injury, and interstitial edema. This improvement in structure was associated with improved hemodynamics, decreased signs of heart failure, and reduced mortality. (*From* Dhalla and coworkers [30]; with permission.)

FIGURE 11-30. Chronic heart failure is associated with impaired endothelium-mediated vasodilation [31]. Recent studies have shown that acute administration of vitamin C improves endothelium-dependent vasodilation in patients with diabetes or coronary artery disease. The acute and chronic effects of vitamin C therapy on nitric oxide (NO)-mediated flow-dependent dilation (FDD) were tested in chronic heart failure (CHF) patients and healthy volunteers. Vascular effects of vitamin C and placebo were determined at rest and during reactive hyperemia before and after intra-arterial infusion of N^G-monomethyl-L-arginine (L-NMMA), an inhibitor of NO synthesis. Shown is the percent change in radial artery diameter during hyperemia that was inhibited by L-NMMA (representing the portion of FDD mediated by NO). Vitamin C restored NO-mediated FDD in patients with heart failure after both acute and chronic administration. (*Adapted from* Hornig and coworkers [32]; with permission.)

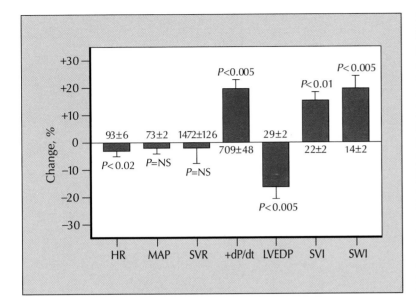

FIGURE 11-31. The hemodynamic effects of an intracoronary infusion of milrinone in patients with severe left ventricular failure. Although phosphodiesterase (PDE) inhibitors are usually thought of as positive inotropic agents, they are also potent vasodilators. In fact, both positive inotropy and vasodilation contribute importantly to the effects of most PDE III inhibitors. Because there is little or no systemic vasodilation when milrinone is infused by this route, the effects of intracoronary milrinone infusion reflect the hemodynamic consequences of the drug's positive inotropic action. When given by this route, milrinone increased $+dP/dt$ and improved pump function, as shown by the higher stroke volume and work indices (SVI and SWI, respectively) at a lower left ventricular end-diastolic pressure (LVEDP). Systemic vascular resistance (SVR) and mean arterial pressure (MAP) were not affected because the drug was infused in only small quantities that did not spill over to the systemic circulation. Interestingly, in contrast to the effect of systemic milrinone administration, heart rate (HR) decreased, apparently because of a reflex withdrawal of sympathetic tone caused by the improvement in pump function. (*Adapted from* Ludmer and coworkers [33].)

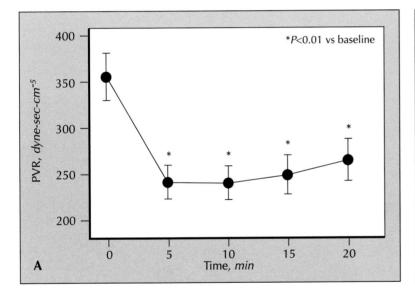

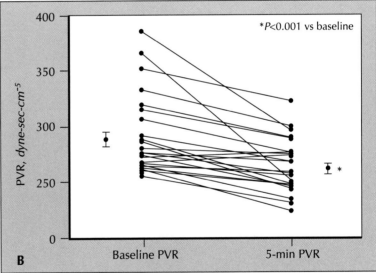

FIGURE 11-32. Fixed pulmonary hypertension is a risk factor for right heart failure and death following cardiac transplantation. An intravenous bolus of milrinone can be used as a rapid test for the reversibility of pulmonary hypertension in patients with heart failure undergoing evaluation for cardiac transplant. The hemodynamic response to a single intravenous bolus of milrinone (50 µg/kg body weight) was measured in 27 patients with severe heart failure and a pulmonary vascular resistance (PVR) greater than or equal to 200 dynes-sec-cm^{-5} Changes in PVR are shown in the group as a whole (A) and in individual patients (B). Milrinone decreased PVR in all patients. The effect was maximal 5 to 10 minutes after the intravenous bolus infusion and persisted for at least 20 minutes. The reduction in PVR at five minutes (31%±4%) was associated with a 42%±4% increase in cardiac output and decreases of 12%±4% and 16%±5% in mean pulmonary artery and pulmonary artery wedge pressures, respectively, but no change in transpulmonary pressure gradient. Milrinone had no effect on heart rate or systemic arterial pressure. (*Adapted from* Givertz and coworkers [34]; with permission.)

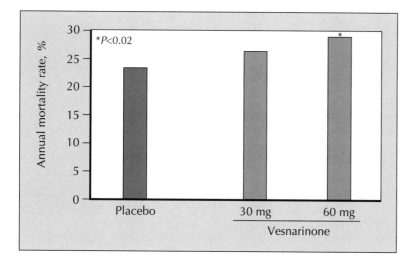

FIGURE 11-33. Vesnarinone is an orally active positive inotropic agent with multiple pharmacologic effects. In addition to being a weak phosphodiesterase inhibitor, vesnarinone inhibits the efflux of potassium by outward rectifying potassium channels and activates sodium channels. In addition, vesnarinone has been shown to inhibit the production of inflammatory cytokines *in vitro* [35]. In an initial chronic study involving 477 patients, vesnarinone reduced mortality compared with placebo at a dose of 60 mg/d but increased mortality at a dose of 120 mg/d [36]. The Vesnarinone Trial (VesT) tested the hypothesis that lower-dose vesnarinone would improve survival in patients with severe heart failure. A total of 3833 patients with functional class III to IV heart failure (mean age, 63; 59% ischemic etiology; mean left ventricular ejection fraction, 21%) were randomized to placebo or vesnarinone 30 mg or 60 mg once daily. The trial was terminated early after the study design endpoint of 233 placebo deaths had occurred. As shown, vesnarinone caused a dose-dependent increase in the annual mortality rate. Further post-hoc adjudication of deaths suggested that the excess mortality in the higher-dose group was attributed to an increase in sudden cardiac death. (*Adapted from* Feldman and coworkers [37].)

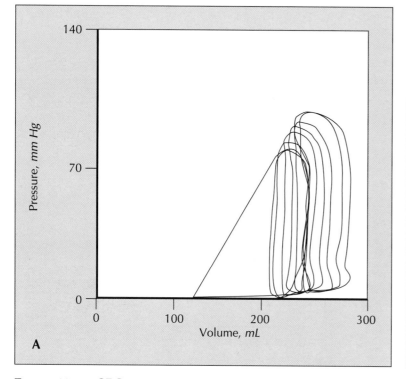

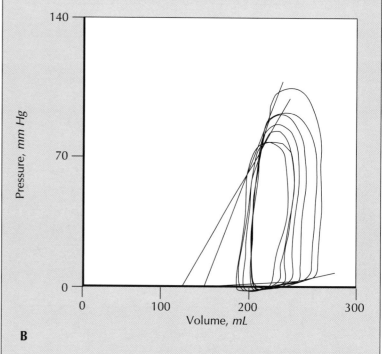

FIGURE 11-34. OPC-18790 is a quinolinone derivative related to vesnarinone that increases cardiac output and lowers filling pressures when administered intravenously. The left ventricular end-systolic pressure-volume (PV) relationship was measured using a conductance catheter in 17 patients with dilated cardiomyopathy. Shown are PV loops for a representative patient receiving a low dose (5 µg/kg/min) of OPC-18790. Data is displayed at baseline (**A**) and after 30 minutes (**B**) and 60 minutes (**C**) of drug infusion. (*continued*)

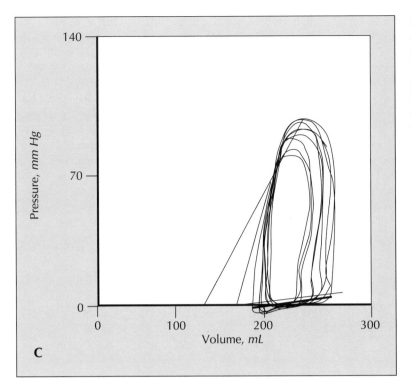

C

FIGURE 11-34. (*continued*) The baseline end-systolic and end-diastolic pressure volume relationships (ESPVR and EDPVR, respectively) are reproduced in *B* and *C* for comparison. OPC-18790 increased the slope of the ESPVR while reducing chamber preload and diastolic pressures. Overall, contractility rose by 25% to 100%. Although isovolumic relaxation shortened, there was no change in the EDPVR. (*Adapted from* Feldman and coworkers [38]; with permission.)

CALCIUM-SENSITIZING AGENTS

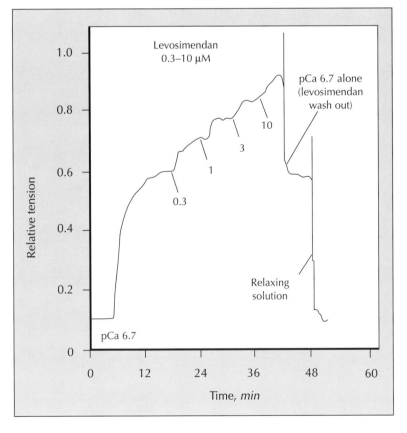

FIGURE 11-35. A limitation of most positive inotropic agents (*eg*, β-adrenergic agonists, phosphodiesterase [PDE] inhibitors) is that they act by increasing intracellular calcium in the myocyte and may thus increase heart rate and arrhythmias. Calcium-sensitizing agents act by directly increasing the sensitivity of the myofilament to calcium so that greater contractile force develops without an increase in calcium level. Levosimendan is a pyridazinone-dinitrile derivative that enhances calcium sensitivity of myofilaments via calcium-dependent binding to troponin C. Other pharmacologic actions observed include mild PDE III inhibition and activation of adenosine triphosphate–dependent potassium channels. Shown is the effect of several concentrations of levosimendan (0.3 to 10 μM) when applied to skinned fibers from guinea pig papillary muscle. Under these conditions, the calcium available to the myofilaments is fixed by the concentration in the bath, and the increase in contractile force therefore must reflect an increase in myofilament sensitivity to calcium. (*Adapted from* Haikala and coworkers [39]; with permission.)

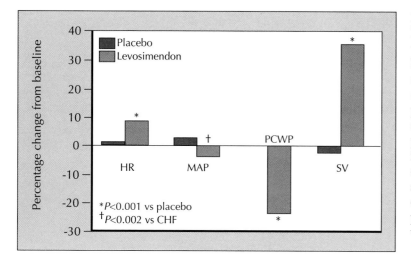

FIGURE 11-36. The acute hemodynamic effects of intravenous levosimendan were studied in 118 patients with functional class III to IV heart failure randomized to levosimendan or placebo. At baseline, the mean left ventricular ejection fraction was 21%, the cardiac index was 1.9 l/min/m², and the mean pulmonary capillary wedge pressure (PCWP) was 27 mm Hg. Shown are the percent change from baseline at 6 hours for heart rate (HR), mean arterial pressure (MAP), mean PCWP, and stroke volume (SV) for placebo and levosimendan. The increase in stroke volume resulted in a 41% increase in cardiac index (data not shown). Hemodynamic effects were maintained for a total of 24 hours. This salutary hemodynamic profile suggests that levosimendan may be of value in the short-term treatment of patients with decompensated heart failure. (*Adapted from* Slawsky and coworkers [40]; with permission.)

NATRIURETIC PEPTIDES

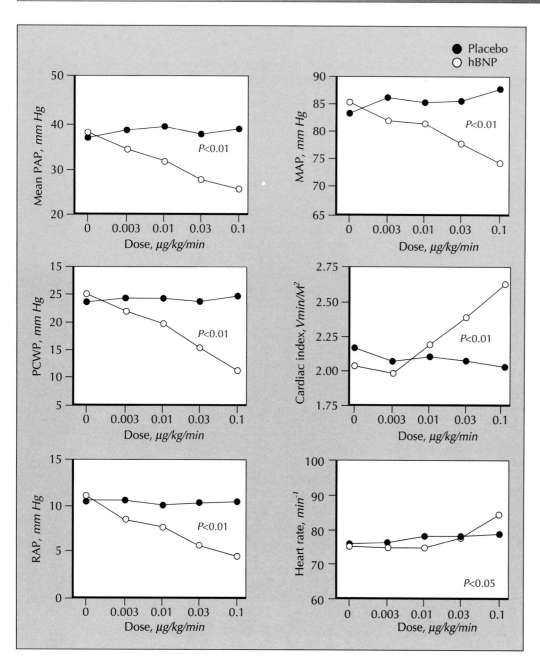

FIGURE 11-37. Synthetic human brain natriuretic peptide (hBNP) is undergoing clinical investigation as a vasodilator and natriuretic agent in patients with heart failure. In one phase II study, 20 patients with functional class II to IV heart failure and a mean ejection fraction of 20% were randomized in a double-blind crossover trial to receive 90-minute infusions of hBNP (0.003, 0.01, 0.03, and 0.1 μg/kg/min) or placebo. hBNP (*open circles*) caused dose-related decreases in mean pulmonary artery pressure (PAP), pulmonary capillary wedge pressure (PCWP), right atrial pressure (RAP), and mean arterial pressure (MAP). It caused an increase in cardiac index compared with placebo (*closed circles*) and a slight reduction in heart rate. Urine volume and sodium excretion also increased significantly during hBNP infusion. (*Adapted from* Marcus and coworkers [41]; with permission.)

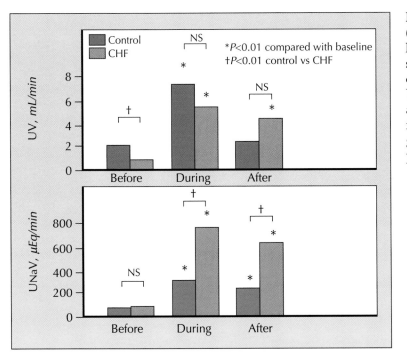

FIGURE 11-38. Effect of synthetic human brain natriuretic peptide (hBNP) on renal function. To determine the effects on renal function, hBNP was infused at a rate of 0.1 µg/kg/min for 60 minutes in seven patients with symptomatic heart failure (CHF) and eight control subjects. hBNP increased urine volume (UV) in both groups. Urinary excretion of sodium (UNaV) also increased in both groups, although the response was greater in patients with CHF. hBNP infusion also decreased plasma aldosterone concentrations in both groups. (*Adapted from* Yoshimura and coworkers [42]; with permission.)

REFERENCES

1. Cohn JN, Levine TB, Olivari MT, *et al.*: Plasma norepinephrine as a guide to prognosis in patients with chronic congestive heart failure. *N Engl J Med* 1984, 311:819–823.

2. Francis GS, Benedict C, Johnstone DE, *et al.*: Comparison of neuroendocrine activation in patients with left ventricular dysfunction with and without congestive heart failure. *Circulation* 1990, 82:1724–1729.

3. Swedberg K, Hjalmarson A, Waagstein F, Wallentin I: Prolongation of survival in congestive cardiomyopathy by β-receptor blockade. *Lancet* 1979, 1:1374–6.

4. Hjalmarson A, Waagstein F: Use of β-blockers in the treatment of dilated cardiomyopathy. In *Heart Failure: Basic Science and Clinical Aspects*. Edited by Gwathmey JD, Briggs GM, Allen PD. New York: Marcel Dekker; 1993:223–251.

5. Hall SA, Cigarroa CG, Marcoux L, *et al.*: Time course of improvement in left ventricular function, mass and geometry in patients with congestive heart failure treated with β-adrenergic blockade. *J Am Coll Cardiol* 1995, 25:1154–1161.

6. Gilbert EM, Anderson JL, Deitchman D, *et al.*: Long-term β-blocker vasodilator therapy improves cardiac function in idiopathic dilated cardiomyopathy: a double-blind, randomized study of bucindolol versus placebo. *Am J Med* 1990, 88:223–229.

7. Doughty RN, Whalley GA, Gamble G, *et al.*: Left ventricular remodeling with carvedilol in patients with congestive heart failure due to ischemic heart disease. Australia-New Zealand Heart Failure Research Collaborative Group. *J Am Coll Cardiol* 1997, 29:1060–1066.

8. Andersson B, Hamm C, Persson S, *et al.*: Improved exercise hemodynamic status in dilated cardiomyopathy after β-adrenergic blockade treatment. *J Am Coll Cardiol* 1994, 23:1397–1404.

9. Waagstein F, Bristow MR, Swedberg K, *et al.*for the Metoprolol in Dilated Cardiomyopathy (MDC) Trial Study Group: Beneficial effects of metoprolol in idiopathic dilated cardiomyopathy. *Lancet* 1993, 342:1441–1446.

10. Anonymous: A randomized trial of β-blockade in heart failure. The Cardiac Insufficiency Bisoprolol Study (CIBIS). CIBIS Investigators and Committees. *Circulation* 1994, 90:1765–1773.

11. Packer M, Bristow MR, Cohn JN, *et al.*: The effect of carvedilol on morbidity and mortality in patients with chronic heart failure. U.S. Carvedilol Heart Failure Study Group. *N Engl J Med* 1996, 334:1349–1355.

12. Heidenreich PA, Lee TT, Massie BM:. Effect of β-blockade on mortality in patients with heart failure: a meta-analysis of randomized clinical trials. *J Am Coll Cardiol* 1997, 30:27–34.

13. Bristow MR, Gilbert EM, Abraham WT, *et al.*: Carvedilol produces dose-related improvements in left ventricular function and survival in subjects with chronic heart failure. MOCHA Investigators. *Circulation* 1996, 94:2807–2816.

14. Colucci WS, Packer M, Bristow MR, *et al.*: Carvedilol inhibits clinical progression in patients with mild symptoms of heart failure. US Carvedilol Heart Failure Study Group. *Circulation* 1996, 94:2800–2806.

15. Swedberg K, Waagstein F, Dickstein K, *et al.*: Moxonidine, a centrally acting sympathetic inhibitor, causes sustained reduction of plasma norepinephrine in heart failure patients [abstract]. *J Am Coll Cardiol* 1997, 29:220.

16. Gottlieb SS, Dickstein K, Fleck E, *et al.*: Hemodynamic and neurohormonal effects of the angiotensin II antagonist losartan in patients with congestive heart failure. *Circulation* 1993, 88:1602–1609.

17. Pitt B, Segal R, Martinez FA, *et al.*: Randomised trial of losartan versus captopril in patients over 65 with heart failure (Evaluation of Losartan in the Elderly Study, ELITE). *Lancet* 1997, 349:747–752.

18. Hamroff G, Blaufarb I, Mancini D, *et al.*: Clinical benefits of long-term angiotensin II receptor blockade in patients with severe symptoms of congestive heart failure despite full angiotensin converting enzyme inhibition [abstract]. *J Am Coll Cardiol* 1998, 31:188.

19. Tsutamoto T, Wada A, Maeda Y, *et al.*: Relation between endothelin-1 spillover in the lungs and pulmonary vascular resistance in patients with chronic heart failure. *J Am Coll Cardiol* 1994, 23:1427–1433.

20. Kiowski W, Sutsch G, Hunziker P, *et al.*: Evidence for endothelin-1-mediated vasoconstriction in severe chronic heart failure. *Lancet* 1995, 346:732–736.

21. Sutsch G, Bertel O, Kiowski W: Acute and short-term effects of the nonpeptide endothelin-1 receptor antagonist bosentan in humans. *Cardiovasc Drugs Ther* 1997, 10:717–725.

22. Sakai S, Miyauchi T, Kobayashi M, *et al.*: Inhibition of myocardial endothelin pathway improves long-term survival in heart failure. *Nature* 1996, 384:353–355.

23. Torre-Amione G, Kapadia S, Benedict C, *et al.*: Proinflammatory cytokine levels in patients with depressed left ventricular ejection fraction: a report from the Studies of Left Ventricular Dysfunction (SOLVD). *J Am Coll Cardiol* 1996, 27:1201–1206.

24. Tsutamoto T, Hisanaga T, Wada A, *et al.*: Interleukin-6 spillover in the peripheral circulation increases with the severity of heart failure, and the high plasma level of interleukin-6 is an important prognostic predictor in patients with congestive heart failure. *J Am Coll Cardiol* 1998, 31:391–398.

25. Deswal A, Seta Y, Blosch CM, Mann DL: A phase I trial of tumor necrosis factor receptor (p75) fusion protein (TNFR:Fc) in patients with advanced heart failure [abstract]. *Circulation* 1997, 96:I–323.

26. Sliwa K, Skudicky D, Candy G, *et al.*: Randomised investigation of effects of pentoxifylline on left ventricular performance in idiopathic dilated cardiomyopathy. *Lancet* 1998, 351:1091–1093.

27. Morrow JD, Hill KE, Burk RF, *et al.*: A series of prostaglandin F2-like compounds are produced in vivo in humans by a non-cyclooxygenase, free radical-catalyzed mechanism. *Proc Natl Acad Sci USA* 1990, 87:9383–9387.

28. Keith M, Geranmayegan A, Sole MJ, *et al.*: Increased oxidative stress in patients with congestive heart failure. *J Am Coll Cardiol* 1998, 31:1352–1356.

29. Mallat Z, Philip I, Lebret M, *et al.*: Elevated levels of 8-iso-prostaglandin F2α in pericardial fluid of patients with heart failure: a potential role for in vivo oxidant stress in ventricular dilatation and progression to heart failure. *Circulation* 1998, 97:1536–1539.

30. Dhalla AK, Hill MF, Singal PK: Role of oxidative stress in transition of hypertrophy to heart failure. *J Am Coll Cardiol* 1996, 28:506–514.

31. Kubo SH, Rector TS, Bank AJ, *et al.*: Endothelium-dependent vasodilation is attenuated in patients with heart failure. *Circulation* 1991, 84:1589–1596.

32. Hornig B, Arakawa N, Kohler C, Drexler H: Vitamin C improves endothelial function of conduit arteries in patients with chronic heart failure. *Circulation* 1998, 97:363–368.

33. Ludmer PL, Wright RF, Arnold JMO, *et al.*: Separation of the direct myocardial and vasodilator actions of milrinone administered by an intracoronary infusion technique. *Circulation* 1986, 73:130–137.

34. Givertz MM, Hare JM, Loh E, *et al.*: Effect of bolus milrinone on hemodynamic variables and pulmonary vascular resistance in patients with severe left ventricular dysfunction: a rapid test for reversibility of pulmonary hypertension. *J Am Coll Cardiol* 1996, 28:1775–1780.

35. Matsumori A, Shioi T, Yamada T, *et al.*: Vesnarinone, a new inotropic agent, inhibits cytokine production by stimulated human blood from patients with heart failure. *Circulation* 1994, 93:474–483.

36. Feldman AM, Bristow MR, Parmley W: Effect of vesnarinone on morbidity and mortality in patients with heart failure. Vesnarinone Study Group. *N Engl J Med* 1993, 329:149–155.

37. Feldman A, Young J, Bourge R, *et al.*: Mechanism of increased mortality from vesnarinone in the severe heart failure trial (VesT) [abstract]. *J Am Coll Cardiol* 1997, 29:64.

38. Feldman MD, Pak PH, Wu CC, *et al.*: Acute cardiovascular effects of OPC-18790 in patients with congestive heart failure: time- and dose-dependence analysis based on pressure-volume relations. *Circulation* 1996, 93:474–483.

39. Haikala H, Nissinen E, Etemadzadeh E, *et al.*: Troponin C-mediated calcium sensitization induced by levosimendan does not impair relaxation. *J Cardiovasc Pharmacol* 1995, 25:794–801.

40. Slawsky MT, Colucci WS, Leier CV, *et al.*: Hemodynamic effects of levosimendan, a novel calcium-sensitizer with vasodilating properties, in severe heart failure: a double-blind placebo-controlled trial [abstract]. *Circulation* 1997, 96:I–712.

41. Marcus LS, Hart D, Packer M, *et al.*: Hemodynamic and renal excretory effects of human brain natriuretic peptide infusion in patients with congestive heart failure: a double-blind, placebo-controlled, randomized crossover trial. *Circulation* 1996, 94:3184–3189.

42. Yoshimura M, Yasue H, Morita E, *et al.*: Hemodynamic, renal, and hormonal responses to brain natriuretic peptide infusion in patients with congestive heart failure. *Circulation* 1991, 84:1581–1588.

CARDIAC TRANSPLANTATION

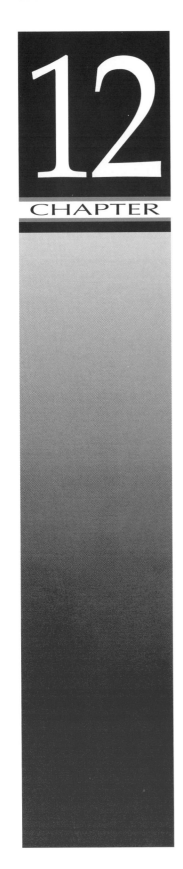

12

CHAPTER

Donna Mancini and Ainat Beniaminovitz

Since the first human heart transplantation in 1967 [1], cardiac transplantation has evolved from a medical curiosity to an accepted therapy for end-stage cardiomyopathy. Initial immunosuppression regimens included high-dose steroids, azathioprine, actinomycin C, and local irradiation, with a 1-year survival of only about 20%. With the subsequent development of endomyocardial biopsy techniques to monitor allograft rejection and the addition of antithymocyte globulin to treat acute rejection episodes [2], 1-year survival increased to 50% by 1970. Improved donor management and refined recipient selection criteria further improved 1-year survival to 70%, with a 5-year survival of 40%. However, it was not until the general availability of cyclosporine in 1986 that 1-year survival improved to more than 80% [3]. This highly effective immunosuppressive agent stimulated the growth of cardiac transplantation, and the number of transplants increased worldwide from 90 in 1981 to 2000 in 1988 [4].

Although remarkable progress has been achieved in cardiac transplantation in the past two decades, significant morbidity still exists following the procedure. Most of the morbidity is due to the consequences of immunosuppression or the side effects of the immunosuppressive drugs. Current immunosuppression includes triple therapy with cyclosporine, prednisone, and azathioprine or mycophenolate mofetil. Early transplantation-related problems include allograft rejection and infection. Chronic clinical problems of hypertension, nephrotoxicity [5], steroid-induced diabetes, obesity, and osteoporosis [6] are frequently observed. Transplantation-related coronary artery disease as a manifestation of chronic rejection is the major long-term morbidity. As the ability to treat acute rejection has improved, transplantation vasculopathy has become the Achilles heel of cardiac transplantation. It currently represents the major limitation to long-term survival after transplantation [7]. Efforts have been directed at prevention of this complication by the identification of risk factors responsible for its development. Once established, this vasculopathy becomes so diffuse and extensive that the only possible treatment is retransplantation.

Development of newer immunosuppressive therapies such as rapamycin and monoclonal antibodies that may be effective in the treatment of both acute and chronic allograft rejection are continually being sought. The agent or biologic technique to induce graft tolerance remains the holy grail of transplantation.

Despite the comorbidities related to transplantation, the quality of life of these patients is frequently dramatically improved. Exercise performance is greatly enhanced, although it remains submaximal compared with normal age-matched subjects [8]. Diastolic dysfunction, chronotropic incompetence, and recipient-donor size mismatch are some potential limitations to exercise performance in transplantation patients [9].

The sustained improvement in survival following heart transplantation has lead to a broadening of recipient selection criteria and an increase in the number of potential transplantation candidates. Current estimates indicate that between 14,000 and 15,000 people per year could benefit from heart transplantation [10]. The continued expansion of heart transplantation is limited by the availability of donor organs, which has remained stagnant at approximately 2000 per year. Public awareness campaigns have minimally increased the donor pool. Improved medical therapy for heart failure and refined risk stratification have helped to defer transplantation in large numbers of patients. Despite these efforts, the waiting lists for transplantation candidates continue to lengthen. Alternatives to transplantation with mechanical-assist devices and other biologic donors such as xenografts are actively being investigated.

POSTTRANSPLANTATION SURVIVAL

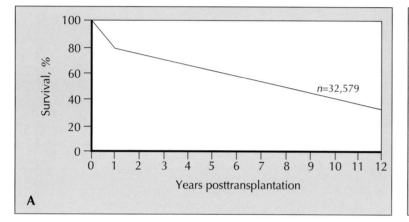

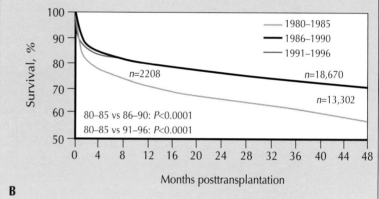

FIGURE 12-1. Heart transplantation actuarial survival. Survival following cardiac transplantation has significantly improved following the addition of cyclosporine to the immunosuppressive regimen. **A,** Actuarial heart transplantation survival for 32,579 heart transplantations performed between 1982 and 1995. **B,** The improvement in actuarial heart transplantation survival for 1980 to 1996, with the patients divided into pre- and post- cyclosporine eras. (Part A *adapted from* Hosenpud [11]; part B *adapted from* Hosenpud [12].)

CANDIDATE SELECTION

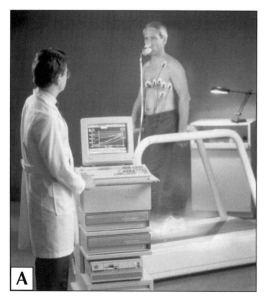

FIGURE 12-2. Cardiopulmonary stress testing. Application of cardiopulmonary stress testing has been an extremely valuable tool for guiding the transplantation selection process in ambulatory patients. **A,** The equipment used to conduct this form of testing. The patient breathes through a disposable pneumotach into a metabolic cart (Medical Graphics 2001, Minneapolis, MN) while exercising on a treadmill or bicycle. The metabolic cart is equipped with rapidly responding CO_2 and O_2 analyzers enabling online measurement of oxygen consumption (VO_2) and CO_2 production. As VO_2 equals the cardiac output times the arterial-venous oxygen difference, peak VO_2 provides an indirect noninvasive assessment of cardiac output response to exercise. (*continued*)

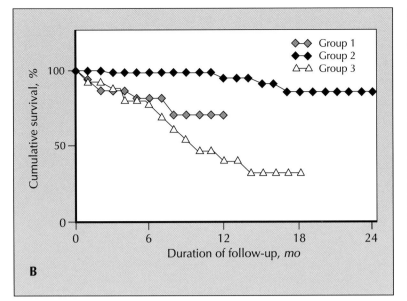

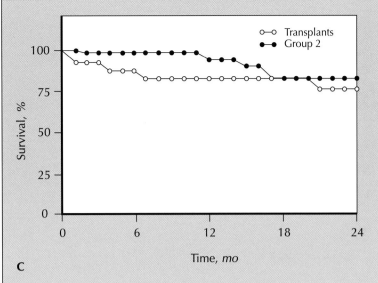

B

C

FIGURE 12-2. (*continued*) Cardiopulmonary stress testing was first used in candidate selection in 1986. **B**, In a study by Mancini *et al.* [13], 114 transplantation candidates were divided into three groups on the basis of exercise capacity. In patients with a VO_2 level greater than 14 mL/kg/min, cardiac transplantation was deferred (Group 2). Patients with a VO_2 of 14 mL/kg/min or less were accepted for transplantation in the absence of any other contraindications (Group 1). Patients with a significant comorbidity that excluded transplantation and with VO_2 less than 14 mL/kg/min constituted a medical control group (Group 3).

Cumulative survival curves for the three groups are shown here. For Group 1, transplant was considered a censored observation. The 52 patients with a preserved exercise capacity (*ie*, peak VO_2 greater than 14 mL/kg/min) had a 1-year survival rate of 94%. This was significantly better than the survival of patients with reduced exercise capacity (*ie*, VO_2 of 14 mL/kg/min or less). **C**, The survival of the heart failure patients with VO_2 greater than 14 mL/kg/min (Group 2) was similar to the survival of patients in Group 1 who underwent cardiac transplantation. (Parts B and C *adapted from* Mancini and coworkers [13].)

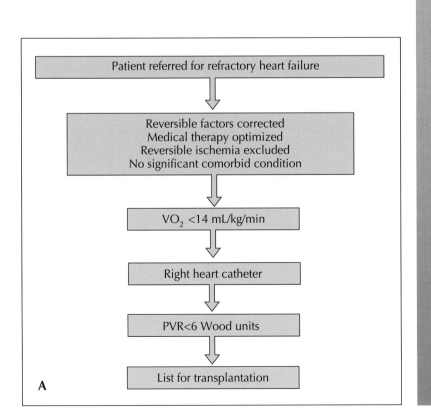

A

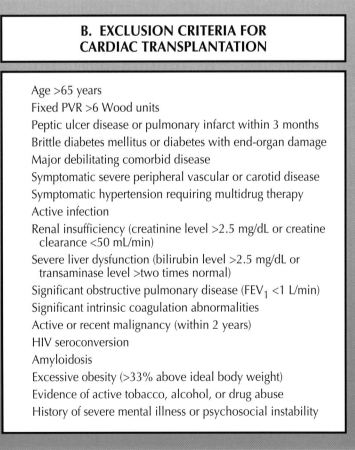

B. EXCLUSION CRITERIA FOR CARDIAC TRANSPLANTATION

Age >65 years
Fixed PVR >6 Wood units
Peptic ulcer disease or pulmonary infarct within 3 months
Brittle diabetes mellitus or diabetes with end-organ damage
Major debilitating comorbid disease
Symptomatic severe peripheral vascular or carotid disease
Symptomatic hypertension requiring multidrug therapy
Active infection
Renal insufficiency (creatinine level >2.5 mg/dL or creatine clearance <50 mL/min)
Severe liver dysfunction (bilirubin level >2.5 mg/dL or transaminase level >two times normal)
Significant obstructive pulmonary disease (FEV_1 <1 L/min)
Significant intrinsic coagulation abnormalities
Active or recent malignancy (within 2 years)
HIV seroconversion
Amyloidosis
Excessive obesity (>33% above ideal body weight)
Evidence of active tobacco, alcohol, or drug abuse
History of severe mental illness or psychosocial instability

FIGURE 12-3. Proposed algorithm for cardiac transplantation recipient selection (**A**). All referred candidates should be New York Heart Association Class III or IV after optimization of

medical therapy. A list of clinical contraindications to transplantation is included here (**B**) [14]. FEV_1—1-sec forced expiratory volume.

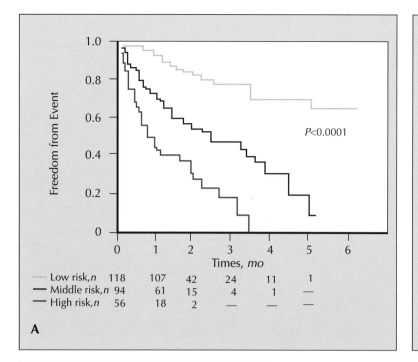

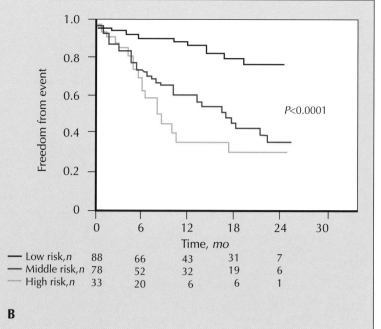

C. CALCULATION OF PROGNOSTIC SCORE

CLINICAL CHARACTERISTIC	VALUE (χ)	COEFFICIENT (β)	PRODUCT
Ischemic cardiomyopathy	1	+0.06931	+0.6931
Resting heart rate	90	+0.0216	+1.9440
LVEF	17	-0.0464	-0.7888
Mean BP	80	-0.0255	-2.0400
IVCD	0	+0.6083	0
Peak VO$_2$	16.2	-0.0546	-0.8845
Serum sodium	132	-0.0470	-6.2040
PROGNOSTIC SCORE	$=\Sigma\beta_1\chi_1+\beta_2\chi_2+...+\beta n\chi n$		
	=SUM OF THE PRODUCTS		=7.2802

Figure 12-4. In an attempt to further refine the use of oxygen consumption (VO$_2$) in the selection of ambulatory transplantation candidates, a clinical index was developed and prospectively validated to predict survival [15]. Multivariable proportional hazards modeling was used to develop the model from 80 clinical characteristics in 268 ambulatory patients with severe heart failure. The statistical model was subsequently validated in 199 patients. The smallest number of prognostic variables that accurately predicted 1-year survival was used to develop the heart failure survival score. The most significant prognostic factors were etiology of heart failure, resting heart rate and mean arterial blood pressure, left ventricular ejection fraction, presence or absence of intraventricular conduction defect, peak VO$_2$ in mL/kg/min, and serum sodium. The heart failure survival score is calculated as the absolute value of the sum of the products of the identified prognostic variables and their computed coefficients. Noncontinuous variables were graded as 1 if present or 0 if absent. Low-risk patients are identified as those with a score of more than 8.10; medium- and high-risk patients have scores below 8.1. Medium- and high-risk candidates are appropriate for listing for transplantation. **A,** Survival curve for the derivation sample. **B,** Survival curve for the validation group. **C,** An example of the calculation of the heart failure survival score for a 55-year-old man with an ischemic cardiomyopathy; resting heart rate of 90 bpm; left ventricular ejection fraction (LVEF) of 17%; mean arterial blood pressure (BP) of 80 mm Hg; absence of an intraventricular conduction defect (IVCD); peak VO$_2$ level of 16.2 mL/kg/min; and a serum sodium level of 132. The prognostic score below 8.1 places the patient in the medium- to high-risk group. In the absence of any major contraindications, the patient should be activated on the transplantation list. (*Adapted from* Aaronson and coworkers [15].)

SERIAL ASSESSMENT

Reevaluation in status 2 patients includes:

Repeat peak VO_2 and LVEF every 6 months; studies are done sooner if major changes have been made in medical regimen

PRA repeated every 2 months if level >20% and after transfusions in all patients

Right heart catheterization with infusion of vasodilators every 6 months if PVR >3 Wood units

Transplantation deferred if:

Peak VO_2 is markedly improved

LVEF >30%

PVR becomes fixed <6 Wood units despite parenteral inotropic therapy and optimization of vasodilators

FIGURE 12-5. Reevaluation of the need for transplantation. Heart failure is a dynamic state and therefore requires periodic reevaluation of the continued need for transplantation. A protocol for reevaluation is listed here. Left ventricular ejection fraction (LVEF) and exercise capacity are reassessed within 3 months of the initial evaluation in patients with major alterations in therapy or with symptomatic improvement. In the majority of patients, reevaluation is performed every 6 months. Patients selected using criteria emphasizing reduced oxygen consumption (VO_2) generally continue to have a high mortality, with few patients being deactivated from the transplantation list. Thus, accumulated time on the list remains a good parameter by which to allocate organs. PRA—panel of reactive antibodies; PVR—pulmonary vascular resistance.

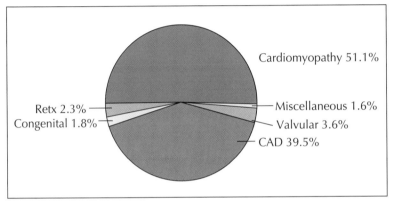

Cardiomyopathy 51.1%
Retx 2.3%
Congenital 1.8%
Miscellaneous 1.6%
Valvular 3.6%
CAD 39.5%

FIGURE 12-6. Indications for adult heart transplantation. In 1996, the most common indication for cardiac transplantation was dilated cardiomyopathy (51.1%) followed by coronary artery disease (CAD) (39.5%). Interestingly, with the advent of high-risk coronary bypass surgery in recent years, the percent of patients with ischemic heart disease undergoing transplantation has been declining. (*Adapted from* Hosenpud and coworkers [12].)

DONOR SELECTION CRITERIA

DONOR CRITERIA

Brain death declared; signed donor consent

Age ≤60 y of age; cardiac catheterization required in all donors >50 y of age

Normal heart

History, physical examination, EKG, ECHO

Inotropic requirement

<10µg/kg/min dopamine with adequate venous pressure

Absence of:

Malignancy (except primary brain tumor)

Cardiac contusion, arrhythmia

Infection (except pneumonia)

HIV, Hep BsAg or hepatitis C–positive

Anticipated ischemic time <4 h

FIGURE 12-7 Donor criteria. The major limitation to the growth of cardiac transplantation has been the scarcity of donor organs. Attempts have been made to expand the donor pool by accepting hearts from older candidates, serologic-positive organs (*ie*, hepatitis C–positive), and even marginal hearts with high inotropic requirements and small segmental wall abnormalities pretransplant. Guidelines for selecting suitable heart donors at Columbia-Presbyterian Medical Center (New York, NY) are shown here. Bs Ag—hepatitis B surface antigen; ECG—electrocardiogram; ECHO—echocardiogram,

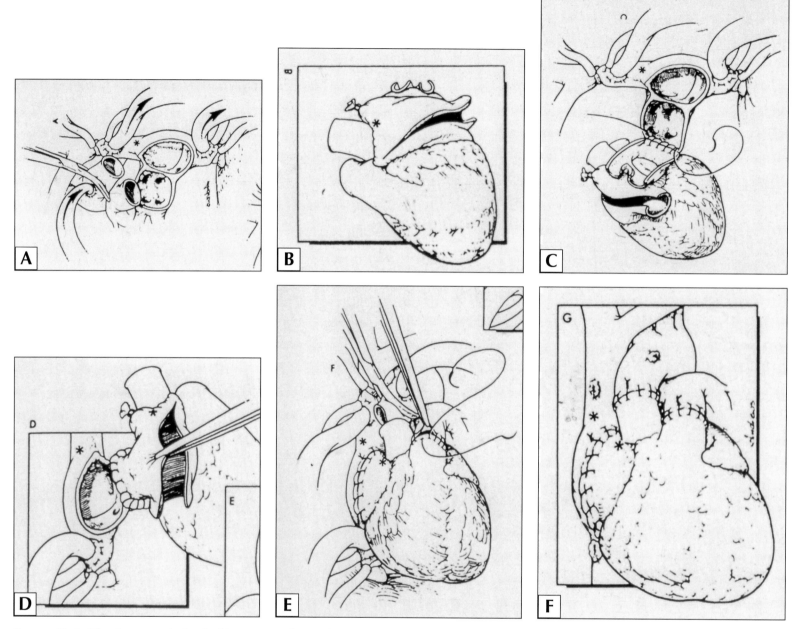

FIGURE 12-8. The three surgical techniques presently used to perform cardiac transplantation. The orthotopic cardiac transplantation developed by Shumway [16] is the most common surgical approach used worldwide. The native heart is removed, leaving biatrial cuffs (**A**). The excised donor heart is prepared with ligation of the superior vena cava. A curvilinear incision into the right atrium is made to protect the donor sinus node (*asterisk*; **B**). Biatrial anastomoses are performed, beginning with the left-to-left atrial anastomoses. This is followed by right atrial anastomoses (**C** and **D**) and finally by the pulmonary (**E**) and aortic (**F**) anastomoses. (*continued*)

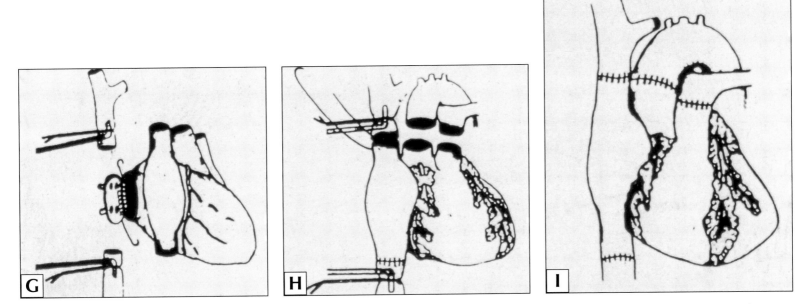

FIGURE 12-8. (*continued*) Preservation of the recipient's native pulmonary veins with biatrial anastomoses is the hallmark of the orthotopic technique; this preservation greatly simplified transplantation surgery. The orthotopic cardiac transplantation has been recently modified in an attempt to improve atrial geometry and function. This modification, the second procedure used for cardiac transplantation, is called the *bicaval technique*. In this modification, the recipient's atria are completely excised, with the exception of one or two small left-atrial cuffs containing the pulmonary veins. Direct anastomoses are then performed between the donor and recipient inferior and superior venae cavae, and then the left atrial cuff on the donor heart is anastomosed to the pulmonary venous cuff on the recipient side (**G**). The aorta and pulmonary artery and then anastomosed (**H**). The completed bicaval transplant (**I**) thus preserves atrial geometry.

The third technique for transplantation currently utilized is the heterotopic technique (not shown), which was the original trans-

plantation performed by Dr. Christian Barnard in 1967. In this technique, the donor organ is "piggybacked" to the recipient heart. The two aortas are anastomosed, and a Dacron graft is interposed between the donor and recipient pulmonary artery. The right and left ventricular circulations are connected parallel. In a recent modification of this technique, the donor pulmonary artery is anastomosed to the recipient right atrium. This modification places the right ventricles in series; the left ventricles remain in parallel circuits. Heterotopic transplantation permits transplantation of patients with fixed elevated pulmonary vascular resistances who are not eligible for orthotopic transplantation. However, this approach is limited by a lower long-term survival, need for chronic anticoagulation, development of arrhythmias, and potential for refractory angina in some patients [17]. (Parts A to G *adapted from* Cooley [18]; parts H to J *adapted from* El Gamel and coworkers [19]; with permission.)

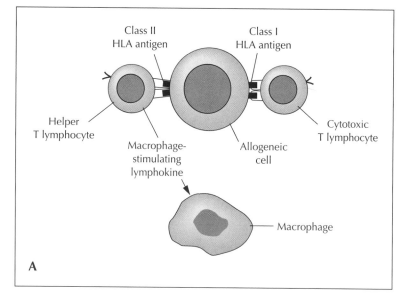

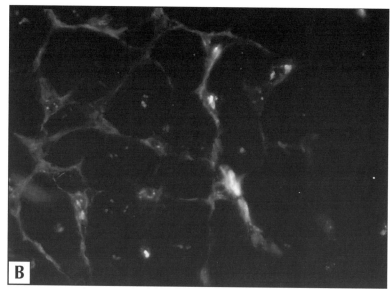

FIGURE 12-9. Allograft rejection. **A,** The rejection of an allograft is primarily determined by the recognition of foreign antigens on the surface of engrafted cells. The major surface histocompatibility antigens are determined by a single complex genetic region called the *HLA region* in humans. The loci are divided into two classes, I and II, based on structure, function, and tissue distribution of their cell surface protein products.

Cell-mediated rejection is the primary cause of rejection. T lymphocytes are crucial to the initiation and execution of cellular rejection. Donor antigens are presented either directly (*ie*, on the surface of a donor cell) or indirectly. The subsequent recognition of foreign or donor HLA antigens by highly specific T-cell receptors remains the critical control element for the immune response. However, the recognition of foreign HLA protein by a T-cell receptor is not sufficient to provoke the rejection response. The interaction between the antigen-presenting cell and the T-cell receptor must be aligned with integrins and adhesion molecules such that a conformational change can occur in the T-cell receptor. T-cell surface molecules that promote adhesion include lymphocyte-associated antigen (LFA-1). LFA1 binds to intracellular adhesion molecule (ICAM I), which is a glycoprotein expressed on endothelial cells, fibroblasts, lymphocytes, and monocytes. Interleukin 2 is the main cytotrophic factor to T lymphocytes that causes allospecific clonal expansion activation of cytotoxic and helper T cells, as well as activation of B lymphocytes. The complexity of the cellular interaction provides many potential targets for immunosuppression. Development of monoclonal antibodies against these cellular molecules has been an active area of research.

Humoral rejection can occur early after transplantation. It is characterized histologically by immunoglobulin and complement deposition in the absence of cellular rejection. It is frequently associated with hemodynamic compromise and occurs in about 10% of cases. **B,** Immunofluorescent staining of a myocardial biopsy with fluorescein-conjugated anti-human immunoglobulin G (IgG). The green fluorescent stain demonstrates the linear deposition of IgG on the endothelial capillaries; the yellow stain represents autofluorescent lipofusion within the myocytes. (Part A *adapted from* Cerilli [20].) (*See Color Plate* for part B.)

A. IMMUNOSUPPRESSIVE DRUGS

DRUG	MECHANISM OF ACTION	DOSE	SIDE EFFECTS
ANTIMETABOLITES			
Azathioprine	Inhibition of purine metabolism	2 mg/kg/d (titrated to WBC count of 5000/cc)	Leukopenia, bone marrow suppression, hepatotoxicity, nausea
Mycophenolate mofetil	Inhibition of purine metabolism	1500 mg bid	Nausea, diarrhea leukopenia
Brequinar sodium*	Inhibition of pyrimidine metabolism	—	Leukopenia, thrombocytopenia, diarrhea
Cytoxan	Inhibition of pyrimidine metabolism	1 g/m^2 every 3–4 wk	Leukopenia, mucositis, thrombocytopenia, hemorrhagic cystitis
ANTIPROLIFERATIVES			
Prednisone	Inhibits macrophage migration factor; inhibits processing and display of antigen; inhibits IL1 release & synthesis of IL1 & 2	0–10 mg/d	Diabetes, osteoporosis, obesity, dyslipidemia, myopathy, cataracts, mood swings
Cyclosporine	Interferes with transcription of IL2 by binding cyclophilin on T cells	4–6 mg/kg/d bid (titrated to trough blood levels)	Nephrotoxicity, headache, tremors, hyperkalemia, photosensitivity, gingival hyperplasia
Tacrolimus	Binds cyclophilin on T cells and interferes with IL2 transcription	0.15–0.3 mg/kg/d bid	Nephrotoxicity, hyperkalemia, seizures, headache, tremor
Rapamycin*	Binds to cyclophin causing IL2 receptor blockade	—	Thrombocytopenia, nausea
ANTIBODY THERAPY			
OKT3	Monoclonal antibody to the CD3 receptor that prevents IL2 release	5 mg/d	Pulmonary edema with cytokine release, fever, myalgias, aseptic meningitis
Daclizumab*	Monoclonal antibody to the IL2 receptor	1 mg/kg on day 1, then every 2 wk for 2 mo	Gastrointestinal disorders
ATGAM	Polyclonal antibody	15–20mg/kg for 14 d	Fever, serum sickness, thrombocytopenia

FIGURE 12-10. Immunosuppressive drugs. The immunosuppressive drugs can be grouped into three categories: antimetabolites, antiproliferatives, and antibodies. **A,** Doses and side effects for the most commonly used drugs. Antimetabolites block purine or pyrimidine synthesis clonal lymphocyte expansion; antiproliferatives inhibit clonal expansion of cell lines that modulate rejection; and antibody therapy includes targeted and specific inhibition of cell lines that modulate rejection. (*continued*)

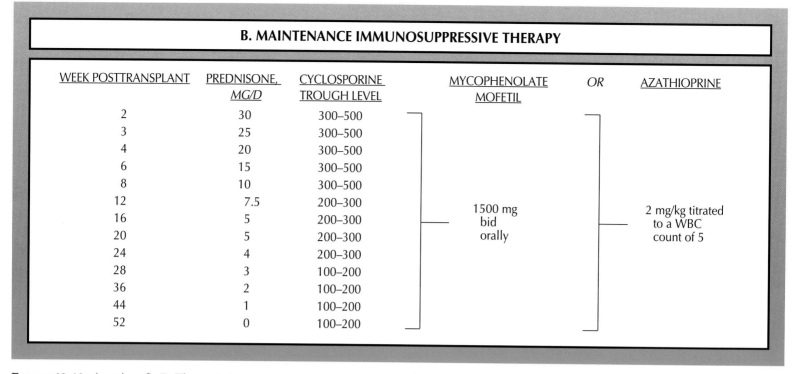

B. MAINTENANCE IMMUNOSUPPRESSIVE THERAPY

WEEK POSTTRANSPLANT	PREDNISONE, MG/D	CYCLOSPORINE TROUGH LEVEL	MYCOPHENOLATE MOFETIL	OR	AZATHIOPRINE
2	30	300–500			
3	25	300–500			
4	20	300–500			
6	15	300–500			
8	10	300–500			
12	7.5	200–300			
16	5	200–300	1500 mg bid orally		2 mg/kg titrated to a WBC count of 5
20	5	200–300			
24	4	200–300			
28	3	100–200			
36	2	100–200			
44	1	100–200			
52	0	100–200			

FIGURE 12-10. (*continued*) **B,** The maintenance immunosuppressive regimen used after cardiac transplantation at Columbia-Presbyterian Medical Center (New York, NY). Rapid withdrawal of corticosteroids is attempted to minimize steroid associated side effects. bid—twice a day; IL—interleukin; WBC—white blood cell.

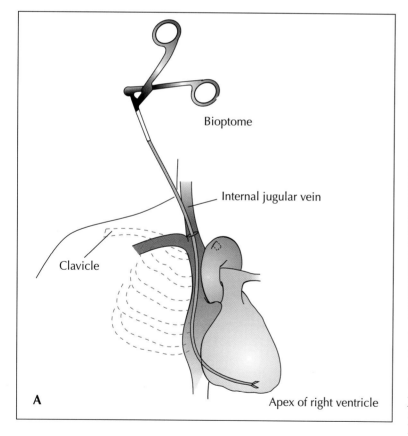

A

B. ISHLT ENDOMYOCARDIAL GRADING SYSTEM

GRADE	HISTOLOGIC DESCRIPTION
0	No rejection
1A	Focal perivascular or interstitial infiltrate without necrosis
1B	Diffuse but sparse infiltrate without necrosis
2	One focus of aggressive infiltration or focal myocyte damage
3A	Multifocal aggressive infiltrates or myocyte damage
3B	Diffuse inflammatory process with necrosis
4	Diffuse aggressive polymorphous infiltrate with necrosis ±edema, ±hemorrhage, ±vasculitis

FIGURE 12-11. Histologic grading of allograft rejection. In order to monitor rejection, periodic endomyocardial biopsies are performed. **A,** The percutaneous technique of endomyocardial biopsy using the Caves bioptome. The bioptome is inserted through the internal jugular vein to the right ventricular portion of the interventricular septum under fluoroscopy. Four to six specimens containing at least 50% myocytes are required for 90% to 95% confidence in the interpretation. **B,** The standardization of histologic biopsy grading according to the International Society for Heart Transplantation (ISHLT). (Part A *adapted from* Unverferth [21].)

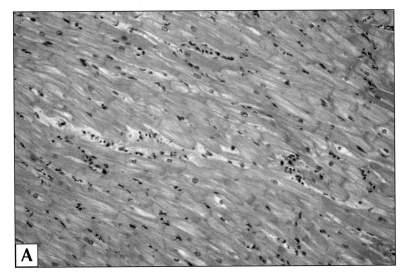

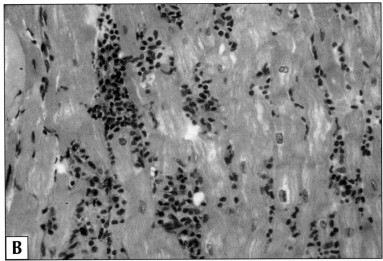

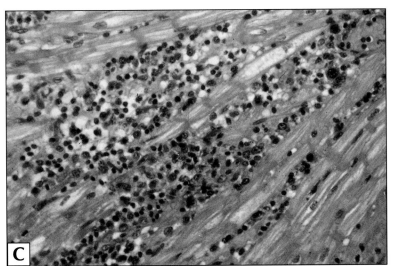

FIGURE 12-12. Hematoxylin and eosin staining of representative endomyocardial biopsies at a magnification of 100 × showing grade 1B rejection with focal lymphocytic infiltrate without evidence of myocardial necrosis (**A**), grade 3A rejection demonstrating more intensive lymphocytic infiltration and myocyte necrosis (**B**), and grade 4 allograft rejection with extensive lymphocyte infiltration, myocyte necrosis, and hemorrhage (**C**).

FIGURE 12-13.
Infections associated with posttransplant immunosuppression. Because of reduced cellular immunity, the cardiac transplantation recipient is subject to development of typical bacterial as well as atypical viral, protozoal, and fungal infections. **A,** The typical posttransplant infections and the times at which they occur. (*continued*)

Conventional Nosocomial Infections	Unconventional or Opportunistic Infections	Community-acquired or Persistant Infections

Viral

├HSV─────┤

────── Onset of CMV──────────┤ ├─CMV retinitis or colitis────

├─EBV, VZW (shingles), influenza, RSV, adenovirus ──────┤

├─Papillomavirus, PTLD─────

├─Onset of hepatitis B or hepatitis C──────────

Bacterial

├──── Wound infections, catheter-related infections, pneumonia

├─Nocardia────────────────

├─Listeria, tuberculosis────────────────

Fungal

├─Pneumocystis────────────────

├─Aspergillus───────┤ ├─Cryptococcus ──────

├─Candida──────┤ Geographically restricted, endemic fungi

Parasitic

├─Strongloides ──────────────

├─Toxoplasma ───────────┤

├─Leishmania

├──── *Trypanosoma cruzi* ──────────

0   1   2   3   4   5   6

Months after transplantation

A

B. ANTIMICROBIAL PROPHYLAXIS

BACTERIAL PROPHYLAXIS

Cefazolin 1.5 g IV preoperatively and 1 g IV every 6 hours for 24 hours

Isoniazid 300 mg and pyridoxine 50 mg orally daily for 1 year for PPD-positive
   candidates and recipients

Pneumococcal vaccine IM pretransplant

VIRAL PROPHYLAXIS (CMV, HSV, INFLUENZA)

Acyclovir 800 mg orally qid for 3 months in all patients; CytoGam 150 mg/kg IV within
   72 hs of transplant, then 100 mg/kg on weeks 2, 4, 6, 8, then 50 mg/kg on weeks 12
   and 16 in all CMV-positive recipients or in all recipients of CMV-positive donor hearts

CMV-positive recipients who receive CMV-negative hearts receive HSV prophylaxis with
   Acyclovir 400 mg orally tid

CMV-negative blood products to all transplant recipients

Influenza A and B vaccine every November to all recipients after year 1

PROTOZOAL PROPHYLAXIS (PCP, TOXOPLASMOSIS)

Trimethaprin-sulfamethoxazole single-strength tablet daily for 1 year or monthly 300 mg
   of aerosolized Pentamidine isethionate in patients with sulfa allergy

Pyrimethamine 50 mg daily and folinic acid 5 mg orally bid for 6 weeks for all recipients
   with negative titers for toxoplasmosis who receive a heart that is positive for toxoplasmosis

FUNGAL PROPHYLAXIS

Mycostatin swish and swallow 5 cc orally qid for 2 months or clotrimazole troches orally
   5 times per day for 2 months

FIGURE 12-13. (*continued*) **B,** In an attempt to prevent the various infections, the antimicrobial prophylactic regimen is implemented. bid–twice a day; CMV—cytomegalovirus; CNS—central nervous system; EBV—Epstein Barr virus; HSV—herpes simplex virus; IM—intramuscular; IV—intravenous; PCP—*Pneumocystis carinii* pneumonia; qid—four times a day; TB—tuberculosis; tid–four times a day; UTI—urinary tract infection; VZV—varicella zoster virus. (Part A *adapted from* Fishman and Rubin [22]; with permission.)

QUALITY OF LIFE AFTER TRANSPLANTATION

A. DETERMINANTS OF DECREASED EXERCISE CAPACITY AFTER CARDIAC TRANSPLANTATION

DONOR

Abnormal LV relaxation or diastolic dysfunction

Reduced systolic performance due to rejection or
   accelerated atherosclerosis

Chronotropic incompetence

RECIPIENT

Effects of immunosuppressive drugs: steroid-induced
   myopathy

Persistent pulmonary abnormalities

Persistent skeletal muscle abnormalities

FIGURE 12-14. Exercise capacity after transplantation. Quality of life after transplantation is generally excellent. Many recipients are able to return to work and an active lifestyle [23]. However, multiple studies have demonstrated that cardiac transplantation recipients exhibit a 30% to 40% reduction in exercise capacity compared with normal individuals [8]. **A,** Determinants of decreased exercise capacity after cardiac transplantation. There are many theories to explain this reduced exercise capacity some that relate to the recipient and others to the donor characteristics. An important determinant of reduced exercise capacity is chronotropic incompetence due to graft denervation [8]. As a consequence of denervation, the heart rate response is determined primarily by the transplanted heart response to circulating cate-cholamines. (*continued*)

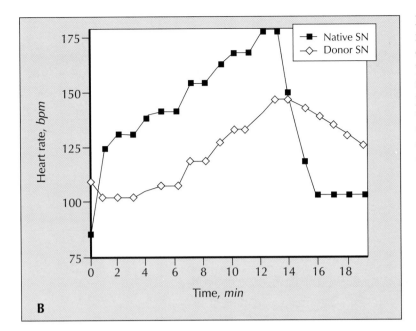

B

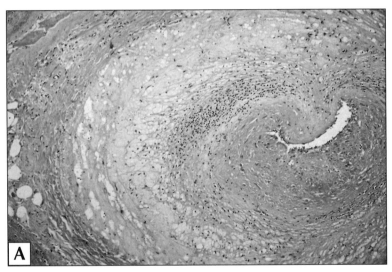

FIGURE 12-14. (*continued*) **B,** Simultaneous esophageal electrode recordings of the remnant native sinus node (SN) and the surface electrocardiogram recordings of donor heart rate from a patient 2 years after transplantation. The heart rate recorded from the native sinus node quickly increases at the onset of exercise and decreases precipitously with its termination. In contrast, the donor heart rate does not increase until minute 8 of exercise, consistent with its cate-cholamine-dependent response. Deceleration is also delayed as cate-cholamines are cleared from the circulation. LV—left ventricular. (*Adapted from* Beniaminovitz and coworkers [24].)

ACCELERATED TRANSPLANTATION ATHEROSCLEROSIS AND RETRANSPLANTATION

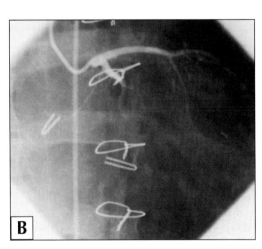

FIGURE 12-15. Transplantation coronary allograft disease (TCAD). The major cause of late death after cardiac transplantation is the development of TCAD, a unique accelerated form of coronary artery disease. By 1 year posttransplant, about 30% of patients demonstrate some TCAD, and the incidence and severity continue to increase with time [25]. The pathogenesis of TCAD is thought to begin with immunologic and nonimmunologic injury to the arterial endothelium, with resultant loss of endothelial integrity [26]. Microthrombi, cellular proliferation, and plasma lipids accumulate at the site of the injured intima. **A,** This leads to further cellular proliferation and finally profound myointimal hyperplasia leading to diffuse coronary artery lumen narrowing. **B,** Selective left coronary angiography from a patient with severe TCAD, which shows diffuse tapering of the left anterior descending and circumflex arteries as well as pruning of all the secondary vessels. Immunologic mechanisms resulting in endothelial injury include both cellular and humoral factors [27]. Nonimmunologic risk factors also contribute to the development of cardiac allograft vasculopathy. Recipient age and gender, donor age and gender, obesity, hyperlipidemia, and donor ischemic time may impact on the development of vasculopathy [28]. An association has also been found between the presence of active cytomegalovirus infection and the development of vasculopathy [29]. Given the diffuse, concentric nature of this disease, percutaneous transluminal coronary angioplasty and coronary artery bypass grafting are not useful strategies for management. Unfortunately, patients with TCAD have a fivefold greater risk of cardiac events such as myocardial infarction, severe refractory heart failure, and sudden death. Presently, retransplantation is the only treatment for severe TCAD; however, survival after repeat transplantation is significantly reduced. Consequently, preventative strategies have assumed clinical importance. Hyperlipidemia management with HMG Co-A (3-hydroxy-3-methylglutaryl-coenzyme A) reductase inhibitors and routine aspirin use are two such approaches.

MECHANICAL-ASSIST DEVICES

PATIENT SELECTION CRITERIA FOR LEFT VENTRICULAR ASSIST DEVICES

Transplant candidate
Hemodynamic parameters
    Cardiac index <2 L/min/m^2
    Systolic blood pressure <80 mm Hg
    Pulmonary capillary wedge > 20 mm Hg
Technical considerations for exclusion
    Body surface area <1.5 m^2
    Aortic insufficiency
    Right to left shunt
    Abdominal aortic aneurysm
    Prosthetic valves
    Left ventricular thrombus
Severe right ventricular failure
Preoperative risk factors
    Right atrial pressure >16 mm Hg
    Prothrombin time >16 s
    Reoperation
    White blood cell count >15
    Urine output <30 cc/h
    Mechanically ventilated
    Temperature >101.5°F

FIGURE 12-16. Selection criteria for insertion of mechanical-assist devices. Approximately 25% of the patients listed for cardiac transplantation die before a suitable donor heart becomes available. Consequently, several types of short-term and more permanent mechanical-assist devices have been developed to bridge patients to transplantation. Commonly used short- and long-term devices are the Abiomed (Danvers, MA), Novacor (Oakland, CA), and Thermocardiac (TCI; Woburn, MA) systems. LVAD—left ventricular assist device.

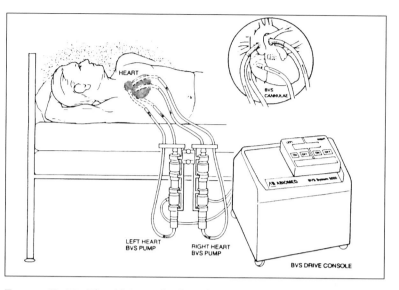

FIGURE 12-17. The Abiomed. The Abiomed is a pulsatile extra-corporeal assist device that can provide univentricular or biventricular support. Cannulae are placed either in the right or left atria, and blood flows into the two-chamber device. An atrial filling chamber connects a trileaflet valve to a ventricular pumping chamber. Each chamber consists of a 100-mL, smooth-surfaced, polyurethane bladder. The atrial chamber fills passively by gravity. The ventricular chamber fills and empties through pneumatic compression of the bladder by a console. Blood flows to an arterial Dacron graft cannula that inserts into the pulmonary artery or the ascending aorta. (*Adapted from* Higgins and coworkers [30].)

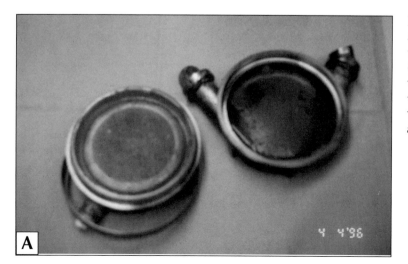

FIGURE 12-18. The Thermocardiac (TCI) device. The TCI device is another commonly used left ventricular assist device that has a textured surface that facilitates formation of a biologic membrane (**A**). The inflow Dacron graft, which is inserted into the left ventricular apex, and the longer outflow graft, which is inserted to the ascending aorta, are connected to the pump with porcine valves. The pneumatic-powered device has received FDA approval. (*continued*)

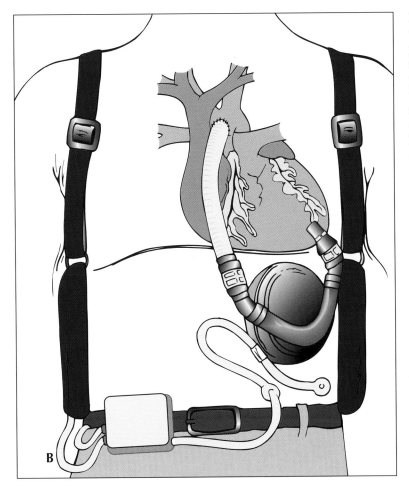

FIGURE 12-18. (*continued*) The electrical-powered device is still undergoing clinical trials (**B**). This device requires an external power source. Two external portable batteries linked via the external drive lines provide 6 to 8 hours of power and thus render patients free to engage in a variety of indoor and outdoor activities while awake. Overnight, the patients are linked to a power base station. The Novacor system (not shown) is the other most commonly used left ventricular assist device (LVAD) bridge. The Novacor system does not contain a textured surface. Despite anticoagulation, the incidence of embolic cardiovascular accidents remain high with the present Novacor system.

At the Columbia-Presbyterian Medical Center (New York, NY), the TCI system has been used in 111 patients as a bridge to transplantation. A total of 72 patients (65%) successfully proceeded to transplantation, 27 patients (24%) died while on left ventricular assist device (LVAD) support, 5 patients (4.5%) were explanted, and the remainder are awaiting cardiac transplantation. Causes of mortality following LVAD insertion include infection, right heart failure, bleeding complications, and embolic events. With refinement of selection criteria for suitable device candidates, mortality continues to decrease. Moreover, because of the rapidly evolving technology, the possibility for completely implantable devices appears promising in the not-too-distant future. (Part A *from* Rose and Goldstein [31]; part B *adapted from* Rose and Goldstein [31]; with permission.)

REFERENCES

1. Barnard CN: A human cardiac transplant: an interim report of a successful operation performed at Groote Schuur Hospital, Cape Town. *S Afr Med J* 1967, 41:1271–1274.

2. Dong E Jr, Stinson EB, Griepp RB, *et al.*: Cardiac transplantation following failure of previous cardiac surgery. *Surg Forum* 1973, 24:150–152.

3. Oyer PE, Stinson EB, Jamieson SW: Cyclosporine A in cardiac allografting: a preliminary experience. *Transplant Proc* 1983, 15:1247–1250.

4. Fragomeni LS, Kaye MP: The Registry of the International Society for Heart Transplantation: Fifth Official Report–1988. *J Heart Transplant* 1988, 7:249–253.

5. Kahan B: Cyclosporine. *N Engl J Med* 1989, 321:1725–1738.

6. Kobashigawa JA, Stevenson LW, Brownfield ED, *et al.*: Initial success of steroid weaning late after heart transplantation *J Heart Lung Transplant* 1992, 11:428–430.

7. Sharples LD, Caine N, Mullins P, *et al.*: Risk factor analysis for the major hazards following heart transplantation: rejection, infection, and coronary occlusive disease. *Transplantation* 1991, 52:244–252.

8. Mandack JS, Aaronson KD, Mancini DM: Serial assessment of exercise capacity after heart transplantation. *J Heart Lung Transplant* 1995, 14:468–478.

9. Young JB, Winters WL, Bourge R, Uretsky BF: 24th Bethesda Conference: Cardiac Transplantation. Task Force 4: Function of the Heart Transplant Recipient. *J Am Coll Cardiol* 1993, 22:31–41.

10. Evans RW, Manninen DL, Garrison LP Jr, Maier AM: Donor availability as the primary determinant of the future of heart transplantation. *JAMA* 1986, 255:1892–1898.

11. Hosenpud JD: The Registry of the International Society for Heart and Lung Transplantation: Thirteenth Official Report–1996. *J Heart Lung Transplant* 1996, 15:655–674.

11. Hosenpud JD: The Registry of the International Society for Heart and Lung Transplantation: Fourteenth Official Report–1997. *J Heart Lung Transplant* 1996, 16:691–712.

13. Mancini DM, Eisen H, Kussmaul W, *et al.*: Value of peak exercise oxygen consumption for optimal timing of cardiac transplantation in ambulatory patients with heart failure. *Circulation* 1991, 83:778–786.

14. Costanzo MR: Selection and treatment of candidates for heart transplantation: a statement for health professionals from the Committee on Heart Failure and Cardiac Transplantation of the Council on Clinical Cardiology, American Heart Association. *Circulation* 1995, 92:3593–3612.

15. Aaronson KD, Schwartz JS, Chen TM, *et al.*: Development and prospective validation of a clinical index to predict survival in ambulatory patients referred for cardiac transplant evaluation. *Circulation* 1997, 95:2597–2599.

16. Shumway NE, Lower RR, Stofer RC: Transplantation of the heart. *Adv Surg* 1966, 2:265–284.

17. Kawaguchi A, Gandjbakhch I, Pavie A, *et al.*: Factors affecting survival after heterotopic heart transplantation. *J Thorac Cardiovasc Surg* 1989, 98:928–934.

18. Cooley DA: *Techniques in Cardiac Surgery*, edn 2. Philadelphia: WB Saunders; 1984:372.

19. El Gamel A, Yonan NA, Grant S, *et al.*: Orthotopic cardiac transplantation: a comparison of standard and bicaval Wythenshawe techniques. *J Thorac Cardiovasc Surg* 1995, 109:721–730.

20. Cerilli GJ: *Organ Transplantation and Replacement*. Philadelphia: JB Lippincott; 1988:120.

21. Unverferth DV: *Dilated Cardiomyopathy*. Mt. Kisco, NY: Futura Publishing Co; 1985.

22. Fishman J, Rubin R: Infection in organ transplant recipients. *N Engl J Med* 1998, 338:1741–1751.

23. Paris W, Woodbury A, Thompson S, *et al.*: Returning to work after heart transplantation. *J Heart Lung Transplant* 1993, 12:46–54.

24. Beniaminovitz A, Coromilas J, Oz M, *et al.*: Electrical connection of native and transplanted sinus nodes via atrial pacing improves exercise performance after cardiac transplantation. *Am J Cardiol* 1998, 81:1373–1377.

25. Michler RE, McLaughlin MJ, Chen JM, *et al.*: Clinical experience with cardiac retransplantation. *J Thorac Cardiovasc Surg* 1993, 106:622–629.

26. Ventura HO, Mehra MR, Smart FW, Stapleton DD: Cardiac allograft vasculopathy: current concepts. *Am Heart J* 1995, 129:791–798.

27. Costanzo-Nordin MR: Cardiac allograft vasculopathy: relationship with acute cellular rejection and histocompatibility. *J Heart Lung Transplant* 1992, 11(suppl):90–104.

28. Johnson MR: Transplant coronary artery disease: nonimmunologic risk factors. *J Heart Lung Transplant* 1992, 11(suppl):124–132.

29. McDonald K, Rector TS, Braunlin EA, *et al.*: Association of coronary artery disease in transplant recipients with cytomegalovirus infection. *Am J Cardiol* 1989, 64:359–362.

30. Higgins RSD, Silverman NA: Status of permanent cardiac replacement for end-stage congestive heart failure. *Heart Failure Reviews* 1996, 1:39–52.

31. Rose EA, Goldstein DJ: Wearable long-term mechanical support for patients with end-stage heart disease: a tenable goal. *Ann Thorac Surg* 1996, 61:399–402.

INDEX

COLOR PLATES

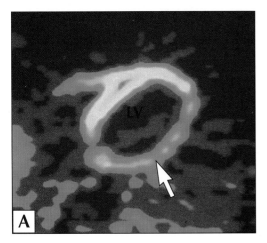

CHAPTER 3, Figure 3-7A, page 3.5

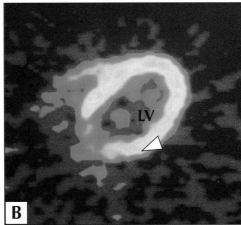

CHAPTER 3, Figure 3-7B, page 3.5

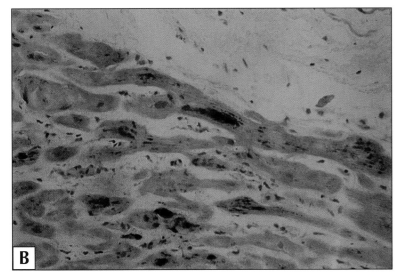

CHAPTER 3, Figure 3-39B, page 3.22

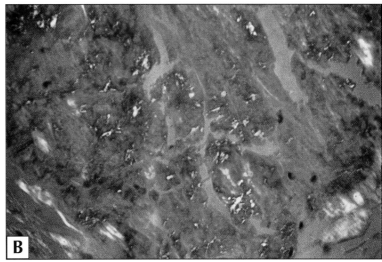

CHAPTER 3, Figure 3-41B, page 3.22

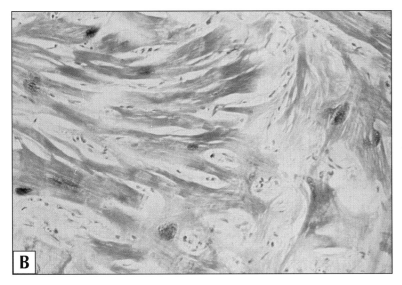

CHAPTER 3, Figure 3-43B, page 3.23

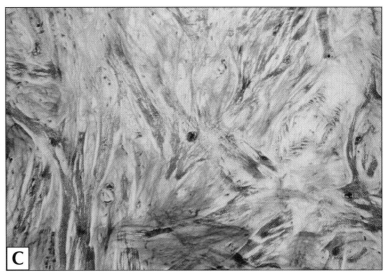

CHAPTER 3, Figure 3-43C, page 3.23

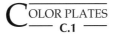

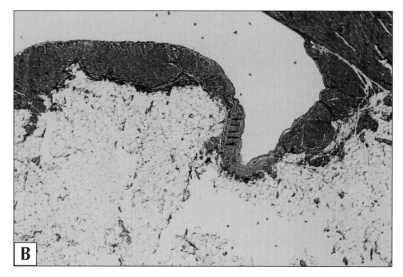

CHAPTER 3, Figure 3-45B, page 3.24

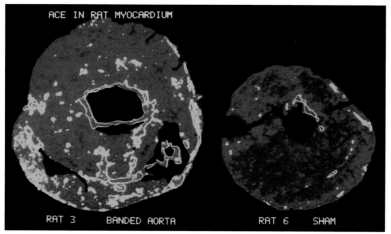

CHAPTER 4, Figure 4-32, page 4.15

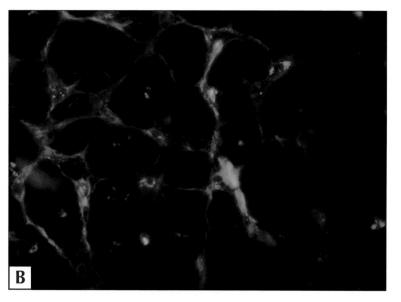

CHAPTER 12, Figure 12-9B, page 12.8